Principles of Biomedical Ethics

Principles of Biomedical Ethics

THIRD EDITION

Tom L. Beauchamp
James F. Childress

New York   Oxford
OXFORD UNIVERSITY PRESS
1989

Oxford University Press

Oxford   New York   Toronto
Delhi   Bombay   Calcutta   Madras   Karachi
Petaling Jaya   Singapore   Hong Kong   Tokyo
Nairobi   Dar es Salaam   Cape Town
Melbourne   Auckland

and associated companies in
Berlin   Ibadan

Copyright © 1979, 1983, 1989 by Oxford University Press, Inc.

Published by Oxford University Press, Inc.,
200 Madison Avenue, New York, New York 10016

Library of Congress Cataloging-in-Publication Data
Beauchamp, Tom L.
Principles of biomedical ethics / by Tom L. Beauchamp,
James F. Childress.—3rd ed.
p. cm.   Bibliography: p.   Includes index.
ISBN 0-19-505901-8; ISBN 0-19505902-6 (pbk.)
1. Medical ethics. I. Childress, James F. II. Title.
[DNLM: 1. Ethics, Medical. W 50 B372p]
R724.B36 1989
174'.2—dc19
DNLM/DLC
for Library of Congress   88-31301   CIP

9 8 7 6 5 4 3 2 1

Printed in the United States of America
on acid-free paper

**To
Georgia, Ruth, and Don**

I can no other answer make but thanks,
And thanks, and ever thanks.

Twelfth Night

Preface to the Third Edition

When the first edition of this book went to press in late 1977, biomedical ethics in its modern form was still an embryonic field. The changes that occurred in the literature of this field between the first edition and the second edition (published in 1983) were immense, and consequently the second edition introduced major changes. The forces of change that convinced us to restructure the first edition have continued, and this third edition involves even more significant changes than did the second.

However, the book retains the same chapter structure and general lines of argument. We have also retained the chapter headings from the second edition, with a few exceptions (for example, "Refusal of Treatment" and "Relevant Properties"). Material under deleted headings has been relocated under different headings. The main innovation is the introduction of large bodies of entirely new material throughout every chapter. Various topics such as AIDS and artificial nutrition and hydration have been included, and our arguments have been extended and deepened throughout.

In order to create more room for our expanded text, we have dropped the appendix of codes and the bibliography of suggested readings, choosing instead to incorporate relevant portions of the codes into the text and to provide bibliographical selections in the notes at the end of each chapter. The appendix of cases has also been expanded through the addition of new cases. Several retained cases have been updated, and numerous cases not in the appendix have been woven into the discussions in the text.

We have received many helpful suggestions for improvements in the previous editions from students, health professionals, and faculty members using the text. Special thanks must be given in this third edition to David DeGrazia, Jeff Kahn, and Courtney Campbell—our outstanding research assistants. We are also grateful to those who prepared cases for or allowed us to use their cases in this edition; they are acknowledged at the end of each case. In addition, Peter Frommer, Michael Rein, and Richard Whitely provided helpful advice in the preparation of certain cases. Denise Brooks, Tanja Hens, Melody Roberts, LaRea Frazier, and Carol Schaffer have shepherded draft after draft of this new edition through our offices—always with patience and often with critical and constructive suggestions.

Several parts of chapters were presented at the seminars of the Kennedy Institute of Ethics. Many arguments were substantially changed as a result of the comments and responses of our critics on these occasions. We are especially grateful to Jorge Garcia and Ruth Faden for some suggestions about virtue theory in Chapter 8. Through the Institute, work on several chapters and cases was supported by the Biomedical Research Support Grant Program, Division of Research Resources, National Institutes of Health (BRSG SO7 RR 0713616). We also acknowledge with due appreciation the support provided by the Kennedy Institute's library and information retrieval systems, which kept us in touch with the most important literature and repeatedly reduced the burdens of library research.

Washington, D.C.   T.L.B
Charlottesville, Va.   J.C.
January 1989

Contents

Principles of Biomedical Ethics

1

Morality and Ethical Theory

Medical ethics enjoyed a remarkable degree of continuity and consistency from the days of Hippocrates until the mid-twentieth century. But recent scientific, technological, and social developments have produced rapid changes in the biological sciences and in health care. These developments have challenged many traditional conceptions of the moral obligations of health professionals and of society. The objective of this book is to provide a moral framework for determining our obligations in the wake of these developments. We do not ignore the history of moral reflection in health care; indeed, we assume its relevance. But we emphasize the development of a theory and a set of principles for the treatment of problems that even the most elevated and ancient forms of medical ethics are ill equipped to handle.

Moral reasoning

These problems of medical ethics may be theoretical—such as whether physicians or nurses may ever legitimately hasten the death of patients—or practical—such as whether a particular patient may be allowed to die. In either form, our perplexity about these matters and our desire for resolution drive us to moral reasoning.

3

Moral dilemmas and moral reasoning

Facing dilemmas and reasoning through them to conclusions is a familiar feature of the human condition. Consider a particular case (Case 1 in the appendix). Under striking conditions, the judges on the California Supreme Court must reach a decision about a possible violation of medical confidentiality. A man killed a woman after confiding to a therapist his intention to commit the act. The therapist attempted unsuccessfully to have the man committed but because of medical confidentiality did not communicate the threat to the woman when the commitment attempt failed. This case reached the California Supreme Court. The majority opinion in the case holds that ''When a therapist determines, or pursuant to the standards of his profession should determine, that his patient presents a serious danger of violence to another, he incurs an obligation to use reasonable care to protect the intended victim against such danger.'' This obligation extends to notification of the police and possibly to a direct warning to the intended victim. The justice argues that health-care professionals generally ought to observe the rule of medical confidentiality but that this rule must yield in this case to the ''public interest in safety from violent assault.'' Although he recognizes that rules of professional ethics have substantial public value, he holds that matters of greater importance, such as protection against violent assault, can override the rules.

In a minority opinion, a second justice disagrees with this analysis. He argues that doctors violate patients' rights when they fail to observe rules of confidentiality. If it were common practice to break these rules, he reasons, the fiduciary nature of the relationship between physicians and patients would begin to erode. Patients would lose confidence in psychiatrists and would refrain from divulging critical information. Violent assaults would then increase, because mentally ill persons would not seek psychiatric aid.

This case presents a straightforward moral dilemma (as well as a legal dilemma), because both judges cite good and relevant reasons to support their conflicting conclusions and directives. In a moral dilemma, an agent morally ought to do X and morally ought to do Y, but the agent is precluded by circumstances from doing both. In a dilemma, the reasons behind alternatives X and Y are weighty, and neither set of reasons is obviously dominant. If one acts on either set of reasons, one's actions will be desirable in some respects but undesirable in others. It is impossible to act on all the reasons, yet each reason is, considered by itself, a good reason.

Moral dilemmas take at least the following two general forms.[1] (1) Some evidence indicates that act X is morally right, and some evidence indicates that act X is morally wrong, but the evidence on both sides is inconclusive. Abortion, for example, is sometimes said to be a terrible dilemma for women who see the evidence in this way. (2) The agent believes that, on moral grounds, he or she both ought and ought not to perform act X. Some have viewed the intentional cessation of lifesaving therapies in the case of permanently comatose patients, such as Karen Ann Quinlan and Paul Brophy (see Case 18), as dilemmatic in this second way.

Many situations involve moral dilemmas created by conflicting moral principles that generate conflicting demands. These dilemmas are often depicted in popular literature, novels, and films about difficult choices. For example, an impoverished person steals in order to save a family from starvation, a mother kills one of her children in order to save a second child, or a person lies to protect a family secret. In such stories, the only way to act in compliance with an obligation is by contravening another obligation; and no matter which course is elected, some obligation must go unfulfilled.

A conflict between a moral obligation on the one hand and self-interest on the other is not a moral dilemma. A moral dilemma arises only if there are *moral* considerations for taking each of two opposing courses of action. Of course, if moral reasons compete with nonmoral reasons, difficult questions about priority can still be posed without creating a moral dilemma. Numerous examples of this type of conflict appear in the work of anthropologist William R. Bascom, who collected hundreds of "African Dilemma Tales" transmitted for decades or centuries in African tribal societies. One traditional dilemma posed by the Hausa tribe of Nigeria is called "cure for impotence":

A friend gave a man a magical armlet that cured his impotence. Later he saw his mother, who had been lost in a slave raid, in a gang of prisoners. He begged his friend to use his magic to release her. The friend agreed on one condition—that the armlet be returned. What shall his choice be?[2]

Hard choice? Yes, but not a hard *moral* choice. The obligation to the mother is moral in character, whereas retaining the armlet is a matter of self-interest. (We are assuming that there is no important moral obligation to another person, such as a wife, in conflict with the man's moral obligation to his mother.)

Some moral philosophers have argued that there are many types of *practical* dilemmas but never genuine *moral* dilemmas. These philosophers do not deny that agents experience moral perplexity, moral conflict, and moral disagreement in difficult cases, but they insist that a genuine moral dilemma is a situation in which two moral *oughts* are in a type of conflict in which an action that one ought to perform cannot be performed without forgoing another action one also ought to perform. The belief that one cannot do what one ought to do seems to these philosophers a confusion about the nature of moral obligation. Some of the major figures in the history of ethics have held this view because they have believed that there is only one supreme moral value and that it overrides all other values, moral and nonmoral, with which it might be in conflict. The only real *ought*, in this theory, is the *ought* generated by the supreme value.[3]

Although certainly respectable, this denial of real dilemmas is not the perspective we adopt in this book. Our argument is that a plurality of moral principles may and do conflict in the moral life. On some occasions the conflict produces a genuine moral dilemma with no supreme principle that allows us to determine an overriding *ought*. We believe, nonetheless, that there are ways of reasoning about what we ought to do in the circumstance of a moral dilemma. In some cases the dilemma can be resolved by moral reasoning; in other cases it may only deepen upon reflection. However, we will not be in an adequate position to defend this viewpoint until we have completed the arguments in Chapter 2.

Moral deliberation and moral justification

The average person has no difficulty, in most circumstances, in making moral judgments such as whether to tell the truth, whether another person has an untenable conflict of interest, and the like. The moral life is composed of a rich mixture of directives, parables, and virtues that we learn as we grow up. Generally these moral guides suffice, because we are not asked to deliberate about or justify either our judgments or the principles that underlie them. But the experience of moral perplexity and of dilemmas leads to moral deliberation and moral justification. When we deliberate about whether a judgment is morally right, we are considering which judgment is morally justified, i.e. which judgment has the strongest moral reasons behind it. Reasons that we use in moral deliberation express the conditions under which we believe an action is morally justified.

Moral justification is appropriate whenever there is a need to defend one's moral convictions. To demonstrate that one is justified requires making explicit the principles that underlie one's judgments or deliberation. But a mere listing of these principles will not suffice. To be justified, one's principles must themselves be defensible. Accordingly, the approach to deliberation and justification accepted in this book can be diagrammed in the form of hierarchical tiers or levels:

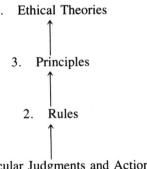

4. Ethical Theories

3. Principles

2. Rules

1. Particular Judgments and Actions

Judgments express a decision, verdict, or conclusion about a particular action (or, as we will see in Chapter 8, about a person's character). Particular judgments are justified by moral rules, which in turn are justified by principles, which ultimately are defended by an ethical theory. For example, a nurse who refuses to assist in an abortion procedure may hold that it is morally wrong to kill an innocent human being intentionally. When pressed, the nurse may justify the moral rule against killing an innocent human being by reference to a principle of the sanctity of human life. Finally, the particular judgment, the rule, and the principle may all be justified by an ethical theory, which may be only implicit and inchoate.

The diagram shows how in moral reasoning we appeal in the top three tiers to reasons of different degrees of abstraction and systematization. The precise nature of the distinction between rules and principles is controversial, because both are generalizations asserting that actions of a certain kind ought (or ought not) to be performed. As we analyze them, *rules* are more specific to contexts and more restricted in scope. A simple example of a rule is "It is wrong to lie to a patient." *Principles* are more general and fundamental than moral rules and serve to justify the rules. For example, a principle of respect for autonomy may support several moral rules of the form "It is wrong to lie." Finally, *theories* are integrated bodies of principles and rules and may include mediating rules that govern choices in cases of conflicts. Utilitarian and deontological theories, which we examine in the next chapter, are prominent types of ethical theory. We will refer to all of these levels or tiers, but especially to principles and rules, as *action-guides.*

Particular moral judgments involve applications of principles and rules to concrete situations and thus also depend on factual beliefs about the world. For instance, if we hold that policy X is wrong because it imposes unjustified risks on a group of people, we express beliefs about the probabilities of harm in the situation. Similarly, judgments about the justifiability of abortion may depend not only on moral rules and principles but also on beliefs about the nature and development of the fetus. Moral disputes thus do not involve only conflicts between moral rules or principles. For example, as we discuss in Chapter 6, many disagreements about the proper allocation of health dollars to preventive programs turn less on disputes over principles of justice than on factual claims about whether such measures prevent illness, promote health, have negative side effects, or are cost-effective.

Broad scientific, metaphysical, or religious beliefs may underlie our interpretation of a situation, and moral debate about a particular course of action may stem not only from disagreements about the relevant moral action-guides and the facts of the case but also from disagreements about the correct scientific, metaphysical, or religious description of the situation. Consider an example that involves various levels of moral justification and an interplay between moral action-guides and descriptive beliefs. Richard McCormick holds that it is morally permissible under some conditions to use children in "nontherapeutic" research—that is, research that does not offer potential medical benefit to the subjects involved, although it may ultimately benefit other pediatric patients.[4] His general rule is that this form of research is justified only if it involves minimal or negligible risk, if there is proxy (second-party) consent, and if the research methods are scientifically sound and suitable. McCormick's basic principle is one of justice: We all ought to bear minimal or negligible burdens for the common good. Such minimal or negligible burdens are not purely charitable, he believes, because they are demanded by justice. Thus we ought to consent to participation in certain forms of research under appropriate conditions.

McCormick further argues that parents (and other proxies) may legitimately consent for children to participate in nontherapeutic research where the child *ought* to consent (if the child were mature enough to be able to consent) because of a moral obligation to participate. A judgment that in a particular case it is morally acceptable to use children in nontherapeutic research depends for McCormick on critical *factual* beliefs about the probable benefits and risks of the research. For example, if the risks are more than minimal, nontherapeutic research on children is not justified. In addition, McCormick's ethical theory, a version of natural-law ethics, depends on certain factual beliefs about human tendencies that allow him to derive principles and rules about what people ought to do. These tendencies, including the human inclination toward community, are ultimately grounded in metaphysics and theology: God has created humankind with identifiable tendencies toward certain values.

As this example suggests, we should distinguish a reason's *relevance* to a moral judgment from its final *adequacy*. Not every proposed reason is relevant, but even relevant reasons are not always determinative. That is, an agent's appeal to a level or tier of justification may be relevant to a position the agent defends but insufficient to justify that position. Even *good* reasons may not be *sufficient* reasons. For example, the presence of dangerous toxic chemicals in a work environment has been offered as a reason to ban pregnant or fertile women from jobs that necessitate exposure to these chemicals. The dangers to health and life constitute a good reason for a ban, but this reason may not be a sufficient reason: Workers have often complained that a ban exclusively directed at women is discriminatory and unfair to those who are qualified. No matter which position is defended, we expect its proponents to give us a further account of why the reasons amount to both good and sufficient reasons. We expect them to cite relevant moral principles or refer to the good or bad consequences of the proposed course of action.

When we engage in argument with others about the justification of a moral judgment, usually in a context of either moral perplexity or moral criticism, we cannot reasonably expect another person's conduct to exceed the conventionally settled norms of morality. However, we can question whether a proclaimed principle is in fact a commonly accepted moral principle, and we can also ask whether an accepted principle should be replaced by another. Much of the concern in ethical theory with justification arises because of questions about which norms are settled norms of common morality and whether we should defend or reject certain generally accepted standards.

Because common morality cannot be invoked to justify itself, many look to ethical theory as an external source to validate moral judgments. However, whether ethical theory can supply the needed forms of justification is a difficult problem that we will need to investigate as we proceed.

Ethical theory and biomedical ethics

Ethics is a generic term for several ways of examining the moral life. Some approaches to ethics are normative, others descriptive.

Approaches to ethics

NORMATIVE ETHICS. The field of inquiry that attempts to answer the question "Which action-guides are worthy of moral acceptance and for what reasons?" may be called *general normative ethics*. It is constituted by the ethical theories placed at the top of our levels of justification. Such theories are studied in Chapter 2. They formulate and defend a system of fundamental moral principles and rules that determine which actions are right and which are wrong. Ideally, an ethical theory will include a complete set of ethical action-guides that meets a series of tests developed below. However, numerous questions would remain unanswered even if a fully satisfactory general ethical theory were available. For example, there would be questions about what the various principles and rules imply for the concrete decisions people must make in everyday life.

The attempts to apply these action-guides to different moral problems can be labeled *applied normative ethics*. The term *applied* refers to the use of ethical theory and methods of analysis to examine moral problems in the professions, technology, public policy, and the like. Often there is no straightforward application of theory in particular judgments in these contexts. Rather, theory is invoked to help develop action-guides that are more specific and fit the context. "Applied ethics" is broader than "professional ethics," but biomedical ethics, political ethics, journalistic ethics, legal ethics, and business ethics are fertile professional areas for such activity. Action-guides developed to handle moral problems in applied areas are generally shaped by moral principles and rules, paradigm cases or models of behavior, empirical data, and reflection on how to put these influential sources into the most harmonious unit.

The focus of this book is on applied normative ethics—specifically biomedical ethics—because we are applying general moral action-guides to biomedicine. *Biomedicine* is here used as a shorthand expression for many dimensions of modern biological sciences, medicine, and health care.

NONNORMATIVE ETHICS. In addition to normative ethics, whether general or applied, there are at least two nonnormative approaches to ethics. First, *descriptive ethics* is the factual investigation of moral behavior and beliefs. It studies not what people ought to do but how they reason and act. Anthropologists, sociologists, psychologists, and historians determine whether and in what ways moral attitudes and codes are expressed by individuals and societies. They study different beliefs and practices regarding sexual relations, codes of professional ethics, the treatment of the dying, the nature of consent obtained from patients, and the like. Second, *metaethics* involves analysis of the language, concepts, thought, and objects of ethics. For example, it studies the meanings of crucial ethical terms such as *right, obligation, virtue,* and *responsibility,* as well as the logic and patterns of moral reasoning and justification.

Descriptive ethics and metaethics can be grouped together as nonnormative because they do not attempt to provide prescriptive guidelines. Their objective is to establish what factually or conceptually is the case, not what ethically ought to be the case.[5] Occasionally in this book we engage in descriptive ethics and metaethics. But when we offer a descriptive analysis—for example, by presenting what professional medical codes say about certain issues—the underlying question is whether the described prescriptions are defensible. We also occasionally deal in metaethics. An example is found in our discussion later in this chapter of the concept of morality, in which we distinguish between moral and nonmoral action-guides. However, both descriptive ethics and metaethics are secondary to normative ethics throughout this book and when we use the term *ethics* without qualification, we mean normative ethics.

Codes of professional ethics

Systematic work in biomedical ethics is a recent phenomenon, despite decades and, in some cases, centuries of discussion by philosophers and theologians. Within the health-care professions the most influential reflection on these problems has evolved through formal codes of medical and nursing ethics, codes of research ethics, and reports by government-sponsored commissions. These writings include specific rules that apply to persons in the relevant professional roles in the practice of medicine and nursing, in health-care institutions, and in research.

We should distinguish between these *particular* moral codes, which govern such groups as physicians, psychologists, and nurses, and *general* moral codes, which govern whole societies and apply to everyone alike. A general moral code consists of the society's cherished moral principles and rules. The word *morality* often refers to this general code and the practices it spawns. An example of a simple rule in a general moral code is "Whenever you have promised to do something, then you have an obligation to do it." By contrast, a special or professional code specifies action-guides for a particular group, such as physicians or nurses. These action-guides should be justified by reference to more general principles and rules, which may not be explicitly identified in the codes themselves. Even if general theories or principles (such as those identified in Chapters 2 through 6) were never considered in the drafting of the codes, the directives in the codes can nonetheless be validly criticized or defended by appeal to general principles, as can many public policies and regulations that have been formulated to guide professionals.

Before we assess the advantages and disadvantages of professional codes, the nature of professions deserves brief discussion. According to Talcott Parsons, a profession is "a cluster of occupational roles, that is, roles in which the incumbents perform certain functions valued in the society in general, and by these activities, typically earn a living at a full-time job."[6] By this definition the circus performer and the exterminator are professionals. This result is not surprising inasmuch as the word *profession* has come, in its broadest sense, to mean any occupation in which a person earns a living. But we need a more restricted meaning for the term as it functions in "professional ethics." The following condition, then, seems essential: Professions control entry into occupational roles by formally certifying that candidates have acquired an essential body of knowledge and skills.

It has sometimes been maintained that the background knowledge of the professional must derive from intellectual training and that a professional must be engaged in an occupation that provides a service to others rather than the pursuit of personal interest. More accurately, these conditions are characteristic of certain learned professions and service professions. Not all professions are either learned or service-oriented.

However, professions do typically specify and enforce primary responsibilities and obligations and thus seek to ensure that people who enter into relationships with their members will find them to be competent and trustworthy. The obligations that professions attempt to enforce are referred to as *role norms*. A professional code represents an articulated statement of role morality as expressed by the members of the profession and thus is to be distinguished from standards imposed by external bodies such as governments. Sometimes codes also specify rules of etiquette and responsibilities to other members of the profession. For example, one historically significant code of the American Medical

Association instructed physicians not to criticize a fellow physician previously in charge of a case and urged all physicians to offer professional courtesy.[7]

Professional codes are beneficial if they effectively incorporate defensible moral principles and rules in the relationships they govern. Unfortunately, some professional codes oversimplify moral requirements or claim more completeness and authority than they are entitled to claim. As a consequence, professionals may suppose that they have satisfied all moral requirements if they have obediently followed the rules of the code, just as many people believe that they have discharged all their obligations when they have met the relevant legal requirements.

The most pertinent question is whether the codes specific to areas of science, medicine, and health care express all essential principles and rules. Many medical codes have much to say about the implications of some principles, such as nonmaleficence and beneficence, and about some rules, such as confidentiality. But only a few have anything to say about the implications of other important principles and rules, such as veracity, respect for autonomy, and justice, which have been the subjects of intense contemporary discussion.[8] Recently there have been efforts to incorporate these principles and rules by formulating statements of patients' rights that invoke the principle of respect for autonomy and rules of veracity.[9] These statements of proper professional conduct differ from earlier codes by focusing on the *rights* of those receiving health services rather than on the *obligations* of health professionals. But such statements are usually incomplete and neither present the whole range of moral principles nor provide an argued defense of the rules that are offered.

There are other reasons for general skepticism about the adequacy of professional codes in biomedicine besides these problems of incompleteness and unclear grounding in principles. Since the time of Hippocrates, physicians have generated narrow codes that involve no scrutiny or acceptance by those whom physicians serve. These codes have rarely appealed to more general ethical standards or to any authority beyond the deliberations of physicians. This history is striking inasmuch as we are ordinarily suspicious of a professional group that provides public services and yet develops its own codes of conduct independent of external warrant or scrutiny.

Another problem is that codes have traditionally been expressed in abstract formulations that dispense vague moral advice and are subject to competing interpretations. This reservation about codes of medical ethics was poignantly expressed in 1972 by psychiatrist Jay Katz in an influential compilation of materials on human experimentation. Originally inspired by his outrage over the fate of Holocaust victims, Katz became convinced that only a persistent educational effort that extended beyond traditional codes could provide meaningful guidance in research involving human subjects:

As I became increasingly involved in the world of law, I learned much that was new to me from my colleagues and students about such complex issues as the right to self-determination and privacy and the extent of the authority of governmental, professional, and other institutions to intrude into private life. . . . These issues . . . had rarely been discussed in my medical education. Instead it had been all too uncritically assumed that they could be resolved by fidelity to such undefined principles as *primum non nocere* or to visionary codes of ethics.[10]

Public policy and formal guidelines

One way of introducing external controls on health professionals and scientists is through regulations and guidelines promulgated by government agencies. Regulation of research involving human subjects provides an instructive example. Since the Nuremberg Code of 1947–48, the U.S. government has promulgated several influential regulations intended to protect research subjects. In 1974, Congress created a national commission to recommend guidelines to the secretary of the Department of Health, Education, and Welfare (now the Department of Health and Human Services), and in 1980 a president's commission was assembled to further examine the issues.[11] Their conclusions and lengthy recommendations, along with other government policies pertaining to biomedicine, raise vital questions explored later in this book about the proper relation between government and professional groups in formulating action-guides.

But what is meant by *public policy,* and how is it connected to ethics? A policy is a set of normative guidelines directed at practice. A public policy is composed of enforceable guidelines, governing a particular area of conduct, that have been accepted by an official public body—such as an agency of government or a legislature. The policies of corporations, hospitals, trade groups, and professional societies may have a deep impact on public policy, but their policies are private rather than public.

Some U.S. federal branches, agencies, and courts often use ethical premises in the development of health policy. These include the Centers for Disease Control (CDC), the National Institutes of Health (NIH), the Office of Technology Assessment (OTA), and the Supreme Court. Although there is an intimate connection between law and public policy, inasmuch as all laws constitute public policies, not all public policies are, in the conventional sense, laws. Public policies need not be explicitly formulated or codified. This occurs, for example, when an official decides not to fund a program that has no prior history of funding. Decisions not to act as well as decisions to act thus can determine public policies.

The making of policy is more complex than applying principles and rules. No ethical theory composed of abstract principles and rules can dictate policy, because it cannot contain enough specific information or guidance. The application of moral principles must take account of problems of efficiency, cultural pluralism, political procedures, uncertainty about risk, noncompliance by patients, and the like. The principles provide the moral background for policy, but the policy itself must be informed by empirical data and by special information available in relevant fields of medicine, biology, law, psychology, and so on. An ethical theory can be used not only as a framework to construct policies but also to criticize those already in place.[12]

When using moral principles to formulate public policies, it is rarely possible to move with assurance from a judgment that *act* X is morally right (or wrong) to a judgment that *law* or *policy* Y is morally right (or wrong). Factors such as the symbolic value of law and the cost of enforcement must be considered. Thus, the judgment that an act is morally wrong does not necessarily lead to the judgment that the government should prohibit it or refuse to allocate funds to support it. For example, one can consistently hold that sterilization and abortion are morally wrong without holding that the law should prohibit them or deny government funds to women who otherwise could not afford these procedures.

Nor does the judgment that an act is morally acceptable imply that the law should permit it. For example, the thesis that active euthanasia may be morally justified if patients face uncontrollable pain and suffering and request death is consistent with the thesis that the government should legally prohibit active euthanasia because it would not be possible to control abuses if it were legalized (see pp. 134–47 in Chapter 4). We are not now defending particular moral judgments about the justifiability of acts of euthanasia. We are maintaining that the connections between moral action-guides and judgments about policy or legal enforcement are complicated and that a judgment about acts does not entail the same judgment in law and policy.

Tests of ethical theories

Several general tests can be used to determine the adequacy of ethical theories. Even if no ethical theory satisfies all of these tests—and we think no currently available theory does—we can legitimately appeal to them when trying to determine which theories or elements of theories are acceptable. In subsequent chapters we will amplify the tests as we use them in analyzing and assessing ethical theories.

First, an ethical theory should be as clear as possible, as a whole and in its parts. Although we can expect only as much precision as is appropriate to a subject matter, there is more obscurity and vagueness in the literature of ethical theory and biomedical ethics than these subjects require.

Second, an ethical theory should be internally consistent and coherent. Parts of a theory should not be inconsistent with each other and should be mutually supportive. Ralph Waldo Emerson dismissed a foolish consistency as "the hobgoblin of little minds." However, we view consistency not as a *sufficient* condition of a good theory, only as a *necessary* one. If a moral account has implications that are inconsistent with other established parts of the account, then at least some aspect will have to be changed. Unless a change can be introduced without further inconsistencies emerging, it is doubtful that such an account qualifies as a theory, because it would not yield similar results when used by different people or even by the same persons in different but relevantly similar circumstances. This is a problem in biomedical ethics because general theories may permit inconsistent solutions of the dilemmas created by conflicts among their principles. (We do not claim to have fully escaped this problem in our theory.)

Third, a theory should be as complete and comprehensive as possible in listing moral principles, rules, and their connections. Although the four principles of respect for autonomy, nonmaleficence, beneficence, and justice presented in this book do not provide a complete system for general normative ethics, they do provide a sufficiently comprehensive framework for biomedical ethics. We do not need additional, *independent principles* such as promise keeping, truthfulness, privacy, or confidentiality.[13] However, we do *justify* rules of promise keeping, truthfulness, privacy, and confidentiality on the basis of the four principles (see Chapter 7).

Fourth, simplicity is a virtue of theories. For example, a theory should have no more principles and rules than are necessary, and no more than people can remember and apply without confusion.

Fifth, a theory must be able to account for the whole range of moral experience, including the principles, rules, and judgments affirmed in common morality. We participate in morality on a daily basis by reaching decisions, making judgments, and offering moral reasons. Ethical theories should build on, systematize, and rationally reconstruct our ordinary action-guides and judgments. However, this test must not be understood as a vindication of all popular judgments. Some may prove unjustified upon careful examination. A good theory consolidates and accounts for its data but need not mirror ordinary judgments; indeed, it should have the power to criticize defective judgments, no matter how widely accepted.

Because of its impact on our theory in this book, this fifth test deserves an extended discussion. Moral experience and moral theories are dialectically related: We develop theories to illuminate experience and to determine what we ought to do, but we also use experience to test, corroborate, and revise theories. If a theory yields conclusions at odds with our ordinary judgments—for example, if it allows human subjects to be used merely as means to the ends of scientific research—we have reason to be suspicious of the theory and to

modify it or seek an alternative theory. As Joel Feinberg suggests, this procedure of reasoning is similar to the dialectical reasoning that occurs in courts of
law. On the one hand, if a principle commits one to an antecedently unacceptable judgment, then one has to modify or supplement the principle in a way
that does the least damage to one's particular and general beliefs taken as a
whole. On the other hand, when a well-founded principle entails a change in a
particular judgment, the overriding claims of consistency may require that the
judgment be adjusted.[14] It seems mistaken, then, to say that ethical theory is
not *drawn from* cases but only *applied to* cases. Rather, cases provide data for
theory and are theory's testing ground as well. Cases lead us to modify and
refine embryonic theoretical claims, especially by pointing to inadequacies in
or limitations of theories.[15]

The theories, principles, rules, and judgments that we propose for acceptance
in this volume have been developed through this dialectical approach, which is
evident in the application of moral principles to concrete cases and the reformulation of the principles in light of those cases. For example, rules about the
disclosure of information in Chapter 3 have been developed by appeal to the
principle of respect for autonomy, clinical cases of medical decision making,
and empirical studies of comprehension and understanding. Principles in our
core framework of respect for autonomy, nonmaleficence, beneficence, and justice all play significant roles in the justification of rules and judgments about
such matters as disclosure and nondisclosure, but psychological information
and clinical experience in the practical problems of the patient-professional relationship are no less important. (A more detailed discussion of our approach
to moral theory is found in Chapter 2, pp. 44–55.)

This broad description expresses not only the authors' general methodology
but also how this book may be used for analysis and reflection well beyond its
theory and cases. The four core principles are intended to provide a framework
of moral theory for the identification, analysis, and resolution of moral problems in biomedicine. Deliberation and justification occur in applying the framework to cases. The reader can use this same approach to test our theory in light
of the above criteria of adequacy. We can also say, without undue paradox,
that the different tiers of justification—judgments, rules, and principles—can
be used to test one another.

Although other general tests could be formulated, the five we have briefly
outlined are the most important for analyzing and appraising various theories.
As we will see in subsequent chapters, a theory may receive a high score on
the basis of one test but a low score on the basis of another. In Chapter 2,
utilitarianism is depicted as consistent, coherent, simple, and comprehensive,
yet its critics claim that it is in tension with our ordinary judgments, especially
with certain judgments about justice and human rights. By contrast, utilitarian
critics of some deontological theories concede that such theories are consistent

with the bulk of our ordinary judgments, but they argue that these ordinary judgments should be modified by a simpler and more consistent, coherent, and comprehensive theory. Thus, a contested and validly criticized moral theory may nonetheless be rationally defensible in light of the different general tests proposed in this section. Although we currently have no perfect or even best moral theory, it does not follow that we have no good moral theories.

Moral and nonmoral action-guides

What makes some principles, problems, and judgments—but not others—*moral?* That is, by what criteria can we say that an action-guide is properly moral rather than economic, religious, legal, or political? Is there a way to distinguish moral standards from society's standards of etiquette, from cultural mores, and from rules of prudential behavior?

The elusive character of answers to these questions can be illustrated by the case of Infant Doe (Case 20), who was born with Down syndrome and other complications that prevented food from reaching the stomach. An operation probably could have saved the baby's life, but the parents and the physicians, ultimately with permission of the courts, did not intervene, and the baby died. Supporters of this decision might hold that parents had the right to make such a decision, that the infant would have been better off dead than alive, or that the burdens of caring for the infant would have been too onerous for the family. Opponents of the decision might claim that the infant had a right to life, that the infant could have anticipated a reasonably good quality of life and thus would have been better off alive than dead, or that the state should help families with such burdens rather than allowing them to withhold treatment from seriously ill and handicapped newborns.

This case exhibited human drama, judicial activity, public policy declarations, federal intervention, medical judgments, hospital practices, institutional rules, religious commitment and consultation, and so on. On the one hand, many medical, legal, and other kinds of judgments made in the case seem to have little to do with morality. On the other hand, they often do have a moral dimension. One problem in distinguishing the moral and the nonmoral is that they can be tightly interwoven in the factual and normative fabric of a case.

Several contemporary philosophers have tried to identify a modest list of criteria to distinguish between moral and nonmoral considerations.[16] They have concentrated on three main conditions of moral action-guides. The first two conditions—supremacy and universalizability—are formal: They refer to the form rather than the content of moral judgments, rules, and principles. Because they do not pertain to content, they would (if used alone) allow too many action-guides to be counted as moral, and thus the third condition—human welfare—is thought to be an essential supplementary condition.

Supremacy

According to the first proposed condition, moral action-guides are those that a person or, alternatively, a society accepts as supreme, final, or overriding. This criterion is appealing, because we expect a person of moral conviction not to be dissuaded by competing interests that would compromise moral belief or lead to moral weakness. Thus, self-interest, political affiliation, religious heritage, and the like seem rightly subordinate to the demands of morality. But, as attractive as this criterion of supremacy may seem, unless it is combined with other conditions, it permits almost anything to count as moral if a person or a society is committed to its overriding pursuit. For example, a person's supreme, overriding commitment to scientific knowledge, to art, or to alcohol could be considered that person's morality. Thus, supremacy is not a *sufficient* condition of morality.

Perhaps supremacy is nonetheless a *necessary* condition and, as such, only one necessary condition in a broader set of sufficient conditions. We think this more modest claim is also untenable. To hold that supremacy is a necessary condition of morality is to prejudge the weight that moral action-guides should have in our deliberations when they conflict with political, legal, and religious action-guides. We cannot without undue narrowness assert that moral considerations, by definition, outweigh or override all other competitive considerations. Nothing about morality demands that it can never be overridden by a competing nonmoral value, unless one stipulatively defines all overriding values of any sort as moral.

A critic might respond that the ultimate justification for following legal, religious, or political action-guides in preference to moral action-guides will always itself be a moral justification, and therefore that moral principles are always supreme. That is, it might be argued that the final justification for allowing a legal or some other obligation to override a moral obligation—such as a judgment to adhere to a law rather than engaging in civil disobedience—would ultimately have to be a moral rather than a legal justification. There is much to be said for this position, but it also needs a non-question-begging formulation that would require more extensive argument than we can present here.

Universalizability

A second and widely accepted condition for moral action-guides is universalizability, the formal principle that a moral standard applies universally, that is, to everyone in relevantly similar circumstances. Proponents of this condition reason as follows. What is right for one person must be right for all persons in relevantly similar circumstances. When we judge an act morally right or wrong we do not believe our declaration is like a judgment of mere taste or preference, which can vary from individual to individual. Ethical judgments transcend individual judgments, holding interpersonally despite the fact that an individual makes the judgment. For example, the rule that experimentation on human subjects requires consent is a universalizable moral rule, not merely a custom preferred in a few countries.

Although we often believe our moral declarations to be universalizable, we also know that many proposed moral declarations cannot justifiably claim such status. There is a gap between believing that one's proposition is universalizable and the proposition's being universalizable. This observation invites a closer examination of the meaning and import of universalizability.

What seems right about the idea of universalizability is the following. If any person judges that X is morally required in circumstance C_1, then that person is thereby committed to the view that X is morally required in circumstance C_2 if C_1 and C_2 are not morally different in any relevant respect. It is also correct to say that moral principles must be formulated in terms of universal rather than particular properties: Morality does not, for example, recognize a relevant difference between *I* and *he* or *she* in formulating what is right or wrong.[17] This is one way in which morality protects against bias, prejudice, and idiosyncratic preference. This explication analyzes universalizability in terms of consistency of moral commitment within a moral system of rules and principles, an analysis that seems to us faultless.

However, universalizability has sometimes been presented in a stronger sense, as if it meant that all moral action-guides apply universally to everyone alike and never apply exclusively to certain groups—irrespective of moral traditions and moral disagreements. If this were so, then North American views about the treatment of handicapped newborns and about access to health-care resources would have to be the same as Chinese views, or one group's views would have to be declared mistaken. Universalizability need not, however, entail that only one moral system of principles and rules is correct and universally applicable regardless of historical tradition and social context. Universalizability makes a formal point about the logic of moral judgment: A moral judgment must, for any person who accepts the judgment, apply to all relevantly similar circumstances. The principle itself does not say, however, what is to count as a relevantly similar circumstance (or whether there are relevantly similar circumstances).

This condition affords limited insight into the nature of morality. Many judgments satisfying this description are not moral judgments. For example, political and legal judgments demand this criterion of consistency. This indicates that universalizability, like supremacy, is not a *sufficient* condition of morality. More importantly, universalizability is suspect as a *necessary* condition of the full range of statements and actions that we call moral. In Chapter 8 we discuss moral ideals and supererogatory actions, which are above and beyond the de-

mands of moral obligation. Charity, exceptional generosity, and heroic interventions are examples. These high moral qualities are not universalizable. We
would not expect everyone to possess such qualities, and we would not judge
a person deficient if he or she failed to live up to such standards. Yet supererogatory acts done from moral ideals are part of the territory of the moral.
Some construals of universalizability as a necessary condition of the moral
would exclude these acts from the domain of morality, when they clearly belong in that domain.

A case study of problems in applying the criterion of universalizability can
be seen in the deliberations and recommendations regarding fetal research of
the aforementioned National Commission for the Protection of Human Subjects
of Biomedical and Behavioral Research.[18] (1) The commission affirmed that in
cases of experimentation in utero, the fetus to be aborted and the fetus to be
brought to term should be treated as equals. It held that "the woman's decision
for abortion does not, in itself, change the status of the fetus for purposes of
protection. Thus, the same principles apply whether or not abortion is contemplated; in both cases, only minimal risk is acceptable." (2) The commission
was otherwise divided, however, because similar treatment is not identical
treatment. Minimal risk for a fetus who will be brought to term is different
from minimal risk for a fetus who will be aborted, if we assume that the woman
will not change her mind. For example, the injection of a drug that crosses the
placenta might not injure a fetus aborted within two weeks after the injection,
but it might injure a fetus two months after the injection. Thus, the commission
agreed that the principle of universalizability (in this case, presented as a principle of equal treatment) is applicable to fetal research, but commission members disagreed about what this principle implies for differently situated fetuses.

Welfare

Some philosophers have proposed a third criterion of the moral. They argue
that it is *necessary* for a moral action-guide to have some reference to protecting or promoting human welfare. This condition of other-regardingness excludes egoistic principles, for example, from the realm of moral action-guides;
and it also excludes certain religious action-guides. However, it is difficult to
maintain that reference to human welfare is *sufficient* to render a judgment moral
in contrast to nonmoral. The fact that buying hogs and playing games are socially beneficial does not place those activities within the domain of the moral.

Whether human welfare is a *necessary* condition of moral action-guides is
more difficult to determine. But most action-guides of interest in biomedicine,
whether moral or not, do involve some direct reference to human welfare. For
example, most of the considerations offered by defenders and opponents of the

decision in the case of Infant Doe meet this condition, although they are also mixed with other considerations.

In conclusion, even if none of the above three conditions is either a necessary or a sufficient condition of morality, each may be *relevant* in any map of the terrain of morality. That is, each may be a marker that helps us identify what is moral, though not an infallible or essential marker. Morality is a complex social institution that draws from law, religion, government, and institutional roles, all of which use general action-guides to prescribe behavior. It is fruitless to seek a precise and decisive set of criteria that will delineate the differences between moral guides and all other action-guides. Part of understanding morality is to appreciate the broad scope of the concept and how pervasively it is infused into the expectations we have for proper social practices and institutional behavior.

Conclusion

While emphasizing the potential contribution of ethical theory, we have sketched an interdisciplinary account of the field of biomedical ethics. Biomedical ethics involves obtaining relevant factual information, assessing its reliability, identifying moral problems, and mapping out alternative solutions to the problems that have been identified. This mapping entails presenting and defending reasons in support of one's factual, conceptual, and moral claims, while at the same time analyzing and assessing one's basic assumptions and commitments. Ideally one should also be able to anticipate and respond to reasonable objections that others might make to one's arguments and solutions.

Far from faulting ethical theory because of its abstractness, our account of biomedical ethics views theory as central. Theoretical examinations of good reasons, moral justifications, moral principles and rules, and moral concepts are ineliminable parts of a balanced and comprehensive approach. One major defect in medical ethics throughout its history has been its distance from such theory.[19] That is, standards developed by the medical profession have suffered from the absence of an external basis for the justification and revision of these standards.[20] At the same time, we believe one of the major defects in contemporary theory in biomedical ethics is its distance from clinical practice and from serious historical work in the traditions of medical and nursing ethics. But this defect cannot be corrected here.

We have not yet discussed the different types of ethical theory that might be invoked in biomedical ethics. This subject is the centerpiece of Chapter 2. The third through sixth chapters then present our theory of basic moral principles— those of respect for autonomy, nonmaleficence, beneficence, and justice.

Notes

1. See John Lemmon, "Moral Dilemmas," *Philosophical Review* 71 (1962): 139–58.

2. William R. Bascom, *African Dilemma Tales* (The Hague: Mouton, 1975), p. 145 (relying on work by Roland Fletcher reported in 1912).

3. For an analysis of the philosophical and theological issues at stake in the debate about whether there are any genuine moral dilemmas, in contrast to situations of moral perplexity and uncertainty, see several essays that generated the recent discussion in Christopher W. Gowans, ed., *Moral Dilemmas* (New York: Oxford University Press, 1987); see also the helpful analysis in Edmund N. Santurri, *Perplexity in the Moral Life: Philosophical and Theological Considerations* (Charlottesville, Va.: University Press of Virginia, 1987).

4. Richard McCormick, S.J., "Proxy Consent in the Experimental Situation," *Perspectives in Biology and Medicine* 18 (Autumn 1974): 2–20; "Experimentation in Children: Sharing in Sociality," *Hastings Center Report* 6 (December 1976): 41–46. See, in reply, Paul Ramsey, *The Patient as Person* (New Haven: Yale University Press, 1970), pp. 1–58; "The Enforcement of Morals: Nontherapeutic Research on Children," *Hastings Center Report* 6 (August 1976): 21–39; "Children as Research Subjects: A Reply," *Hastings Center Report* 7 (April 1977): 40–42. See also the National Commission for the Protection of Human Subjects of Biomedical and Behavioral Research, *Report and Recommendations: Research Involving Children* (Washington, D.C.: DHEW Publication No. OS 77-0004, 1977), esp. chap. 8.

5. For discussion on whether such a sharp distinction can be drawn between metaethics and normative ethics, see Philippa Foot, "Goodness and Choice," and J. R. Searle, "How to Derive 'Ought' from 'Is,' " in *The Is/Ought Question*, ed. W. D. Hudson (London: Macmillan, 1969); see also Alan Gewirth, *Reason and Morality* (Chicago: University of Chicago Press, 1978).

6. Talcott Parsons, *Essays in Sociological Theory*, rev. ed. (Glencoe, Ill.: Free Press, 1954), p. 372.

7. The American Medical Association Code of Ethics of 1847, largely adapted from Thomas Percival's *Medical Ethics* (1803), was a response to a crisis in public and professional confidence. See Donald E. Konold, *A History of American Medical Ethics 1847–1912* (Madison, Wis.: State Historical Society of Wisconsin, 1962), chaps. 1–3; and Chester Burns, "Reciprocity in the Development of Anglo-American Medical Ethics," in *Legacies in Medical Ethics*, ed. Chester Burns (New York: Science History Publications, 1977).

8. See Sissela Bok, "The Tools of Bioethics," in *Ethics in Medicine: Historical Perspectives and Contemporary Concerns*, ed. Stanley J. Reiser, A. J. Dyck, and William J. Curran (Cambridge, Mass.: MIT Press, 1977), pp. 137–41.

9. See Chapter 2 for a discussion of one specific statement, "The Patient's Bill of Rights." In general for this history, see Ruth R. Faden and Tom L. Beauchamp, *A History and Theory of Informed Consent* (New York: Oxford University Press, 1986), chap. 3.

10. Jay Katz, ed., *Experimentation with Human Beings* (New York: Russell Sage Foundation, 1972), p. ix.

11. See Public Law 93–348 and the numerous publications of the National Commission for the Protection of Human Subjects of Biomedical and Behavioral Research. See

also the several volumes published by the President's Commission for the Study of Ethical Problems in Medicine and Biomedical and Behavioral Research.

12. See Dennis Thompson, "Philosophy and Policy," *Philosophy and Public Affairs* 14 (Spring 1985): 205–18. For an insightful discussion of the contributions and limitations of philosophy, especially ethical theory, in the formation of public policy, based on the experience of the President's Commission for the Study of Ethical Problems in Medicine and Biomedical and Behavioral Research, see the symposium on "The Role of Philosophers in the Public Policy Process: A View from the President's Commission," intro. by Daniel Wikler and essays by Alan Weisbard and Dan Brock, in *Ethics* 97 (July 1987): 775–95.

13. For two prominent views to the contrary, see Robert M. Veatch, *A Theory of Medical Ethics* (New York: Basic Books, 1981); and H. Tristram Engelhardt, Jr., *The Foundations of Bioethics* (New York: Oxford University Press, 1986). Veatch holds that there are more basic principles than we propose, and Engelhardt believes that there are fewer.

14. Joel Feinberg, *Social Philosophy* (Englewood Cliffs, N.J.: Prentice-Hall, 1973), p. 34. Chaim Perelman's account is also insightful: "In morals absolute preeminence cannot be given either to principles—which would make morals a deductive discipline—or to particular cases—which would make it an inductive discipline. Instead, judgments regarding particulars are compared with principles and preference is given to one or the other according to a decision that is reached by resorting to the techniques of justification and argumentation." *The New Rhetoric and Humanities: Essays on Rhetoric and Its Applications* (Boston: D. Reidel, 1979), p. 33.

15. See Judith Jarvis Thomson, *Rights, Restitution and Risk: Essays in Moral Theory* (Cambridge, Mass.: Harvard University Press, 1986), pp. 251–60.

16. For an early and influential set of papers, see *The Definition of Morality,* ed. G. Wallace and A. D. M. Walker (London: Methuen, 1970). See also William K. Frankena, *Perspectives on Morality,* ed. K. E. Goodpaster (Notre Dame, Ind.: University of Notre Dame Press, 1976), chaps. 10, 15. For discussion of some of the issues and major positions by the present authors, see James F. Childress, "The Identification of Ethical Principles," *Journal of Religious Ethics* 5 (Spring 1977): 39–68; and Tom L. Beauchamp, *Philosophical Ethics* (New York: McGraw-Hill, 1982), chap. 1.

In our analyses, we often use the terms *moral* and *ethical* interchangeably, although some distinctions can be drawn between them. Cicero apparently formed the Latin word *moralis* (from *mores*) to translate the Greek term *ethikos*. Etymologically their meanings are similar and stress manners, character, and customs. Contemporary usage suggests some rough but not precise distinctions between them. *Ethics* often refers to reflective and theoretical perspectives, whereas *morality* often refers to actual conduct and practice. Our use of the terms *ethics* and *morality* in this book respects this rough distinction, although we use the adjectives *moral* and *ethical* interchangeably.

17. See R. M. Hare, *Moral Thinking: Its Levels, Method and Point* (Oxford: Clarendon Press, 1981), p. 223.

18. The National Commission for the Protection of Human Subjects of Biomedical and Behavioral Research, *Report and Recommendations: Research on the Fetus* (Washington, D.C.: U.S. Department of Health, Education, and Welfare, 1975), p. 66.

19. With due respect, we acknowledge the philosophical acumen and erudition of such

prominent historical figures in medical ethics as John Gregory, Thomas Percival, Worthington Hooker, and Richard Clarke Cabot.

20. By proposing the need for an *external* basis for justification in ethics, we do not embrace foundationalism in moral justification, in the sense of holding that moral theories are rooted in some ahistorical domain rather than in history and tradition. To the contrary, we would support (if we could develop the argument here) a robust historicism in preference to foundationalism. Nonetheless, moral standards do transcend the insights and beliefs of many particular groups and traditions, and these standards are often useful for critically examining and restructuring past moral thinking and present moral perplexity.

2

Types of Ethical Theory

A well-developed ethical theory provides a framework of principles within which an agent can determine morally appropriate actions. In light of the tests developed in the previous chapter, we will now consider which type of ethical theory, if any, is most satisfactory. This chapter concentrates on two types of ethical theory: consequentialist and deontological (derived from the Greek word *deon,* meaning ''duty''). This distinction was introduced in this century in order to bring ancient and modern theories into a unified classification scheme.[1] Consequentialism is the moral theory that actions are right or wrong according to their consequences rather than any intrinsic features they may have, such as truthfulness or fidelity. The most prominent consequentialist theory is utilitarianism, and we concentrate exclusively on this form of consequentialism.

The classical origins of utilitarianism are found in the writings of David Hume (1711–1776), Jeremy Bentham (1748–1832), and John Stuart Mill (1806–1873). Utilitarians maintain that the moral rightness of actions is determined by their consequences, in particular by the maximization of the nonmoral value produced by the action. The value produced—such as pleasure, friendship, knowledge, or health—is said to be *nonmoral* because it is the general goal of many human activities, such as art, athletics, and academics, and thus is not a distinctly moral value like fulfilling a moral obligation. A common feature of these theories is that standards of obligation and right conduct depend on and are subordinated to standards of the good.

Deontological theories deny much that consequentialist theories affirm. Their classical origins are more diverse and include, for example, some religious traditions that concentrate on divine commands. However, the ethical theory of Immanuel Kant (1734–1804) is generally regarded as the first unambiguous formulation of a deontological ethical theory. Deontologists maintain that the concepts of obligation and right are independent of the concept of good and that right actions are not determined exclusively by the production of good consequences. Whereas the consequentialist (and thus the utilitarian) holds that actions are determined to be right or wrong by only one of their features, namely their consequences, the deontologist contends that even if this feature sometimes determines the rightness and wrongness of acts, it does not always do so. Other features of an action may also be relevant, such as the fact that it involves telling a lie or compromising one's integrity.

In this chapter we consider these two types of ethical theory as ways of accounting for rightness and wrongness. We begin with utilitarianism and then examine a small set of deontological theories.

Utilitarian theories

Utilitarianism is a familiar term, but its popular usage can be confusing and misleading. It is said, for example, to be the theory that "The end justifies the means" and that "We ought to promote the greatest good of the greatest number." Because *utility* can mean "usefulness," the theory is also sometimes expressed as "What is right is what is most useful." In some respects each of these popular characterizations is accurate, but utilitarianism is considerably more sophisticated and refined than these explications suggest. We shall use *utilitarianism* to refer to the moral theory that there is one and only one basic principle in ethics, the principle of utility, which asserts that we ought always to produce the greatest possible balance of value over disvalue (or the least possible balance of disvalue, if only undesirable results can be achieved).

An example of utilitarian thinking is the following. It is universally agreed that physicians should minimize the medical costs and the suffering of their patients. This maxim does not require physicians never to charge fees to patients or never to allow any suffering or risk of harm to patients. But it does require that whenever there is a choice between different but equally efficacious methods of treatment, patients' benefits should be maximized and their costs and risks minimized. This example and similar ones from everyday life—such as designing a family budget to meet the family's needs or creating a new national park in a wilderness region—can reflect a utilitarian method of calculating what should be done by balancing resources and comparing the needs of everyone affected. According to this method, an action is justified if it produces more good than any alternative action.

Utilitarians do not regard this method of calculating as unusual in the moral life. They maintain that utilitarianism renders explicit and systematic what is already implicit in ordinary deliberation and justification, whether in individual judgments or in public policy. Case 33 in the appendix provides a typical example. It describes a policy decision announced by the twelve lay trustees of the Massachusetts General Hospital. These trustees voted not to permit heart transplants at that institution "at the present time" (1980) because "in an age where technology so pervades the medical community, there is a clear responsibility to evaluate new procedures in terms of the greatest good for the greatest number." They decided that the resources necessary for heart transplantation could be deployed elsewhere to greater advantage.

The concept of utility

All utilitarians share the conviction that human actions are to be morally assessed in terms of their production of maximal nonmoral value. But how are we to determine what value should be produced in any given circumstance? Here we encounter disputes among utilitarians concerning how the theory is best characterized, as well as disputes over which values are most important. Some grasp of these internal disputes is required in order to understand utilitarian ethics.

Many utilitarians agree that ultimately we ought to look to the production of agent-neutral or intrinsic values, those that do not vary from person to person.[2] That is, what is good in itself, not merely what is good as a means to something else, ought to be produced. For example, neither undergoing nor performing an abortion is intrinsically good. However, many people would consider an abortion as extrinsically good in some circumstances—for instance, as a means to the end of protecting a pregnant woman's life and health, which are intrinsic goods. Many utilitarians believe that we ought to produce those conditions in life that are good in themselves without reference to their further consequences and that all actions are ultimately to be gauged in terms of these intrinsic values. Health and freedom from pain are often included among such values. From this perspective, the whole point of the institution of morality is to promote these values by maximizing benefits and minimizing harms.

Within utilitarian theories of intrinsic value a major distinction is drawn between hedonistic and pluralistic utilitarians. Bentham and Mill are said to be hedonistic because they conceive utility entirely in terms of happiness or pleasure, two broad terms they treat as synonymous. Bentham, for example, views utility as that aspect of any object or event whereby it tends to produce different pleasures in such forms as benefit, advantage, and the prevention of pain.[3] Mill insists that happiness does not refer merely to "a continuity of highly pleasurable excitement" but rather encompasses the pleasurable moments afforded in life, whether they take the form of tranquillity or passionate excitement.[4] The principle of utility for Bentham and Mill thus demands courses of action that produce the maximum possible happiness. That is, an action ought to be performed if the sum of the happiness of all affected individuals would be maximized by the performance of that action.

Mill and Bentham appreciate that many human actions do not appear to be performed merely for the sake of happiness. For example, they understand that highly motivated professionals—such as research scientists—can work themselves to the point of exhaustion for the sake of knowledge they hope to gain, even though they might have chosen different and more successful routes to happiness or pleasure. Mill's explanation of this phenomenon is that these persons are initially motivated by success or money, both of which promise pleasure. Along the way, either the pursuit of knowledge itself makes them happy or such persons never stop associating their hard work with the success, money, or prestige they hope to gain (despite not actually deriving much, if any, pleasure from it). Mill also believes that there are qualitatively different kinds of pleasure, some worth cultivating more than others because they are intrinsically more valuable. This claim is difficult to sustain, but Mill's problems with it cannot be considered here. The main point is that for some utilitarians, including two of its leading proponents, happiness or pleasure is the sole form of intrinsic value, even though it may be analyzed into different subtypes.

Later utilitarian philosophers have not always looked favorably on this monistic conception of intrinsic value. They have argued that other values besides happiness possess intrinsic worth; among these values are friendship, knowledge, health, and beauty. According to G. E. Moore, even some states of consciousness can be valuable apart from their pleasantness.[5] The idea that there are several basic kinds of intrinsic value eventually received widespread acceptance among utilitarians. Its proponents held that the greatest aggregate good, as well as all moral rightness or wrongness, is to be assessed in terms of the total range of intrinsic values ultimately produced by an action.

However, both hedonists and pluralists have been challenged on grounds that individual preferences rather than agent-neutral values should determine utility. For this approach, the concept of utility refers not to experiences or states of affairs but rather to individuals' actual preferences. Utility is thus translated into the satisfaction of those desires that individuals prefer to have satisfied.

This approach to value has seemed to many more defensible than its predecessors for two main reasons. First, a person's choice of values seems deeply affected by personal experiences and desires—a problem preference utilitarianism avoids because personal preference defines value in the theory. Second, to make utilitarian calculations, it is necessary to measure values. In the monistic theory espoused by Bentham and Mill, for example, we must be able to measure states of pleasure and then compare one person's with another's in order to decide which is greater. Yet it is uncertain how to measure and then compare values such as pleasure, health, and knowledge. As Alasdair MacIntyre observes, "The happiness which belongs peculiarly to the way of life of the cloister is not the same happiness as that which belongs peculiarly to the military life. For different pleasures and different happinesses are to a large degree incommensurable."[6] In response, preference utilitarians argue that it is possible to develop a utility scale that numerically measures strengths of individual and group preferences and devises an order of preferences.[7]

The preference approach is not trouble-free, however. A major problem of utilitarianism arises when individuals have what are judged by the common morality to be morally unacceptable preferences. For example, if a skillful researcher derived supreme satisfaction from inflicting pain on animals or on human subjects in experiments, we would condemn and discount this person's preference and would seek to prevent it from being actualized. Utilitarianism based on subjective preferences is a defensible theory only if a range of acceptable preferences can be formulated, where "acceptability" is agent-neutral and thus not a matter of preferences. But this task seems inconsistent with a pure preference approach, because that approach logically ties human values to preferences, which are by their nature not agent-neutral.

One utilitarian response is that unacceptable desires can and should be identified and discounted. On the basis of past experience we can know which preferences undermine utilitarian social objectives by creating conditions adverse to the production of human value. These desires would not be permitted to count in the utilitarian calculus. For example, we would refuse to acknowledge preferences to taunt and abuse aged citizens, not only because these preferences obstruct the preferences of the aged but because more generally such preferences destroy or undermine the achievement of human aspirations (themselves determined by firmly established preferences). Thus, some preferences deserve on utilitarian grounds to be obstructed in a calculus of goods. In this account the principle of utility allows us to exclude some preferences on more general utilitarian grounds, once an experiential basis has been established. However, this exclusion of preferences does not seem consistent with a theory based entirely on preferences. Agent-neutral values must be adopted in order for the reply to have force. This widened utilitarianism requires a second-level set of agent-neutral values that constrains a pure-preference calculus.

Despite these problems, it is easy to overestimate the demands of the utilitarian moral theory, and many critics have distorted it. The utilitarian readily admits that accurate measurements of outcomes and of the preferences of others can seldom be provided because of limited knowledge and time. The utilitarian need not demand that all future consequences or even all avoidable consequences be anticipated. Often it is enough to anticipate only what one can bring about in a relatively narrow context. In everyday affairs we must act on severely limited knowledge of the consequences of our actions. The utilitarian does not condemn any sincere attempt to maximize value merely because the consequences of the attempt turn out to be less than maximal. What is important, in judging the agent of the action, is that the agent conscientiously attempts to produce the best utilitarian outcome. Because common sense and careful deliberation will generally suffice for these calculations, utilitarians cannot be fairly accused of demanding more than is humanly possible.

Act and rule utilitarianism

Another significant distinction is between act and rule utilitarians. For all utilitarians the principle of utility is the ultimate source of appeal for the determination of morally right and wrong actions. Controversy has arisen, however, over whether this principle is to be applied to *particular acts* in particular circumstances in order to determine which act is right, or whether it is to be applied instead to *general rules* that determine which acts are right and wrong. Using the schema of ascending levels of justification introduced in Chapter 1, we may outline how utilitarians attempt to justify moral actions and, at the same time, illustrate how act and rule utilitarians differ:

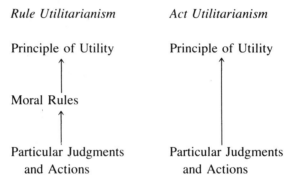

According to this schema, the rule utilitarian justifies particular judgments about actions by appealing to rules such as "Do not steal" and "Do not lie," which in turn are justified by the principle of utility. An act utilitarian simply skips the level of rules and justifies actions by appealing directly to the principle of utility. The act utilitarian thus considers the consequences of each particular act, while the rule utilitarian considers the consequences of rules and kinds of acts. The act utilitarian asks, "What good and bad consequences will result from this action in this circumstance?" and not "What good and bad consequences will result from this sort of action in general in these sorts of circumstances?" The act utilitarian sees rules such as "You ought to tell the truth" as useful rules of thumb in guiding human actions, but not as binding prescriptions. For the rule utilitarian, by contrast, an act's conformity to a rule makes it right; beneficial consequences of individual acts do not alone make them right.

One of the major nineteenth-century figures in academic medicine and medical ethics, Dr. Worthington Hooker, was a rule utilitarian who paid particularly close attention to the importance of rules of truth telling in medicine. In a trenchant analysis of deception by physicians, Hooker argues as follows:

The good, which may be done by deception in a *few* cases, is almost as nothing, compared with the evil which it does in *many,* when the prospect of its doing good was just as promising as it was in those in which it succeeded. And when we add to this the evil which would result from a *general* adoption of a system of deception, the importance of a strict adherence to the truth in our intercourse with the sick, even on the ground of expediency, becomes incalculably great.

Hooker was aware that a patient's health may sometimes maximally be advanced through deception, but he did not believe that a physician can successfully predict the beneficent outcomes in particular cases, and he held that the use of deception will have an incremental effect over time and cause more harm than good. He therefore defended the rule that deception not be practiced at all in medicine.[8]

Act utilitarians affirm a contrary position because they think observance of a general rule such as truth telling would not always maximize the general good and therefore can be no more stringent than a rule of thumb. They regard rule utilitarians as unfaithful to the demands of the principle of utility, which requires that we maximize value. In some circumstances, abiding by a generally beneficial rule will not prove most beneficial to the persons affected by the action, even in the long run. Why, then, ought a rule be obeyed in individual cases if obedience will not maximize value in these cases?

A contemporary act utilitarian, J. J. C. Smart, has argued that the rule utilitarian cannot reply to this criticism that it would be better to require that everybody should obey the rule than that nobody should be required to do so. This objection fails, according to Smart, because there is a third possibility between never obeying a rule and always obeying it, namely that it should *sometimes* be obeyed.[9] From this perspective, physicians do not and should not always tell the truth to their patients. They sometimes withhold information and even lie in order to give hope to a patient. They do so because they think it is better for the patients and for all concerned, and they do not think their acts undermine general observance of moral rules. Smart's position seems in the end to rely on the empirical prediction that we will be better off in the moral life if we sometimes obey and sometimes disobey rules, because this selective obedience will not erode either moral rules or our general respect for morality. Rules, then, are stabilizing but nonbinding guides in the moral life; that is, they are useful rules of thumb that are dispensable in some circumstances.

ASSESSMENT OF ACT UTILITARIANISM. A case of research in the social sciences illustrates act-utilitarian thinking. In order to observe homosexual behavior, a sociologist posed as a lookout for male homosexuals using isolated public facilities (so-called tearooms).[10] His desire to provide a thorough study of this form of life-style led him to record the automobile license plate numbers of the participants so that he could subsequently locate their residences. By misrepresenting himself as a researcher pursuing a different and innocuous kind of study, he gained entrance to their homes and obtained data on family background, marital status, and the like. This research methodology has been heavily criticized not only because it put the subjects studied at risk (e.g., the police might have obtained damaging personal data) but also because it involved outright deception, including a set of lies to gain entrance to private homes. The research thus violated a number of standard moral rules prohibiting deception, lying, invading privacy, and placing other persons at risk. The sociologist involved defended his research on act-utilitarian grounds. He argued that his study would provide a valuable understanding of the motives and general behavioral patterns of those who perform homosexual acts and that it would also help others to appreciate the social pressures that can lead to homosexual activity. He thus attempted to justify the violation of standard moral rules by citing the value of the otherwise unattainable data produced by his research.

Act utilitarianism has been justifiably subjected to sharp criticism in recent moral philosophy. One form of criticism relies on examples of wrong but undetectable actions. For example, suppose a physician, at the patient's request, kills by an undetectable means a rapidly deteriorating dialysis patient, who would have died in two to three months anyway, because the patient's death would maximize utility in the circumstances. Now imagine a second physician who performs the identical action under the identical circumstances, except that the action is detected. It would seem that, according to act utilitarianism, the second action is morally wrong, whereas the first is right. The first action maximizes utility in the circumstances. After all, the dialysis patient has little life left and is a severe financial and emotional burden to the family. In addition, the first doctor does not suffer the consequences of public criticism, professional sanctions, or even imprisonment. In the second case, however, the doctor may suffer imprisonment, and the families of both the patient and the physician may suffer the embarrassment, guilt, and anguish that usually accompany such events. (Compare this hypothetical case with the reported case of Debbie in Chapter 4, p. 143.)

This outcome of act-utilitarian reasoning is odd and unacceptable, for at least two reasons. First, the killing (if wrong) seems to be equally wrong in both cases; the second action does not appear more blameworthy simply because of a chain of unpleasant consequences. Second, some consequences of the physician's act—such as some of the negative consequences in the second case—do not seem relevant to a proper moral assessment of the act. Act utilitarianism seems to make some consequences relevant so as to change our moral assessment of the act when these consequences should be irrelevant.

A similar and standard form of counterexample to act utilitarianism is captured in the following imagined sequence of events. Suppose you are mountain climbing with your closest friend, a person you admire and respect and from whom you have received many favors. Now suppose you lose your grip on a rope while your friend is descending a sheer cliff. He falls. By the time you reach him, he is dying. In these dying moments he asks that you make a promise to be kept in strictest confidence, and you agree. He reveals a financial secret he has been harboring. Through years of hard work and careful investments he has accumulated several million dollars. He asks you to deliver this money to an uncle who has helped him in the past. But you know that this uncle is a rich gambler who will squander the money. No one else knows about either the promise or the secret cash. On act-utilitarian principles, you should not carry out your promise to your dying friend, because you could put the money to much better utilitarian use by giving it to charitable institutions. You would neither disappoint the man to whom you made the promise nor weaken faith in the socially useful institutions of promise making and promise keeping.

The point of these counterexamples is to show that act utilitarianism is inconsistent with our common convictions about moral rightness. We saw in Chapter 1 that one test of an ethical theory is its congruence with these common, well-considered, ethical convictions. The act utilitarian would no doubt reply that although promises usually should be kept in order to maintain a climate of trust, this consideration fails to apply in some cases in which more good is produced by breaking the promise. The act utilitarian might also argue that making exceptions to standard rules is consistent with the common moral consciousness, because we often do so without any sense of committing a moral wrong. Alternatively, the act utilitarian might agree that there is sometimes an inconsistency with ordinary moral convictions in these cases but might respond that (1) our common judgments are not entirely settled in these cases, and (2) in at least some cases we need to revise our ordinary convictions rather than discard act utilitarianism.

An example of the act utilitarian's point is found in a comment by Colorado governor Richard Lamm, who once observed that in light of increasing financial costs of medical care the terminally ill have ''a duty to die and get out of the way with all of our machines and artificial hearts and everything else.'' There was an outcry of indignation and shock that a public official should defend a position so inconsistent with general moral beliefs. Lamm had chosen an unfortunate word when he landed on ''duty,'' but in context he was giving an act-utilitarian answer to what he correctly referred to as an ''ethical question.'' His point was that we cannot continue public funding for medical technology without assessing costs and trade-offs, even if some people will eventually die because a technology is not available. The act utilitarian is confident that many questions posed by technological developments cannot be handled by traditional moral rules and that we will thus inevitably give some moral answers that seem counterintuitive. The important matter from the act utilitarian's point of view is not congruence with past or current judgments but conformity to the goal of maximizing favorable consequences. Those who favor congruence over concern for unprecedented consequences for the larger society have, from this point of view, an inappropriate set of tests of moral theories in the first place.

Another example of the way act utilitarianism sometimes challenges our ordinary convictions appears in Case 35, which features two researchers who became interested in facts and policies pertaining to high blood pressure in American society. These investigators wanted to determine the most cost-effective way to address the problem of controlling hypertension in the American population. As they developed their research, they discovered that it is most cost-effective to target three groups in the attempt to reduce the general public health problem of high blood pressure: younger men, older women, and patients with exceptionally high blood pressure. When they combined these results with findings that large-scale, communitywide screening and informational programs are not medically effective and not cost-effective, they concluded:

A community with limited resources would probably do better to concentrate its efforts on improving adherence to known hypertensives, even at a sacrifice in terms of the numbers screened. This conclusion holds even if such proadherence interventions are rather expensive and only moderately effective, and even if screening is very inexpensive. . . . Finally, screening in the regular practices [of physicians] is more cost-effective than public screening.

If acted on by the government, this recommendation would exclude the poorest sector of the country, which has the greatest general need of medical attention, from the benefits of high-blood-pressure education and management. Public screening would be sacrificed in order to produce the greatest good for the entire community, because only persons known to have high blood pressure and already in contact with a physician about their problem would be recontacted.

The investigators were concerned because of the apparent injustice in excluding the poor and minorities by a public health endeavor aimed at the economically better-off sector of society. Yet their statistics were compelling: No matter how carefully planned the efforts, nothing worked efficiently except programs directed at known hypertensives already in contact with physicians. They knew that in light of other health needs there would be no new federal allocations of public health money to control high blood pressure. Yet it would take massive new allocations to begin to affect the poorer population. The investigators therefore recommended what they explicitly referred to as a "utilitarian" set of criteria for allocation. This case is among the most challenging presented by act utilitarianism for testing our ordinary moral convictions.

ASSESSMENT OF RULE UTILITARIANISM. The objections thus far considered affect act utilitarianism but cannot be used without modification to criticize rule utilitarianism. The term *rule* here encompasses both general principles and general rules. According to rule utilitarians, principles and rules cannot be disregarded because of the exigencies of particular situations (except when other moral rules require a different action; see pp. 51–54). Because of the substantial contributions made to society by the general observance of such rules as truth telling, the rule utilitarian would not compromise them in a particular situation. Such a compromise would threaten the integrity and existence of either the individual rules or the system of rules.

Some rule utilitarians propose that we consider the utility of whole codes or systems of rules rather than assess each rule independently. Among the defenders of different versions of the latter position are David Hume, an eighteenth-century Scottish philosopher, and Richard Brandt, a contemporary American philosopher.[11] According to this approach, the rightness or wrongness of individual acts is determined by reference to moral rules that have a place in a general code or system of rules. The system is assessed as a whole in terms of its overall consequences, and individual moral rules are evaluated as parts of an entire network of rules. The scheme of ascending levels of justification introduced in Chapter 1 again illustrates this version of rule utilitarianism:

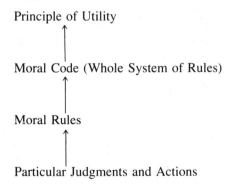

Principle of Utility

Moral Code (Whole System of Rules)

Moral Rules

Particular Judgments and Actions

This whole-code approach has advantages over single-rule utilitarianism. We are more likely to be able to maximize utility across an entire society with a whole system of rules than with single rules that are isolated from the consequences of other rules in the system. Most of us already understand and accept morality—and also law—in the form of an integrated body of rules, none of which stands in isolation.[12]

From the utilitarian's perspective only the principle of utility has an absolute status. No moral action is absolutely wrong in itself, and consequently no rule in the system of rules is unrevisable. A rule's acceptability depends strictly on its consequences. Even rules against killing may be revised or substantially overturned. For example, we will often have occasion in this book to mention the recent discussions in biomedical ethics of the possibility that some seriously suffering patients may or should be killed rather than "allowed to die." The rule utilitarian argues that we should support rules *permitting* such killing if those rules would maximize value; but the rule utilitarian also insists that there should be rules *against* such killing if those rules would maximize value.

This utilitarian approach seems shocking and outrageous to some, because in theory it would permit radical shifts in our present system of moral rules. But utilitarians are not persuaded by this tradition-based objection. They point to the reason why we have the rules against killing that we now have. They argue that we currently do not permit the killing of patients because of the adverse consequences that would be produced for those directly and indirectly affected by such actions. But if these adverse consequences did not generally occur, then the utilitarian would see no reason in principle why mercy killing should be prohibited. This conclusion indicates how utilitarianism is a conse- quentialist theory and also how utilitarians view their theory as responsive to the need for social change.

Deontological theories

By contrast to consequentialist theories, deontological theories hold that some features of acts other than, or in addition to, their consequences make them right or wrong and that the grounds of right or obligation are not wholly de- pendent on the production of good consequences. The essence of the deonto- logical perspective is that some actions are right (or wrong) for reasons other than their consequences.

If a therapist deceives a patient by substituting a placebo (see Case 5), a deontologist might point to both the feature of deception itself (not merely the effects of the act or of a general practice of deception) and the therapist's motives. For many deontologists deception is a wrong-making characteristic for reasons independent of its consequences. A deontologist need not hold that deception or any other type of action is absolutely wrong and never justifiable, but to qualify as a deontologist, one must hold that at least some acts are right and others wrong, not because of their consequences but because of right-making characteristics such as fidelity to promises, truthfulness, and justice.

Versions of deontology

Different deontological theories compete with each other, as well as against consequentialist theories. These theories exhibit more diversity than utilitarian theories, and thus it is possible to analyze them from several perspectives.

GROUNDS OF DEONTOLOGY. First, deontologists try in different ways to vindicate their judgments that certain acts are right or wrong. Some writers in religious traditions appeal to divine revelation (e.g., to God's promulgation of the Ten Commandments), whereas others appeal to natural law and natural right, which they contend can be known by human reason. Some philosophers, including W. D. Ross, find intuition and common sense sufficient. Still others, such as John Rawls, develop a contractarian theory by deriving their principles from a hypothetical social contract; they ask which principles rational contractors would adopt if they were blinded to their particular talents, abilities, and conceptions of the good life.[13]

Perhaps the two most prominent forms of deontology in recent philosophy have been contractarian theories (e.g., Rawls's) and rights-based theories (e.g., Robert Nozick's). However, to further analyze and assess these diverse deontological warrants for moral judgments would lead us through an unnecessary detour into discussions of forms of justification (which have parallels in justifications of utilitarian theories that we did not consider earlier). Most of the principles and rules adopted in this book are accepted by most deontological theories and can also be discovered in the "common moral consciousness."

MONISTIC AND PLURALISTIC THEORIES. Like utilitarian theories, deontological theories may be monistic or pluralistic. A monistic theory holds that there is a single principle or rule from which all other rules or judgments about right and wrong can be derived. Thus, a deontologist could affirm a single basic principle such as care or respect for persons or "the Golden Rule" and then derive rules such as truth telling and fidelity from it. An example appears in Alan Donagan's *The Theory of Morality*. Donagan tries to locate the "philosophical core" of the morality of the "Hebrew-Christian tradition," a part he believes is not dependent on explicitly theistic beliefs. He identifies the fundamental principle of this moral tradition as "It is impermissible not to respect every human being, oneself or any other, as a rational creature."[14] Donagan believes that all other moral principles and rules of the common morality in the Hebrew-Christian tradition are derivative from this fundamental action-guide.

Donagan and many contemporary deontologists are indebted to Immanuel Kant's classic proposal of a single "categorical imperative" for testing all rules of action. Kant held that the moral worth of an agent's action depends exclusively on the moral acceptability of the rule on which the person is acting; or, as Kant prefers to say, moral acceptability depends on the rule that determines the agent's will. An action has moral worth only if performed by an agent who possesses what Kant calls a good will; and a person has a good will only if moral duty based on a valid rule is the sole motive of action.

As an example of Kant's thesis, consider a man who desperately needs money and knows that he will not be able to borrow it unless he promises repayment in a definite time, even though he also knows that he will not be able to repay it within this period. He decides to make a promise that he knows he will break. According to Kant, when we examine the maxim of this man's action— "When I think myself in want of money, I will borrow money and promise to pay it back, although I know that I cannot do so"—we discover that it cannot pass the basic test of what he calls the categorical imperative, which requires that maxims be universalizable. (The categorical imperative is *categorical* because it admits of no exceptions and is absolutely binding. It is *imperative* because it gives instruction about how one morally must act.)

This test of universalizability is richer and more complicated than the formal test of universalizability introduced in Chapter 1. To be universalizable, according to Kant, a maxim must be capable of being conceived and willed without contradiction as valid for everyone. The above maxim about misleading promises cannot be conceived as universally valid, because it is contradictory. As Kant writes, such a maxim is not consistent with what it presupposes:

. . . "How would things stand if my maxim became a universal law?" I . . . see straight away that this maxim can never rank as a universal law of nature and be self-consistent, but must necessarily contradict itself. For the universality of a law that everyone believing himself to be in need can make any promise he pleases with the intention not to keep it would make promising, and the very purpose of promising, itself impossible, since no one would believe he was being promised anything, but would laugh at utterances of this kind as empty shams.[15]

Various examples illustrate Kant's thesis. For example, rules of lying are inconsistent with the practices of truth telling they presuppose, and rules permitting cheating on tests are inconsistent with the practices of honesty on exams they presuppose.

Although few philosophers would hold, as Kant appears to, that the universalizability of a rule is both necessary and sufficient for determining the moral acceptability of rules, many concur that universalizability is a necessary condition of the validity of ethical judgments, rules, and principles. Kant himself may actually have had more than one basic principle, because the several formulations he offers of the categorical imperative do not seem to be equivalent. Neither Kant nor others who have proposed monistic deontological theories have worked out a compelling account of a single fundamental principle.

Pluralistic deontologists, by contrast, affirm more than one basic rule or principle. For example, Ross holds that there are several basic and irreducible moral principles, such as fidelity, beneficence, and justice. This pluralistic approach at first seems more plausible than monistic approaches because it is more closely attuned to our commonsense judgments, but it encounters the difficulty—as Ross recognized—of what to do when these principles or rules come into conflict.

Case 3 provides an example of this problem. A physician has to determine whether to tell the truth or break a confidence. He cannot do both, yet each of two moral rules commands his allegiance. The pluralistic deontologist may give little guidance about which rules or principles take priority in such cases of conflict. For example, Ross holds that the principle of nonmaleficence (noninfliction of harm) takes precedence over the principle of beneficence (production of benefit) when they come into conflict, but he gives no account of the priorities among the other principles except to say that several duties (such as keeping promises) have "a great deal of stringency." Ultimately, as he quotes Aristotle, "The decision rests with perception."[16] While we intuit moral principles, according to Ross, we do not intuit what is right in the situation; rather, we have to find "the greatest balance" of right over wrong.

If a pluralist deontological theory cannot provide some ordering of its principles and rules or some method of determining the relative weight of moral claims, it seems to offer little guidance for making hard decisions. One recent attempt to overcome this and other difficulties of pluralistic theories is Rawls's *A Theory of Justice,* which arranges general principles of justice (not the whole of morality) in a serial or lexical order. This lexical order reduces the need for a pluralistic deontologist to appeal to intuition or to balance every single principle against every other principle.

Rawls argues that rational contractors in a fair bargaining situation behind a "veil of ignorance" would accept the following principles of justice: (I) the principle of equal liberty; (IIa) the difference principle, which permits inequalities in the distribution of social and economic goods only if those inequalities will benefit everyone, especially the least advantaged; and (IIb) the principle of fair equality of opportunity (see Chapter 6, pp. 271–75). According to Rawls, it is not necessary or permissible to balance these principles, because we must satisfy I before we can consider IIa or IIb. Thus, the principle of equal liberty has absolute priority over the second principle. Moreover, within the second principle, IIb has priority over IIa. Rawls does not, however, propose that this rigid ordering can be extended to the arranging of all moral principles in a hierarchy.[17] Many philosophers, including the authors of this work, remain skeptical that any orderings or hierarchical arrangements of principles can be sustained. However, we go beyond Ross in offering a procedure of moral reasoning that reduces—but does not eliminate—intuition (see pp. 52–55).

ACT AND RULE DEONTOLOGY. Finally, like utilitarians, deontologists may focus on acts or on rules that cover classes of acts. However, few philosophers or theologians have tried to defend act deontology, despite traces of it here and there. It has been held, for example, that an individual can immediately and directly perceive what he or she ought to do by intuition, conscience, or faith in God's revelation and grace. All forms of act deontology are problematic for several reasons (some of which also apply to act utilitarianism). First, we seldom have firm grounds for confidence in our own or others' intuition, conscience, or faith to perceive right and wrong in the situation, particularly in the light of immediate pressures, lack of time for deliberation, and the capacity of self-interest to distort perception. Second, a judgment that a particular act is wrong in the situation implicitly appeals to a rule. If we say that act X is wrong, we are acknowledging that all relevantly similar acts in relevantly similar circumstances are wrong. If so, to say it is wrong to lie to a patient who asks a direct question about his or her prognosis is to say that it is wrong to lie in all similar circumstances. Such a statement is at least an incipient rule.

The act deontologist as well as the act utilitarian may recognize some rules without accepting those rules as binding. For the act utilitarian, rules are suggestive generalizations from past experience that alert us to possible consequences of acts; they are not binding, either absolutely or even in most circumstances. For the act deontologist, rules identify what people have previously viewed as required, dictated by conscience, or commanded by God in past, quite particular situations. Such rules do not, however, bind the agent in new situations, because intuition, conscience, or God may prompt new decisions. Even though it too is ultimately unsatisfactory, act utilitarianism is, we suggest, a more plausible theory than act deontology because it requires agents to try to calculate the good that might be produced by alternative actions. In act deontology, the agent's response to the situation is more mysterious.

For rule deontologists, by contrast, the heart of morality is a set of binding principles and rules that classify acts as right, wrong, obligatory, or prohibited. Kant, for example, held that several rules could be derived from the basic categorical imperative. According to Ross, there are several independent duties that can be formulated as rules or principles. Some of these duties rest on previous acts. For example, promises and implicit promises give rise to duties of fidelity, and previous wrongful acts engender duties of reparation. Other duties rest on the previous acts of other persons. When they render services to us, for example, we have duties of gratitude. Ross goes on to develop duties of self-improvement, nonmaleficence, beneficence, and justice.[18] Several of these duties will be central to discussions in later chapters, but here we are illustrating how one version of rule deontology regards some classes of acts as right or wrong without regard to their consequences.

Rule deontology is widely represented in contemporary biomedical ethics.

Major controversies among rule deontologists often stem from their different judgments regarding which principles or rules are primary or more stringent. For example, Paul Ramsey's rule deontology affirms that various principles and rules can be derived from love or covenant fidelity, and his derivative principles include the sanctity of life. Because of this derivative principle, it is permissible in his system to override even a competent patient's refusal of lifesaving medical treatment when there is a medically indicated reason. Ramsey thus recognizes the legitimacy of strong paternalism (which we discuss in Chapter 5). By contrast, both Robert Veatch and H. Tristram Engelhardt, Jr., defend the priority of the principle of respect for autonomy: A competent patient has the right to refuse even lifesaving medical treatment, and strong paternalism is never justified. However, when Veatch and Engelhardt consider the allocation of health-care resources, a further division is evident among these two deontologists. Veatch argues for the priority of the principle of equality, while Engelhardt again opts for the priority of the principle of respect for autonomy (in particular, our autonomy rights protect us from coercion through the tax system to cover the health needs of others, unless everyone consents freely to an arrangement of tax collection).[19]

A comparison of deontological and utilitarian theories

What are the major characteristics, strengths, and weaknesses of deontological theories when compared to utilitarian theories? First, utilitarians hold that only one moral relationship between persons, as determined by the principle of utility, is fundamental: the relationship of benefactor and beneficiary. This conclusion follows from the premise that all obligations are determined by the goal of maximizing the good. Deontologists, however, take various relationships between people as more or equally basic. For them it is not sufficient to say that we should maximize the good and that each person counts as one and only one. They claim that we do not encounter other people merely as benefactors and beneficiaries; rather, we are related to them in various ways by previous acts and histories. For example, the physician does not confront each sick person merely as a stranger needing attention and care. If the physician has already been treating a patient, the relationship to that person is different from the relationship to another person who appears at the office door at the same time with the same ailment. The physician makes an implicit commitment to a patient by accepting care of the patient and generally does not have the right to abrogate that relationship in order to maximize good for others.

The texture of the moral life seems to a deontologist richer and more complicated than the utilitarian model suggests, because numerous relationships with others have special moral significance—for example, parent and child, friend and friend, promisor and promisee, as well as physician and patient.

Parents assume obligations to their children, and children incur obligations to their parents. Utilitarians do not deny the existence of these obligations, but they justify them by invoking the principle of utility. For deontologists, these obligations have a moral significance that is independent of the principle of utility.

A second and closely connected point of comparison concerns the role of past actions in our moral assessments. With its orientation toward the present and the future, utilitarianism seems to leave little room for the past in moral judgments. If utilitarianism considers the past at all, the reason must pertain to the maximization of present and future consequences. For example, to reward people for their past accomplishments tends to encourage them and others to act in similar ways in the present and the future, just as punishment discourages negative behaviors. But for a rule deontologist such as Ross, the performance of certain acts by itself creates obligations, independent of the consequences of the acts in general for human welfare. For example, if a physician has made a promise to a patient, the physician's obligation to fulfill the promise is independent of the consequences of doing so (although the obligation might in some cases be overridden by certain consequences).

The debates of the late 1960s and early 1970s concerning kidney dialysis illustrate these points about the moral significance of interpersonal relationships and past actions. Some utilitarians held that we should distribute this scarce lifesaving resource by choosing (after the appropriate medical and psychiatric judgments) the patients who bear the most burdensome social responsibilities and who show promise of being the most productive for society. However, this standard was usually applied only to *admission* to dialysis treatment. With a few exceptions, the utilitarians held that once a commitment had been made to a patient, it would be morally improper to *remove* that patient from treatment to make room for a patient who showed promise of contributing comparatively more to society. Utilitarians were not willing to call for a reassessment every few weeks or months of the patients already on dialysis.

The rule-utilitarian justification of this position is that rules calling for fidelity and care to those to whom we have made implicit if not explicit commitments will ultimately maximize value. To justify this rule, one could argue that a practice of reassessing patients and breaking commitments to some would tend to destroy the morale of patients, undermine their trust in health professionals, and thereby reduce the program's success rate. The rule deontologist, by contrast, would concentrate directly on the commitment itself, apart from the consequences of respecting that commitment. Here, as elsewhere, the rule utilitarian and the rule deontologist may accept similar or even identical rules, but for different reasons.

As a third point of comparison, utilitarianism conceives the moral life in terms of means-to-ends reasoning. It asks, "How can we most effectively and efficiently realize the objective of the greatest possible good?'' This conception of the moral life in terms of means and ends is congruent with the forms of reasoning found in the empirical sciences and in economics, where efficiency and the maximization of value are prized. Deontologists, by contrast, hold that it is a fundamental mistake to conceive the moral life in terms of means and ends; the starting point is wrong in part because it presupposes a greater capacity to predict and control outcomes than we can muster. Deontologists also insist that the utilitarian model of choosing effective means to good ends fundamentally distorts the moral life. Antony Flew reflects this deontological view: ''To do one's duty, or to discover what it is, is rarely if ever to achieve, or to find a way to achieve, an objective. Rather and typically, it is to meet, or to find a way to meet, claims; and also, of course, to eschew misdemeanors. Promises must be kept, debts must be paid, dependents must be looked after; and stealing, lying, and cruelty must be avoided.''[20] The argument is that we are not merely agents who initiate acts for good ends; we also directly encounter the moral claims of others.

Fourth, the deontologist's standard and perhaps most effective objection is that utilitarianism in principle sanctions morally unacceptable conclusions. One test of moral theories, as we saw earlier, is their congruence with our ordinary moral convictions. Deontologists pose the following situation against act utilitarians. Suppose we have two acts, A and B, which appear to yield the same utilitarian score when we balance their respective good and evil results. But suppose that A involves lying to a patient, whereas B does not. In the end, the result is the same: The patient can be expected to get well. The consistent act utilitarian must say that the acts are equally right. Now suppose that act A, which involves lying to a patient about his or her condition, is preferable on utilitarian grounds because it offers a greater chance of success in restoring the patient's health, whereas act B, which does not involve lying, has a slightly smaller chance of success. According to act utilitarianism, A is right and obligatory, and the physician should therefore lie to the patient because it is in the patient's interest. (This judgment assumes that the patient's overriding interest is in health rather than autonomy and that one can reliably predict in the circumstances that other consequences, such as a loss of confidence in the physician, will not occur.) The deontologist claims that in both cases act utilitarianism leads to morally unacceptable judgments.[21]

The rule utilitarian can avoid these difficulties by holding that a fuller analysis of the consequences, including the remote or long-term consequences, leads to the assignment of a greater weight to the rule of truth telling. But although rule utilitarianism thus appears to be more congruent with our ordinary judgments, it does not, according to its critics, adequately account for claims of some moral principles and rules, particularly those of justice. On the basis of utility, it is possible to determine that *some* standards of justice are necessary to maximize human welfare, but it is not clear, critics charge, that utility can indicate *which* standards should be adopted. Even though utilitarianism requires that each person count as one and only one, it cannot avoid a standard of justice that would assign major benefits to some people and major burdens to others if that distribution scheme would produce the greatest good for the greatest number. Such a scheme could, for example, justify nontherapeutic research on a small number of people in order to maximize the health of the society as a whole. Although most rule utilitarians either oppose such outcomes or specifically constrain the use of distribution schemes by rules such as those requiring consent, critics maintain that these hedging arguments rest on an independent, unacknowledged standard of fairness that is not itself reducible to utility.

Selecting an ethical theory

On balance, which ethical theory, if any, is to be preferred? For one author of this volume, a form of rule utilitarianism is more defensible than any available deontological theory; for the other, a form of rule deontology is more acceptable than any version of utilitarianism. We come to these different conclusions after testing available theories for their consistency and coherence, their simplicity, their completeness and comprehensiveness, and their capacity to take account of and to account for our moral experience, including our ordinary judgments. Still, for both of us the most satisfactory theory is only slightly preferable, and no theory fully satisfies the tests explicated in Chapter 1.

The idea of common ground

Whether one takes the utilitarian or the deontological standpoint no doubt makes a significant difference in the moral life, especially for the theory of justification. Nevertheless, the differences between these two types of theory are exaggerated when they are presented as two warring armies locked in endless combat. We find that some (not all) forms of rule utilitarianism and rule deontology lead to virtually identical principles and rules and recommended actions. It is possible from both utilitarian and deontological standpoints to defend the same principles (such as respect for autonomy and justice) and rules (such as truth telling and confidentiality) and to assign them roughly the same weight in cases of conflict. These two types of theory can be drawn still closer if utilitarians take a broad view of the values underlying the rules and include indirect as well as direct and remote as well as immediate consequences of classes of acts, and if deonotologists agree that moral principles such as beneficence and nonmaleficence require us to maximize good and minimize evil outcomes and to trade off some values for the sake of other values.

An indication that those utilitarians and deontologists who accept a conception of the moral life as rule-governed can and sometimes do develop similar or even identical rules, rather than fragment into disagreement, is found in the writings of Richard Brandt. As we have seen, he argues that morality should be conceived as an ideal code consisting of a set of rules that function to maximize utility. The following statement by Brandt is revealing:

[The best code] would contain rules giving directions for recurrent situations which involve conflicts of human interests. Presumably, then, it would contain rules rather similar to W. D. Ross's list of prima facie obligations: rules about the keeping of promises and contracts, rules about debts of gratitude such as we may owe to our parents, and, of course, rules about not injuring other persons and about promoting the welfare of others where this does not work a comparable hardship on us.[22]

That Brandt appeals to utility and that Ross appeals to intuition to justify their similar sets of rules is a significant difference on the level of the theory of moral justification, but it may turn out to be a trivial difference in specifying the material action-guides that must be followed and in making particular moral judgments.

We agree, of course, that at least one important theoretical difference always remains, no matter how closely a deontological theory matches a utilitarian theory. The rule utilitarian believes that the principle of utility justifies all other principles and rules, which have their rationale in the prediction that they will maximize utility over time. By contrast, the rule deontologist believes that some principles and rules are justified for reasons other than utility and are binding even if they cannot be reliably predicted to maximize utility. The rule deontologist may hope and expect that such principles and rules will maximize good, but that hope or expectation of maximization does not justify the principles and rules. The rule deontologist may even believe that having moral rules will maximize utility, but will not believe that we can always determine which rules we ought to have by their utility.

How important is the utilitarian/deontological distinction?

In ethics, law, public policy, and other normative contexts, agreement among persons of widely varying value commitments can often be reached about what action should be taken in a particular case or what policy should be espoused. Agreement may even be reached over the principles and precedent cases that justify an action or policy. For example, in the deliberations of institutional review boards (IRBs), it is common for committee members to agree about the unacceptability of particular research protocols on grounds that the risks they present are, like those in certain past precedent cases, too great. There may, of course, be underlying disagreements over the justification and status of a principle of avoiding harm in moral theory; and thus, a manifest agreement that suffices for the purpose at hand may only conceal an underlying disagreement. Nevertheless, deep disagreements in the theory of moral justification do not necessarily lead to disagreements in practical moral deliberation.

Theoretical differences can, of course, eventuate in practical disagreements and in different general policies. For example, we shall see throughout this volume that utilitarians tend to support various types of research involving human subjects on grounds of the social benefits of the research for future patients. Deontologists, by contrast, tend to be skeptical of some of this research on grounds of its actual or potential violation of individual rights, which are grounded in principles of respect for autonomy and protection against harm. But deontologists and utilitarians often cross over these lines of demarcation and agree that any adequate ethical approach to research involving human subjects must include some of the constraints and considerations that have been highlighted by proponents of both types of theories (and that are now embedded in most codes and regulations of research involving human subjects).[23]

The fact that no currently available theory, whether rule utilitarian or rule deontological, adequately resolves all moral conflicts points to their incompleteness. But this incompleteness may reflect the complex and sometimes dilemmatic character of the moral life rather than inherent defects in the theories. Each of our most celebrated types of ethical theory has made a substantial contribution to our understanding of ethics, but none has successfully shown that it alone presents a valid and complete system. The thesis that our best moral systems may be substantially incomplete may seem odd in light of the argument in Chapter 1 that one test of any moral theory is its completeness and comprehensiveness. Our present point, however, is only that no available moral theory *fully* satisfies the ideal set forth by this criterion.

In reference to consequentialist theories, Alan Donagan has correctly observed that "In all the vast and imposing body of work on consequentialist moral theories, there are many sketches and projects for constructing moral systems. But none has been constructed."[24] This assessment applies as well to deontological theories. The most complete and comprehensive of the latter theories tend to focus on special subjects, such as justice, rather than providing a comprehensive and integrated account of the moral life. (Some would contest these claims in the instance of Kant or others.)

There are, then, reasons for holding that the consequentialist/deontological or utilitarian/deontological distinctions are not as significant for moral theory as they have sometimes been taken to be. It is a mistake to suppose that a single great divide separates all moral theorists neatly into consequentialists and nonconsequentialists. Moreover, consequentialists sometimes disagree with their fellow consequentialists over the defining characteristics of consequentialist theories, and the same is true of deontologists in conflict with other deontologists. These theories are often described, even by their proponents, in terms that would not be acceptable to other proponents of the same general type of theory. For example, as we have seen, many utilitarians describe utilitarianism so that it is restricted to an agent-neutral perspective on the nature of value. That is, they require that a utilitarian accept a theory of intrinsic value that is independent of what any particular agent subjectively values. Preference utilitarians obviously cannot accept this characterization.

We can safely say that the descriptions that we (and all other writers) have given of both "utilitarian" and "deontological" types of ethical theory would not be acceptable to some proponents of these general theories, because our characterizations are, from their perspectives, either too narrow or too broad. There is no way to eliminate this problem, because any general description will be either too narrow or too broad or both from the perspective of some current proponents of the theories. This suggests that "utilitarianism" and "deontology" are such general labels that they cannot reasonably be expected to characterize any single utilitarian or deontological account. Rather, the labels point to major trends and identify families of theories.

This range of variation prompts questions about whether the distinction between deontological and consequentialist theories is more fundamental than many other distinctions that are used to differentiate types of moral theory. We have investigated this distinction at length because of its high visibility and its profound significance for contemporary moral theory. The distinction does, in a useful form, collect major elements of two quite different perspectives on the moral life. We can nonetheless place too much of a burden on this distinction, overlooking that some deontological theories are (as Brandt implicitly notices) closer in substantive principles and rules to some utilitarian theories than to other deontological theories.

In later parts of this and subsequent chapters we argue that other distinctions between ethical theories also deserve serious consideration. For example, we introduce distinctions between different theories of rights, different theories of the place of rules, and different accounts of the virtues. These differences may in the end be as important as the contrast between utilitarians and deontologists. Each type of theory offers an important moral perspective from which we stand to learn, and there is no reason why only one type of theory must be selected as preeminent.

The place of rules and principles

Rules and principles as rules of thumb

In defending a rule-governed concept of morality, we have implicitly rejected situation ethics. All pure forms of situation ethics—whether act utilitarianism or act deontology—face difficult problems of coordination, cooperation, and trust. The following encounter between act utilitarians in a medical setting, as envisioned by G. J. Warnock, expresses some salient reasons for rejecting situation theories:

Suppose that I, a simple Utilitarian, entrust the care of my health to a simple Utilitarian doctor. Now I know, of course, that his intentions are generally beneficent, but equally that they are not uniquely beneficent towards me. Thus, while he will not malevolently kill me off, I cannot be sure that he will always try to cure me of my afflictions; I can be sure only that he will do so, unless his assessment of the "general happiness" leads him to do otherwise. I cannot of course condemn this attitude, since it is the same as my own; but it is more than possible that I might not much like it and might find myself put to much anxiety and fuss in trying to detect, as successive consultations, what his intentions actually were. But conspicuously, there are two things that I could not do to diminish my anxieties: I could not get him to promise, the style of the Hippocratic Oath, always and only to deploy his skills to my advantage; nor could I usefully ask him to disclose his intentions. The reason is essentially the same in each case. Though he might, if I asked him to, promise not to kill me off, he would of course keep this promise only if he judged it best on the whole to do so; knowing that, I could not unquestioningly rely on his keeping it; and knowing that, he would realize that, since I would not do so, it would matter that much less if he did not keep it. And so on, until his "promise" becomes perfectly idle. Similarly, if I ask him what his intentions are, he will answer truthfully only if he judges it best on the whole to do so; knowing that, I will not unqualifiedly believe him; and knowing that, he will realize that, since I will not do so, it will matter that much less if he professes intentions that he does not actually have. And so on, until my asking and his answering become a pure waste of breath. And this is quite general; if general felicific beneficence were the only criterion, then promising and talking alike would become wholly idle pursuits. At best, as perhaps in diplomacy, what people said would become merely a part of the evidence on the basis of which one might try to decide what they really believed, or intended, or were likely to do; and it is not always obvious that there is much point in diplomacy.[25]

Although situational or act-oriented theories recognize rules, they treat them as summary rules or rules of thumb that are expendable. Their hypothesis is that moral rules summarize the wisdom of the past by expressing better and worse ways to handle recurring problems. Such rules assist deliberation but can be set aside at any time according to the demands of the situation. For example, an investigative reporter seeking facts about a potential political scandal might believe that he must lie, invade privacy, and breach confidentiality in order to get the story. From the perspective of a situational theory, if the reporter's acts are justified by the importance of the story, they should not be viewed as violations of binding rules.

Moral and legal action-guides are thus treated in these theories as rules that give guidance but do not prescribe with authority by establishing firm obligations. A rule of thumb in baseball is analogous: "Don't bunt on third strike" is a prudent general maxim, but in some situations it would be advisable for the batter to bunt despite having two strikes. The rule is jettisoned when it does not serve the purpose at hand. For act deontology, act utilitarianism, and other situational theories, all moral rules approximate this sort of rule. We have argued against this interpretation of moral rules, even though we have agreed that some moral rules—such as some rules in professional codes—resemble rules of thumb. We shall now provide further support for a stronger conception of rules in moral theory.

Rules and principles as absolute

We need to consider first whether binding principles and rules are absolute—that is, whether fundamental principles and rules cannot be overridden or infringed under any circumstances. There are good reasons for being suspicious of this interpretation. Absolute rules disallow the discretion for moral agents that we believe is essential in the moral life, and an overly rigid adherence to rules can produce moral victims. It seems to us undeniable that in some cases, such as emergencies, the consequences of following some moral rules would be so unacceptable that those rules must be understood as overridable by competing moral considerations. But before we settle on this conclusion, we need to consider whether some rules can legitimately claim to be absolute.

There are several classes of candidates for the status of "absolute rule." The first class appears in what we have described as monistic ethical theories, those with a single ultimate principle. It is hard to understand how a supreme principle in a monistic theory could be anything but absolute. For example, the principle of utility is not a principle that, for utilitarians, competes with other principles, because only utilitarian considerations are relevant to moral decision making. The principle of utility is the principle from which all other principles are derived or validated. The same monistic approach is present in Kant's categorical imperative. Thus, the best known and most discussed moral theories during the last two hundred years—Mill's utilitarianism and Kant's deontology—both advance absolute principles. In neither of these theories can there be genuine moral dilemmas because both retain an absolute rule that serves, in Mill's words, as a "common umpire" in all instances of conflicting obligations.

Other types of moral rules refer to traits of character that are always good, and such rules may also be absolute. To exhort a physician colleague to "Be caring" or "Be conscientious" is to call for the development and expression of traits of character that are good. Of course, one may obscure important aspects of one's responsibilities by misconstruing or too narrowly construing the demands of care or conscientiousness, but this does not detract from the possibility of a well-formulated absolute rule. (In the final chapter we will closely examine these traits of character as virtues.)

Rules of action formulated explicitly to include all exceptions may also be absolute. An example might be "Always obtain the oral or written informed consent of your competent patients *except* in emergency or low-risk situations.'' There might still be considerable debate about what constitutes an emergency or a low risk, but this rule could be absolute if all legitimate exceptions could be included in its formulation.

Finally, some rules that do not specify or even permit exceptions may be absolute. If murder is taken to mean ''unjustified killing,'' then its prohibition would be absolute; and the prohibition of cruelty can likewise be considered absolute if it means ''Do not inflict suffering for the sake of suffering.'' In medical contexts, especially in some therapeutic settings, there might at first appear to be exceptions to this second prohibition; but if a therapist intentionally makes a patient suffer in order to make the patient angry and to motivate the patient to assume responsibility for his or her decisions, this act does not fall under the prohibition of cruelty. The infliction of suffering is here strictly a means to the valuable end of getting the person to assume responsibility.

These examples indicate that the debate about whether some rules can be defended as absolute hinges in important respects on the definition of moral terms such as *murder, cruelty,* and *lying.* Suppose Nazi soldiers investigating a hospital in Germany in the late 1930s had asked the administrator whether there were Jewish patients in the hospital. If the administrator insisted that the hospital had no Jewish patients, although knowing there were several, how should we describe this exchange? Consider two possibilities. (1) The administrator's statement is a lie, but the lie is justified because it is intended to save the lives of innocent patients. (2) The administrator's statement is not a lie, because the questioners have no right to the truth. In the first description, *lying* may be defined as intentionally telling a person what one believes to be false in order to deceive him or her. In the second description, *lying* may be defined as not making truthful statements to a person to whom the truth is due.

The first definition involves a ''neutral and relatively definite description'' of lying; the second involves a ''nonneutral and relatively indefinite description.''[26] The first definition indicates what counts as lying or truth telling but not how much moral weight lying or truth telling has. The second definition indicates how much lying or truth telling counts but not what is to count as lying or truth telling. Although the second approach holds that lying is always wrong, it leaves open the question of when the truth is due someone. The first approach admits the possibility that the moral life involves doing the lesser of two evils and that it is thus sometimes necessary to lie in order to prevent a worse evil. Proponents of the second approach may stress the harmony rather than the conflict among various principles and rules once we appreciate their meaning and range of applicability.

The importance of the meaning of moral terms may be illustrated by Case 3, in which a father decided that he did not want to donate a kidney to his five-year-old daughter. His reasons are complex and include an uncertain prognosis for his daughter, who had been on chronic renal dialysis for three years. He asked the physician to tell the other family members that he was not histocompatible, because he feared that the truth would lead to recriminations against him and would wreck the family. The physician informed the family that "medical reasons" prevented the father from being a donor.

One could hold that the physician told a lie by intentionally deceiving the wife but that it was justified because of the evil it prevented. Alternatively, one could hold that the lie was justified because, in a conflict of obligations, the protection of confidentiality to the patient takes precedence over telling the truth to another person, and the father had entered into a relationship of confidentiality with the physician. Or one could hold that the lie was justified because the physician had no obligation to tell the wife the truth; if what transpired between the father and the physician was confidential, the wife had no right to that information, and deceiving her was not an act of lying. Finally, one could argue that "medical reasons" include psychological reasons and thus that the physician's statement was not a lie, even if it deceived (and was intended to deceive) the wife. However, it would have been a lie if the physician had said that the father was not histocompatible when in fact he was.

In this analysis of the case, we do not exclude the possibility that the statement to the wife was an unjustified lie. The present point is that different approaches to moral dilemmas and rules may hinge on different definitions or interpretations of the relevant moral terms as well as on their weight and stringency. On some interpretations, some moral rules are absolute. However, we will now argue that the model of absoluteness for moral rules is the wrong model.

Rules and principles as prima facie binding

In addition to the two possibilities that moral rules and principles are either rules of thumb or absolute rules, a third possibility is to conceive them as binding but not absolutely binding. We defend this thesis throughout this book by treating principles and rules as prima facie binding. The theory we defend may be called a composite theory. It stands in opposition to monistic or absolutistic theories such as act utilitarianism, Kantianism, and libertarianism (a monism based on the principle of respect for autonomy). A composite theory permits each basic principle to have weight without assigning a priority weighting or ranking. Which principle overrides in a case of conflict will depend on the particular context, which always has unique features.[27]

W. D. Ross, whose pluralistic deontology we outlined previously, offered a useful, and we think essential, approach to this problem of conflict and judgment. His list of independent principles of duty includes some that resemble those in our Chapters 3 through 6. Ross maintained that the overriding duty is found by locating "the greatest balance" of right over wrong in the circumstance of conflict between these principles. Ross believes that each basic duty is a "self-evident" part of common morality. However, when two or more of these duties conflict and a balancing of them is necessary, Ross does not claim that judgments about what should be done are self-evident. Here, he says, we have only probable opinion, which is a matter of making judgments about the weight of rules rather than judgments that apply rules.

Ross's metaphor of weights moving on a scale is graphic but misleading without an additional explanation. Ross sought greater precision for his ideas through a distinction between prima facie duties and actual duties. *Prima facie duty* indicates that duties of certain kinds are on all occasions binding unless they are in conflict with equal or stronger duties. An agent's actual duty in the situation is determined by an examination of the weight of all the competing prima facie duties. Duties such as beneficence, fidelity, and reparation are thus not absolute, because they can be overridden under some conditions. Yet they are more than expendable rules of thumb. Because they are always morally relevant, they constitute strong moral reasons for performing the acts in question, although they may not always prevail over other prima facie duties. One's actual duty is thus determined by the balance of the respective weights of the competing prima facie duties in the situation. One might say that prima facie duties count even when they do not win.

For example, Ross considered nonmaleficence—noninfliction of harm—as a prima facie duty. (All of the moral principles taken as primary in Chapters 3 through 6 in this book state prima facie *duties* in Ross's sense, but we use the language of prima facie *obligations*.) Although it is plausible, as we have seen, to hold that murder is absolutely prohibited because of the meaning of *murder*, it is not plausible in most moral theories to hold that killing is absolutely prohibited. Even the prohibition against killing in the Ten Commandments is more accurately translated as the prohibition of "murder" or "unjustified killing," because the Hebrew people recognized killing as valid in self-defense, in war, and as punishment for some crimes. Killing persons nonetheless is prima facie wrong, because it is an act of maleficence.

The different features or characteristics of acts often generate moral conflicts. The duty not to kill someone may, for example, come into conflict with a duty of justice that protects innocent persons from aggression. The duty not to kill may also come into conflict with the duty of beneficence—the duty to benefit others—as mercy killing illustrates. Killing a person in order to alleviate or prevent that person's terrible pain or suffering is not always wrong. (We provide an example in Chapter 8, on p. 377.) Indeed, Ross's view that nonmaleicence has greater stringency than beneficence is a thesis we reject in Chapter 4. The crucial point to notice about prima facie duties is that insofar as an act involves a wrong-making feature such as killing, there is a moral reason to avoid it. It is always prima facie wrong and always actually wrong unless justified by another overriding prima facie duty. Yet killing may be the only way to meet some other prima facie duties; and, if so, then killing can become an actual duty.

If a prima facie duty is outweighed or overridden, it does not simply disappear or evaporate. It leaves what Robert Nozick calls "moral traces." [28] The agent should approach such a decision conscientiously and should expect to experience regret and perhaps even remorse at having to override and infringe this prima facie duty. This method of "overriding" prima facie duties seems to some philosophers too intuitive and flexible—as though moral theory lacks a rigid backbone if it allows us to make "situational" judgments of overridingness. Although we earlier conceded that there is no escape from having to exercise such judgment, we can now add that the logic of prima facie duties does contain moral conditions that prevent just any judgment based on a grounding principle from being acceptable in a moral conflict. For example, the following are all requirements for justified infringements of a prima facie principle or rule:

(1) the moral objective justifying the infringement must have a realistic prospect of achievement;
(2) infringement of a prima facie principle must be necessary in the circumstances, in the sense that there are no morally preferable alternative actions that could be substituted;
(3) the form of infringement selected must constitute the least infringement possible, commensurate with achieving the primary goal of the action; and
(4) the agent must seek to minimize the effects of the infringement.

The first three conditions have already been evident in our discussion of cases, but it may be useful to give an example of the fourth condition. In Case 5, a therapist deceives a patient by giving a placebo. The deception may damage the patient's self-conception and his confidence in and reliance on the therapists, just as Warnock envisions in his example of a "simple utilitarian" doctor. The overridden duties of veracity and respect for autonomy call for the therapist to give an explanation and an apology to the patient, as well as to provide the kind of counseling that could be reasonably expected to reduce the residual harms.

One final point deserves attention. A rule-governed theory must, on the interpretation of nonabsolute, prima facie rules that we have defended, allow that any rule may theoretically be validly overridden in a circumstance by a competing moral rule. The question then emerges of whether our theory differs significantly from act-oriented or situational theories. In practice, the differences may be minimal, because both oppose absolutist theories and both may reach the same conclusions in particular situations. However, important theoretical differences remain and affect their respective approaches to moral reasoning. Act theories recognize cases or moral perplexity and uncertainty, but they cannot admit conflicts of binding rules (and principles) of the sort we have seen to characterize many moral dilemmas. Hence they neglect the kind of moral reasoning required by our account of prima facie obligation. It is not necessary for them to override rules of thumb, because they are only advisory, not morally obligatory. By contrast, a prima facie rule is binding or obligatory unless overridden by a competing prima facie rule. Of course, if an ''act'' or ''situational'' theory were to give an interpretation of rules of obligation identical to the one we have defended, there would be no substantive difference in the theories. But it is difficult to see how a theory with binding rules could constitute an act or situational theory.

We have argued in effect that any acceptable theory would be a rule-governed and not an act-governed theory. (Here again, *rule* includes principles.) However, we are not bent on an ideological rejection of act-governed theories. Our main objective is a clarification of crucial terms and a precise expression of the commitments of our moral theory. Just as we earlier argued that the consequentialist/deontological distinction may not be as significant for moral theory as it has sometimes been taken to be, so we might reasonably conclude now that the distinction between act and rule theories can, without careful analysis, create more obscurity than insight.

Some limitations of rule-governed morality

We have been arguing in favor of rule-governed moral theories, but we note in conclusion some limitations inherent in these theories (beyond the problems noted above in discussing prima facie and absolute rules).

First, it can be unclear whether a case falls under a rule. For example, it may be unclear whether a physician's partial disclosure to a patient is or is not deceptive under the circumstances. Even a rule that unqualifiedly bans deception in the patient-physician relationship cannot determine one's precise moral obligation in all circumstances. Among the strongest arguments advanced by situational and act theories is that rules can be so abstract or their applicability so ambiguous that we are forced to call upon nonrule resources such as feelings, intuition, or conscience. We agree that rules can conflict without mediating rules being available to resolve the conflict and that there will be times when we are uncertain whether a rule applies. But this concession does not support a pure situation ethics. To acknowledge these problems of applying principles and rules to particular cases is not to deny the binding character of the principles and rules when they do apply.

Second, the analysis of principles and rules as prima facie allows some circumstances in which a single principle or rule directs a person to two competing and equally attractive alternatives, only one of which can be pursued. For example, the principle of beneficence when applied to problems of disclosing information to patients could be correctly invoked to require both disclosure and nondisclosure, because both options could (on some occasion) lead to equally beneficial, although different results. Whether the conflict arises from the application of a single principle or rule or from two or more distinct principles or rules, we need to recognize that there may be no single right action in some circumstances, because two or more morally acceptable actions may prove of equal weight in those circumstances.

Third, moral rules are not constructed to take account of competing factors (including nonmoral factors) that no moral system could reasonably anticipate. Religious convictions and professional obligations may on occasion compete with moral obligations. No system of rules can make these problems vanish. It does not follow that we can or must dispense with general action-guides or treat them as mere rules of thumb. The question to be asked is where discretion rightly enters and how such rules are to be understood and applied, not whether they apply at all.[29]

Rights in moral theories

We have primarily been using the following terms from moral discourse: *right, wrong, obligatory, morally justified, unjustified, obligation,* and *duty*. We have examined how principles and rules in deontological and utilitarian theories establish obligations and determine the rightness and wrongness of acts. It may seem odd that we have not employed the language of rights, especially in light of the recent explosion of rights language in contexts from applied ethics to foreign policy. Many moral controversies in biomedicine and public policy involve debates about rights such as a right to die, a right to reproduce, a right of privacy, and a right to life. In discussions of health-care delivery, proponents of a broad extension of medical services often appeal to the "right to health care," whereas opponents commonly appeal to the "rights of the medical profession." These moral, political, and legal debates sometimes appear to presuppose that no arguments or reasons can be persuasive unless they can be stated in the language of rights.

Rights language is congenial to the liberal individualism pervasive in our society. At least since Thomas Hobbes, liberal individualists have employed the language of rights to buttress moral, social, and political arguments, and the Anglo-American legal tradition has incorporated this language. In the tradition of liberal individualism, the language of rights has served on occasion as a means to oppose the status quo, to assert claims that demand recognition and respect, and to promote social reforms. Historically it was also instrumental in securing certain freedoms from established orders of religion, society, and state, such as freedom of the press and freedom of religious expression.

An instructive recent example of the development and continuing importance of rights language is found in the "Patient's Bill of Rights" of the American Hospital Association (AHA).[30] In 1969, the Joint Commission on Accreditation of Hospitals, a private association drawing its membership from medical and hospital groups, issued a policy document that scarcely mentioned problems of patients. Various consumer groups active at the time asked the commission to redraft the document with closer attention to the needs and perspective of patients. The National Welfare Rights Organization drafted a statement in June 1970 with twenty-six proposals for the rights of patients. This document proved to be a major contributing cause of the so-called patients' rights movement. The AHA then began to debate the issue of patients' rights and adopted its Bill of Rights in late 1972 (published in 1973). This document contains a potentially revolutionary departure from traditional Hippocratic benevolence, because the physician is required, by claim of right, to incorporate patients into the decision-making process and to recognize the rights of patients to make authoritative decisions. In effect, patients' rights of autonomy are given formal recognition.

Rights language is important in our society because of its symbolic significance and because of its legitimate role in ethical theory. It is difficult, however, to explicate the status and content of rights, as we shall now see.

The nature and status of rights

Rights should be defined in terms of claims that demand respect. In our framework, rights are justified claims that individuals and groups can make upon others or upon society. A right is thus analogous to property over which one has control, so that rights contrast with privileges, personal ideals, optional acts of charity, and the like. Legal rights are claims that are justified by legal principles and rules, and moral rights are claims that are justified by moral principles and rules. A moral right, then, is a justified claim, or entitlement, validated by moral principles and rules.[31]

Are rights, so defined, absolute? Here we need to recall the analysis of prima facie obligations and their conflicts in the previous section on rules. The same conflicts can and do occur among rights, as when the fetus's right to life may conflict with the woman's right to privacy. Even the right to life cannot be plausibly maintained to be absolute, irrespective of competing claims or social conditions, as is evidenced by common moral judgments about killing in war and killing in self-defense. We have only a right not to have our lives taken without sufficient justification, not an absolute right to life. This and any right can be legitimately exercised and can create actual obligations on others only if the right overrides rights that compete with it. Rights such as a right to give an informed consent or refusal, a right to die, and a right to lifesaving medical technology must compete with other rights in many situations—producing protracted controversy and a need to balance with great care the competing rights. Thus rights, exactly like obligations, are prima facie.[32]

We need also to distinguish a violation of a right from an infringement of a right.[33] *Violation* refers to an unjustified action against a right, whereas *infringement* refers to a justified action overriding a right. When a (prima facie) right is justifiably overridden, it is infringed but not violated. The conditions that must be met to justify overriding a prima facie right are identical to those that must be met to justify overriding a prima facie obligation (see pp. 51–54).

The correlativity of rights and obligations

The analysis thus far proposes that moral rights express morally justified claims that others should (prima facie) respect. A modest extension is that a right entails an obligation on others either not to interfere or to provide something—both the obligation and the right being justified by the same overarching principle or rule. In this section we defend a firm although untidy correlativity between obligations and rights.[34] This relation makes it possible to analyze both obligations and rights in terms of principles and rules.

According to the correlativity thesis, a right entails that someone else has an obligation to act in certain ways, and an obligation similarly entails a right. For example, if a physician agrees to take John Doe as a patient and commences treatment, the physician incurs an obligation to Doe, and Doe has correlative rights against the physician. There may be rights to a certain level of care and rights in care, such as the right to refuse treatment. The moral issues in the relationship between the physician and Doe can be analyzed equally well either by examining the physician's obligations or by examining the patient's rights, because the correlativity thesis implies that it is possible to start from a right and infer a correlative obligation, and vice versa.

The thesis of the correlativity of rights and obligations is untidy because one use of the words *requirement, obligation,* and *duty* suggests that obligations do not always imply correlative rights. For example, we sometimes refer to requirements, obligations, and duties of love, charity, and self-sacrifice, and these do not seem to be restatable in terms of rights. A person cannot claim another person's love or charity as a matter of right. The problem is that some obligations express what we ought to do because of personal ideals and actions that exceed obligation. These "obligations" are best treated as self-imposed rules that are not strictly required by morality—such as when we believe that we ought to contribute substantially to charity, even though we do not believe that morality requires it.

A somewhat different perspective on rights and duties is found in a traditional distinction between duties of perfect obligation and duties of imperfect obligation. John Stuart Mill, who rightly says that the terms *perfect* and *imperfect* are "ill-chosen" for this distinction, analyzes the difference as follows: "Duties of perfect obligation are those duties in virtue of which a correlative *right* resides in some person or persons; duties of imperfect obligation are those moral obligations which do not give birth to any right."[35] Mill thus argues that duties of perfect obligation are duties of justice and entail rights, whereas duties of imperfect obligation belong to other spheres of morality: "Justice implies something which is not only right to do, and wrong not to do, but which some individual person can claim from us as his moral right. No one has a moral right to our generosity or beneficence, because we are not morally bound to practise those virtues towards any given individual."[36]

For Mill, duties such as beneficence and generosity are real duties, but no particular persons can claim by right to have these duties discharged toward them. Justice, promise keeping, and the like are duties to particular persons, who can make claims based on their rights. Thus far we largely agree with Mill: Duties of justice have correlative rights and are perfect duties; and, as we explicate beneficence in Chapter 5, many obligations of beneficence conform to his description. But we need to distinguish still further between the following. (1) Some obligations of beneficence are *perfect* (e.g., the obligations of rescue discussed in Chapter 5). (2) Some obligations of beneficence and charity are *imperfect,* just as Mill describes them. (3) Some "obligations" of beneficence are *self-imposed* requirements and therefore are beyond the bounds of moral obligation. The latter, ideal "obligations" are only in a weak sense moral requirements at all. Thus, if an obligation of either type 1 or type 2—perfect or imperfect—is required by the system of moral principles and rules, the correlativity thesis always holds; self-imposed requirements, by contrast, are optional and never entail rights. We discuss these ideals and self-imposed requirements in Chapter 8. Which obligations are enforceable general obligations is still under serious dispute, as we will see in Chapter 5.

So interpreted, the correlativity thesis indicates how both rule utilitarianism and rule deontology, as obligation-oriented theories, can incorporate the language and substance of rights. This claim may appear surprising, because some utilitarians have opposed certain conceptions of rights, and many of the strongest supporters of rights have appealed to deontological frameworks. The rights of individuals and groups are also often stated in opposition to social utility, and many moral philosophers now maintain that moral theory or some part of moral theory must be "right-based."[37] Nevertheless, we may doubt both that these efforts have been successful[38] and that traditional thinkers have generally denied that rights should play an important role in moral theory. The quotation from Mill indicates how easily he accommodated rights within his utilitarian framework, and others have argued that the objectives of a theory of rights and a consequentialist theory are mutually supportive.[39] It follows from the doctrine of the logical correlativity of rights and obligations that both rule utilitarianism and rule deontology, being obligation-oriented theories, can be equally committed to rights.[40]

It remains controversial in contemporary theory whether rights are the basis of obligations or vice versa, and whether either forms the basis of the other. We believe these controversies can be circumvented by making principles and rules the basis of both rights and obligations. If principles are our general action-guides for promoting and protecting basic human interests, then it is hard to see how rights can be justified on any other basis.[41] In using the language of "principles," we do not seek to evade substantive questions about whether principles are more fundamental to a moral framework than obligations, rights, or virtues. But, as this chapter and Chapter 8 together make clear, we believe there is a correlativity or correspondence among obligations, rights, *and* virtues; and each category may be understood as having its basis in principles.

Positive rights and negative rights

The distinction in moral theory between positive rights and negative rights is based on the difference between the right to be provided with a particular good or service by others and the right to be free from some action taken by others. A person's positive right entails another's obligation to do something for that person; a negative right entails an obligation to refrain from doing something.[42] Either kind of right may be directed against other individuals or against a society as a whole. Examples of both sorts or rights can be found in biomedical practice, research, and policy. If there is a right to health care, for example, it is a positive right to goods and services grounded in the principle of justice (see Chapter 6, pp. 275–80); the right not to be operated on without one's consent is a negative right grounded in the principle of respect for autonomy. The liberal individualist tradition has generally found it easier to justify negative rights, especially those that call for noninterference in others' affairs, than positive rights; but the recognition of welfare rights in modern societies has extended the range and power of positive rights.

Confusion in moral discourse about public policies governing biomedicine can often be traced to a failure to distinguish positive rights from negative rights. One example comes from the controversy surrounding U.S. Supreme Court decisions on abortion.[43] Some who contend that the abortion decisions are inconsistent fail to see that the Court recognized a negative right in 1973 and refused to recognize a positive right in 1977. In *Roe* v. *Wade* and *Doe* v.

Bolton (both 1973), the Court ruled that a woman's right to privacy gives her a right to abort her fetus, within certain limits. If the decision is made within the first trimester of the pregnancy, the state may not intervene. The state, however, may regulate abortions for the protection of maternal health in the second trimester; and in the third trimester it may prohibit abortions, except in cases of a threat to the pregnant woman's life or health. The constitutionally protected right of privacy is here construed exclusively as a negative right. It identifies a sphere of general noninterference and limits state interference to specified circumstances. This right was interpreted in the *Danforth* decision (1976) to exclude a husband's veto of his wife's and her physician's decision to terminate her pregnancy. Again, the Court recognized a right of noninterference. In these cases the Court established a right of unimpeded access to an abortion within limits but not a right to the services or resources required for an abortion.

Many people thought the Court had recognized a positive right in these cases, namely a right to receive aid and assistance. They were therefore surprised when the Court in 1977 ruled that the federal and state governments do not have obligations to provide funds for nontherapeutic abortions. The Court held that governments do not have an obligation to provide financial assistance, and pregnant women who are seeking nontherapeutic abortions therefore do not have a correlative right to financial assistance. The Court's reasoning is consistent: It affirmed a negative right in some decisions and denied a positive right in others. Some opponents of the most recent decisions have charged that these decisions embody a different order of inconsistency in that they affirm (in some instances) a positive right to financial assistance for bringing a pregnancy to term while they deny a positive right to the services necessary to terminate a pregnancy. This, however, is a separate issue.

This controversy, and rights claims more generally, may also be analyzed by reference to the distinction between the statements (1) "X has a right to do Y" and (2) "X acts rightly in doing Y." The distinction is between rights (or a right) and right conduct, as well as between rights and their right exercise.[44] Sometimes when we say that a person "has a right to do X," we mean that he or she does not do wrong in performing X. But often our statement that someone "has a right to do X" implies nothing about the morality of the act; it means only that others have no right to interfere with the act. Thus, one can consistently affirm that a woman has a moral or a legal right to have an abortion and that she is not acting rightly in having an abortion. Perhaps her reasons are not strong enough to warrant an abortion, or perhaps she acts on false information.

The enforceability of rights and obligations

Because of the correlativity between rights and obligations, everything true of positive rights is true of positive obligations, and everything true of negative rights is true of negative obligations. If a person has a positive right to goods or services such as medical care, then others have a positive obligation to provide them. If a person has a negative right against interference, then another person has an obligation to abstain from interference. Also important is that both obligations and rights are *enforceable*. That is, one who is bound by an obligation may be imposed upon to discharge it; and the valid claim that constitutes a right is an enforceable claim. Whether the mechanism of enforcement is a legal system with threats and penalties or a moral system with other forms of disapproval, the thesis holds that some pressure is justified. One distinction between law and morality hinges in part on the nature of their respective sanctions for enforcing compliance with their principles and rules. The sanctions in morality tend to involve contempt, social ostracism, criticism, blame, attempts to induce shame, and the like; and they are applied more informally than legal sanctions.[45]

From the perspective of moral theory, the most important classes of obligations and rights are general negative rights and obligations and general positive rights and obligations. They are *general* in that they are enforceable requirements that bind all members of the moral community because they are members of that community. *Special* rights and obligations hold only in virtue of special relationships, such as those between physicians and patients. Because general negative rights are rights of noninterference, their direct connection to liberal individualism is apparent, with its typical emphasis on freedom from government and protection of zones of privacy. Because general positive rights require that all members of the community yield some of their resources to advance the welfare of others by providing social goods and services, there is a natural connection in theories that emphasize general positive rights to a communitarianism that limits the scope of individualism. To generalize the point, the broader the scope of positive rights in a theory, the more likely that theory is to emphasize a scheme of social justice that confers positive rights to redistributions of resources (as we see in Chapter 6).

The main import of these distinctions for this book is that a moral system composed of a powerful set of general negative obligations and rights is antithetical to a moral system composed of a powerful set of general positive obligations and rights, just as a strong individualism is opposed to a strong communitarianism. Rights of privacy and the pursuit of one's autonomous projects will inevitably conflict with enforceable obligations to assist or provide resources for others. Many of the conflicts we encounter throughout this book spring from these basic differences over the existence and scope of negative and positive rights and obligations—especially regarding the number, types, and weight of positive rights and obligations.

Conclusion

In this chapter we have surveyed broad types of ethical theory and delineated their strengths and weaknesses. We have offered reasons for affirming a conception of morality that is oriented to principles and rules and for viewing obligations and rights as correlative. We have argued that the distinction between consequentialist (especially utilitarian) and deontological theories, while important, can be and has been overestimated. There are major differences within each type of theory—regarding the grounds of the theory, the number of its principles, and whether the theory's principles apply directly to acts or are mediated through rules. But there are also major similarities across certain rule-oriented theories. In particular, some rule-utilitarian and rule-deontological theories (where "rule" includes principles) converge on the same principles and rules.

Rule-oriented theories allow room for discretionary judgment when rules are conceived, as we propose, as prima facie binding rather than as absolute or as rules of thumb. Nevertheless, when prima facie principles and rules conflict, agents are not left with only intuition as a guide. We have proposed a process of reasoning that is consistent with both a rule-utilitarian and a rule-deontological theory. This process will be evident when we explore the content and conflicts of the four basic principles (Chapters 3 through 6) and several derivative rules (Chapter 7), all of which are prima facie obligatory.

Notes

1. In 1930, C. D. Broad introduced a distinction between teleological and deontological theories in order to classify ancient and modern theories in a systematic form. See *Five Types of Ethical Theory* (London: Routledge and Kegan Paul, 1930), pp. 206, 278. A 1958 article by Elizabeth Anscombe gave the term *consequentialism* wide currency; see G. E. M. Anscombe, "Modern Moral Philosophy," *Philosophy* 33 (January 1958): 1–19. For a more contemporary treatment of consequentialism, see Samuel Scheffler, ed., *Consequentialism and Its Critics* (Oxford: Oxford University Press, 1988).
2. For critical explorations of this utilitarian thesis, see Thomas Nagel, "The Limits of Objectivity," *Tanner Lectures on Human Values*, ed. S. McMurrin (Cambridge: Cambridge University Press, 1979), p. 119; Samuel Scheffler, *The Rejection of Consequentialism* (Oxford: Clarendon Press, 1982).
3. See Jeremy Bentham, *An Introduction to the Principles of Morals and Legislation* (New York: Hafner, 1948), esp. Principle 1.3.
4. John Stuart Mill, *Utilitarianism, On Liberty, and Essay on Bentham*, ed. with intro. by Mary Warnock (New York: New American Library, 1974), pp. 256–78.

5. G. E. Moore, *Principia Ethica* (Cambridge: Cambridge University Press, 1962), pp. 90 ff.

6. Alasdair MacIntyre, *After Virtue* (Notre Dame, Ind.: University of Notre Dame Press, 1981), p. 62. For still sterner criticisms of utilitarianism and incommensurable values, see Bernard Williams, *Morality: An Introduction to Ethics* (Baltimore: Penguin Books, 1973), pp. 94–103.

7. See James Griffin, "Are There Incommensurable Values?" *Philosophy and Public Affairs* 7 (Fall 1977): 39–59, esp. his example of the preferences of geriatric patients on p. 55, and *Well-Being: Its Meaning, Measurement, and Importance* (Oxford: Clarendon Press, 1986), pp. 89–102.

8. Worthington Hooker, *Physician and Patient; or a Practical View of the Mutual Duties, Relations and Interests of the Medical Profession and the Community* (New York: Baker and Scribner, 1849), pp. 357ff, 378–81; see also 375, 377.

9. J. J. C. Smart, *An Outline of a System of Utilitarian Ethics* (Melbourne: University Press, 1961); and "Extreme and Restricted Utilitariansim," *Philosophical Quarterly* VI (1956), as reprinted in *Contemporary Utilitarianism*, ed. M. Bayles (Garden City, N. Y.: Doubleday Anchor Books, 1968), esp. pp. 104ff.

10. See Laud Humphreys, *Tearoom Trade: Impersonal Sex in Public Places* (Chicago: Aldine, 1970).

11. David Hume, *A Treatise of Human Nature,* ed. L. A. Selby-Bigge (Oxford: Oxford University Press, 1888), Book III, Parts I and II, esp. pp. 494–500. Richard B. Brandt, "Toward a Credible Form of Utilitarianism," in *Contemporary Utilitarianism,* ed. Bayles, pp. 143–86. Brandt's later views are found in *A Theory of the Good and the Right* (Oxford: Clarendon Press, 1979), esp. chaps. 14 and 15.

12. Moral-code utilitarianism also may provide a way of circumventing a prominent objection against the act/rule distinction advanced by David Lyons in *Forms and Limits of Utilitarianism* (Oxford: Clarendon Press, 1965). He argues that whatever would count for an act utilitarian as a reason for breaking a rule would count equally for a rule utilitarian as a good reason for amending a rule, and hence the two amount, in practice, to the same theory. It would be difficult and perhaps impossible to amend rules in an entire code with the frequency with which a rule could be validly broken by act utilitarians.

13. See W. D. Ross, *The Right and the Good* (Oxford: Clarendon Press, 1930), and *The Foundations of Ethics* (Oxford: Clarendon Press, 1939); and John Rawls, *A Theory of Justice* (Cambridge, Mass: Harvard University Press, 1971). The general outlines of Ross's so-called intuitionist theory were anticipated by eighteenth-century philosopher Richard Price. Although we discuss only Ross, there are striking similarities between the two.

14. See Alan Donagan, *The Theory of Morality* (Chicago: University of Chicago Press, 1977), p. 66.

15. Immanuel Kant, *Groundwork of the Metaphysic of Morals,* trans. H. J. Paton (New York: Harper and Row, 1964), pp. 90–91.

16. Ross, *The Right and the Good,* pp. 22, 41–42.

17. Rawls, *A Theory of Justice,* §§ 8, 11, 46, 51.

18. See Ross, *The Right and the Good* and *The Foundations of Ethics.*

19. See Paul Ramsey, *The Patient as Person* (New Haven: Yale University Press, 1970), and *Ethics at the Edges of Life: Medical and Legal Intersections* (New Haven: Yale University Press, 1978); and Robert Veatch, *Death, Dying and the Biological Revolution* 2nd ed. (New Haven: Yale University Press, 1988), and *A Theory of Med-*

ical Ethics (New York: Basic Books, 1981). Among the writings of H. Tristram Engelhardt, Jr., see *Foundations of Bioethics* (New York: Oxford University Press, 1986), and "Health Care Allocations: Responses to the Unjust, the Unfortunate, and the Undesirable," in *Justice and Health Care,* ed. Earl E. Shelp (Dordrecht: D. Reidel, 1981), pp. 121–37.

20. Antony Flew, "Ends and Means," in *The Encyclopedia of Philosophy,* ed. Paul Edwards (New York: Macmillan and Free Press, 1967), Vol. II, p. 510.

21. See William Frankena, *Ethics,* 2d ed. (Englewood Cliffs, N.J.: Prentice-Hall, 1973).

22. Brandt, "Toward a Credible Form of Utilitarianism," p. 166.

23. For research involving human subjects to be ethically justified, it is now generally agreed that the research must satisfy several ethical principles and rules. For instance, the research must be designed to offer a high probability of generating knowledge, its probable benefits must outweigh its risks, the selection of subjects must be just, the subjects (or their proxies) must give informed consent, and their rights to privacy and confidentiality must be respected. See LeRoy Walters, "Some Ethical Issues in Research Involving Human Subjects," *Perspectives in Biology and Medicine* (Winter 1977): 193–211; National Commission for the Protection of Human Subjects of Biomedical and Behavioral Research, *The Belmont Report* (Washington, D.C.: DHEW Publication No. 0578-0012, 1978); and President's Commission for the Study of Ethical Problems in Medicine and Biomedical and Behavioral Research, *Protecting Human Subjects* (Washington, D.C.: U.S. Government Printing Office, 1981), and *Implementing Human Research Regulations* (Washington, D.C.: U.S. Government Printing Office, 1983).

24. Donagan, *The Theory of Morality,* p. 191.

25. G. J. Warnock, *The Object of Morality* (London: Methuen, 1971), p. 33.

26. Donald Evans, "Paul Ramsey on Exceptionless Moral Rules," *American Journal of Jurisprudence* 16 (1971): 184–214. See also Sissela Bok, *Lying: Moral Choice in Public and Private Life* (New York: Pantheon Books, 1978), pp. 13–16.

27. This theory is sometimes labelled intuitionism because it involves a balancing of the various moral considerations and precludes the possibility of deductions from fixed, preweighted principles. Although we eschew the label *intuitionism,* we accept the premise that intuitive judgments in the sense of fallible and rebuttable applications of rules are inevitable in ethics. For a "pluralistic theory" in biomedical ethics that has much in common with our composite theory, see Baruch Brody, *Life and Death Decision Making* (New York: Oxford University Press, 1988), chaps. 1 and 2.

28. See Robert Nozick, "Moral Complications and Moral Structures," *Natural Law Forum* 13 (1968):1–50.

29. In Stephen Toulmin's vigorous article, "The Tyranny of Principles," *Hastings Center Report* 11 (December 1981): 31–39, it is unclear whether he is opposed to principles and rules in our sense, as his language suggests, or only to absolute principles and rules, as his argument generally seems to indicate. For a defense of casuistry in "clinical ethics," see Albert R. Jonsen, Mark Siegler, and William J. Winslade, *Clinical Ethics,* 2d ed. (New York: Macmillan, 1986). The factors or categories Jonsen, Siegler, and Winslade present as substitutes for principles reflect or are restatable in terms of the principles presented in this book. Those categories are medical indications, patient preferences, quality of life, and external factors such as family wishes or social allocations.

30. American Hospital Association (AHA), "Statement on a Patient's Bill of Rights," *Hospitals* 47 (February 1973): 41.

31. See Joel Feinberg, *Social Philosophy* (Englewood Cliffs, N.J.: Prentice-Hall, 1973), p. 67. Feinberg prefers the narrower term *validity* to the broader term *justification*, because validity "is justification of a peculiar and narrow kind, namely justification within a system of rules."

32. This thesis is instructively argued, for different reasons, by James Griffin, "Towards a Substantive Theory of Rights," in *Utility and Rights*, ed. R. G. Frey (Minneapolis: University of Minnesota Press, 1984), esp. pp. 155–58.

33. See Rex Martin and James W. Nickel, "Recent Work on the Concept of Rights," *American Philosophical Quarterly* 17 (July 1980): 172–74. See also the discussion of rights in Theodore M. Benditt, *Rights* (Totowa, N.J.: Rowman and Littlefield, 1982).

34. We have drawn on David Braybrooke, "The Firm but Untidy Correlativity of Rights and Obligations," *Canadian Journal of Philosophy* 1 (March 1972): 351–63.

35. Mill, *Utilitarianism*, p. 305.

36. Ibid. It is still largely undecided whether we should ascribe rights to nonpersons, such as trees and animals. We have an obligation not to be cruel to animals, but is it appropriate to ascribe rights to them? The answer to this question will depend on one's theory of rights and their foundation. According to one theory, only entities capable of having interests can have rights, and therefore trees and vegetables cannot have rights. However, both animals and persons in future generations can be said to have interests, and therefore they can be said meaningfully to have rights.

37. Ronald Dworkin argues that political morality is right-based in *Taking Rights Seriously* (London: Duckworth, 1977); see p. 171. John Mackie has applied this thesis to morality generally. See "Can There Be a Right-Based Moral Theory?" *Midwest Studies in Philosophy* 3 (1978): esp. 350.

38. For a penetrating criticism, see Joseph Raz, "Right-Based Moralities," in *Utility and Rights*, ed. Frey, pp. 42–60.

39. See L. W. Sumner, *The Moral Foundation of Rights* (Oxford: Clarendon Press, 1987).

40. Act utilitarians, by contrast, seem committed to the translation of rights into interests and needs in order to facilitate utilitarian calculation; but rule utilitarians need not resort to this maneuver. The utilitarian critique of natural rights offered by Bentham is well known: "Natural rights is simple nonsense: natural and imprescriptible rights, rhetorical nonsense—nonsense upon stilts." That critique, however, was aimed at the epistemology of natural rights, not at all uses of the language of rights or at all developments of a theory of moral rights. Bentham's invectives were directed against "naturalistic" theories rather than "rights." Jeremy Bentham, "Anarchical Fallacies," in *The Collected Papers of Jeremy Bentham*, ed. John Bowring (Edinburgh, 1843), Vol. II, as reprinted in A. I. Melden, ed., *Human Rights* (Belmont, Calif.: Wadsworth, 1970), p. 32. See also Jeremy Waldron, ed., *Nonsense upon Stilts* (London: Methuen, 1987), which contains the material by Bentham as well as other nineteenth-century works on rights.

41. See T. M. Scanlon, "Rights, Goals, and Fairness," in *Public and Private Morality*, ed. Stuart Hampshire (Cambridge: Cambridge University Press, 1978), pp. 93–111.

42. See Feinberg, *Social Philosophy*, p. 59. The distinction between positive and negative rights and obligations is carefully explored in several essays in Eric Mack,

ed., *Positive and Negative Duties* (New Orleans: Tulane University, 1985). The relevant distinctions are situated in the context of contemporary political affairs by Henry Shue, *Basic Rights: Subsistence, Affluence, and U.S. Foreign Policy* (Princeton: Princeton University Press, 1980), pp. 5ff, 35ff.

43. The relevant decisions are *Roe* v. *Wade*, 410 U.S. 113 (1973); *Doe* v. *Bolton*, 410 U.S. 179 (1973); *Planned Parenthood of Missouri* v. *Danforth*, 423 U.S. 52 (1976); *Beal* v. *Doe*, 432 U.S. 438 (1977); *Maher* v. *Roe*, 432 U.S. 464; *Poelker* v. *Doe*, 432 U.S. 519 (1977); *City of Akron* v. *Akron Center for Reproductive Health* (June 1983).

44. See A. I. Melden, *Rights and Right Conduct* (Oxford: Basil Blackwell, 1959).

45. See the insightful analysis in H. L. A. Hart, *The Concept of Law* (Oxford: Clarendon Press, 1961), pp. 175–76.

3

The Principle of Respect for Autonomy

Diverse philosophers have held that morality requires autonomous actors. Their philosophies are often different because they select different themes from a family of ideas associated with autonomy. These different and sometimes inconsistent accounts suggest a need to examine the concept of autonomy before delineating a moral principle of respect for autonomy and its implications for biomedical ethics.

The concept of autonomous decision making is used in this chapter to examine informed consent, informed refusal, and many other forms of decision making. We argue that rules requiring consent in medicine and research are rooted in concerns about protecting and enabling autonomous choice by patients and subjects. An account of autonomous choice adequate to express what is respected or protected by rules of informed consent is therefore essential to the objectives of this chapter. However, the problems of autonomy in biomedical ethics stretch well beyond the problems of consent.

The concept of autonomy

Autonomy is a term derived from the Greek *autos* (''self'') and *nomos* (''rule,'' ''governance,'' or ''law''). It was first used to refer to self-rule or self-governance in Greek city-states, where citizens made their own laws rather than having them imposed. *Autonomy* has since been used to refer to a set of diverse notions including self-governance, liberty rights, privacy, individual choice, liberty to follow one's will, causing one's own behavior, and being one's own person. In light of this semantic uncertainty, it is doubtful that autonomy is a univocal concept in either ordinary English or contemporary philosophy. If there are but families of ideas constituting the concept of autonomy, we need to refine the concept in light of the particular analytical objectives of a theory of autonomy—a task sometimes called a reconstruction of the concept. Autonomy, we believe, is so imprecise in its ordinary meaning that restructuring is required before it can be used in moral theory.

As a beginning, the core idea of personal autonomy is an extension of political self-rule to self-governance by the individual: personal rule of the self while remaining free from both controlling interferences by others and personal limitations, such as inadequate understanding, that prevent meaningful choice.[1] The autonomous person acts in accordance with a freely self-chosen and informed plan, just as a truly independent government acts to control its territories and policies. A person of diminished autonomy, by contrast, is in at least some respect controlled by others or incapable of deliberating or acting on the basis of his or her plans. For example, institutionalized persons such as prisoners and the mentally retarded may have diminished autonomy. Psychological incapacitation affects the autonomy of the retarded; a severely restricted social environment limits the autonomy of prisoners.

Autonomous persons and autonomous choices

Some ethical theories have featured the traits of the autonomous person, but our interest in acts such as consenting and refusing leads us to focus on *autonomous choices*. Consents and refusals are actions, not persons. Moreover, autonomous persons sometimes make nonautonomous choices because of temporary constraints imposed by illness or depression or because of ignorance or coercion. An autonomous person who signs a consent form without reading or understanding the form is qualified to give an informed consent but has nonetheless failed to do so because of a failure to act autonomously. Similarly, some persons who in general are not autonomous can at times make autonomous choices. For example, some patients in mental institutions who are generally unable to care for themselves and have been declared legally incompetent may still be able to make autonomous choices such as stating preferences for meals and making phone calls to acquaintances.

In some theories of autonomy both persons and their actions must meet rigorous standards or else fail of autonomy. For example, a theory may demand that the autonomous person be consistent, independent, in command, resistant to control by authorities, and the source of his or her own basic values, beliefs, and life plans.[2] One of the problems with this theory of autonomy is that few choosers, and also few choices, would be autonomous if held to such demanding standards, which in effect present an aspirational ideal of autonomy. An ideal theory of this sort reaches beyond the criteria needed for a theory of autonomous actions. Instead of this demanding account, we will delineate what is and should be meant in moral and legal theory by expressions such as "respect for autonomy" and "exercise of autonomy," which refer to normal choosers and their choices rather than ideal choosers.

Accordingly, we analyze autonomous action in terms of normal choosers who act (1) intentionally, (2) with understanding, and (3) without controlling influences that determine the action.[3] The first condition is a matter of planning on the agent's part and is not a matter of degree: Acts are either intentional (and therefore potentially autonomous) or nonintentional (and therefore nonautonomous). By contrast, the conditions of understanding and absence of controlling influences can both be satisfied to a greater or lesser extent. Actions can be autonomous by degrees, as a function of satisfying these two conditions to different degrees. Thus, the conditions of understanding and noncontrol are analyzed here in terms of a broad continuum from fully present to wholly absent.

For an action to be autonomous we should only require a substantial satisfaction of these conditions, not full or even nearly full understanding or complete absence of influence (see pp. 100–105, 107–111). To chain adequate decision making by patients to fully or completely autonomous decision making strips the rules of informed consent of any meaningful place in the practical world, where people's actions are rarely, if ever, fully autonomous. A person's appreciation of information and independence from controlling influences in the health-care setting need not exceed a person's information and independence in making a financial investment, hiring a new employee, or attending a particular college. The goal, realistically, is only that such consequential decisions be substantially autonomous.

The line between what is substantial and what is insubstantial might seem arbitrary, and therefore our entire approach and theory might seem imperiled by arbitrariness. However, thresholds marking substantially autonomous decisions can be carefully reasoned in light of specific goals. Substantial autonomy should be a reasonable and achievable goal for decision making about research and medical interventions no less and no more than substantial degrees of autonomous action are achieved elsewhere in life. For example, it is difficult in the abstract to say exactly what a physician or a nurse needs to know and be able to do in order to be licensed, but we are not without resources for specifying the proper threshold of information and training that they must possess. Accordingly, the criteria of substantiality and substantial autonomy in particular will be treated throughout this book as a matter that is best addressed in a particular context, rather than pinpointed through a general theory of what is a "substantial amount."[4]

Autonomy and authority

It is sometimes held that autonomous action is incompatible with the authority of church, state, or other groups that function to direct the decisions of moral agents. One argument for this position is that autonomous persons must act on their own reasons and thus should never submit to another person or authority simply because the other utters an imperative. Because this conclusion might seem to follow from our analysis of autonomous action, it is worth considering whether autonomy is radically inconsistent with authority in the way some suggest.[5]

We think there is no fundamental inconsistency, because the notions of autonomy and authority that underlie this suggestion are eccentric and indefensible. Common conceptions of nondictatorial political and social practices assume that the provision of justifying reasons is part of, not distinct from, the process of legitimate authoritative command. Dutiful citizens are not expected to comply with authoritative commands without provision of reasons and merely because authorities have spoken. The legitimacy of any order is contingent upon its not exceeding the limits set by those citizens, from whom the authority to command ultimately derives.

Individuals may also exercise their autonomy in choosing to submit to the authoritative demands of an institution or tradition. They exercise their autonomy in accepting the legitimacy of the institution or tradition as a source of guidelines.[6] For example, in accepting the authority of his or her religious institution, a Jehovah's Witness may agree not to consent to a blood transfusion even in medical emergencies (see Case 12 and 13), or a Roman Catholic may agree not to consent to an abortion. It may be tempting to view a refusal of a blood transfusion by a Jehovah's Witness or a refusal of an abortion by a Roman Catholic as heteronomous—as rule by others—but such a view is not warranted if the individual in question autonomously accepts the authority of the institution or tradition.

Moral principles should not be interpreted as disembodied personal rules, cut off from their social and cultural setting. To interpret autonomy in morality as entailing the reign of subjective principles involves a misunderstanding of both moral belief and ethical theory. This conception wrongly portrays moral principles as formulated by agents disengaged from society. As we argued in Chapter 1, "morality" emerges from shared experiences and social arrangements (tacit or otherwise). That we share accepted principles in no way prevents them from being an individual's personal principles. Virtuous conduct, role responsibilities, acceptable forms of loving, charitable behavior, respect for autonomy, and many other moral notions are autonomously accepted by individuals but usually derive, in some part, from cultural traditions.

How could a principle be a moral principle and stand outside minimal social arrangements that form the terms of cooperation in society? What would make such a principle more than the belief or policy of an individual? Could the moral requirement that we respect autonomy be merely a personal creation, or could it be valid if accepted only by one single individual? And what of rules or codes of professional ethics? By their nature they do not permit individual authorship, yet their character in no way renders them incompatible with autonomy.[7]

This conclusion about the compatibility of autonomy and both delegated authority and moral tradition holds for medical contexts as well as for political ones. We shall encounter some paradoxes of autonomy in medical contexts because of the dependent condition of the patient and the authoritative position of the medical professional. On occasion we may doubt that authority and autonomy are compatible, but this doubt does not arise because the two concepts are intrinsically incompatible. It arises because in the context under consideration authority has not been properly delegated or is itself of questionable legitimacy.

It also does not follow from the fact of an action's being autonomous that it is morally acceptable or morally principled. One can reject morality or act against morality and still act autonomously. Autonomy is compatible on the one hand with immorality and on the other hand with moral authority and tradition. Autonomy is thus a concept that is properly linked to reflective individual choice but should not be thought to require a rejection of authority, tradition, or social morality.

The principle of respect for autonomy

Being autonomous and choosing autonomously are not the same as being respected as an autonomous agent. To respect an autonomous agent is, first, to recognize that person's capacities and perspective, including his or her right to hold views, to make choices, and to take actions based on personal values and beliefs. But respect involves more than taking this attitude. It involves treating agents so as to allow or to enable them to act autonomously. That is, true respect includes acting to respect, not the mere adoption of a certain attitude.

Such respect has historically been connected to the idea that persons possess a value independent of particular circumstances. Two philosophers who have shaped the modern understanding of respect for autonomy were examined in Chapter 2: Immanuel Kant (a deontologist) and John Stuart Mill (a utilitarian). In various writings, Kant argued that respect for autonomy flows from the recognition that all persons have unconditional worth, each having the capacity to determine his or her own destiny.[8] To violate a person's autonomy is to treat that person merely as a means, to treat that person in accordance with one's own goals and without regard to that person's goals. To reject that person's goals and considered judgments or to restrict his or her freedom to act on those goals and judgments is to fail to respect autonomy.

Mill was more concerned about the autonomy—or, as he preferred to say, the individuality—of action and thought. He argued that social control over individual actions is legitimate only if it is necessary to prevent harm to other individuals and that citizens should be permitted to develop their potential according to their personal convictions, as long as they do not interfere with a like expression of freedom by others. Mill held that a person with true character is one of genuine individuality, whereas a person "without character" is under an oppressive, controlling influence by church, state, parents, or family.[9]

It is doubtful that a utilitarian theory that follows Mill and a deontological theory in the Kantian tradition require significantly different courses of action. Although Mill's view most obviously requires noninterference with autonomous expression and Kant's view entails a moral imperative to frame certain attitudes of respect, in the end these two profoundly different philosophies can both be invoked in support of what we will call the principle of respect for autonomy.

This principle can be stated in its negative form as follows: *Autonomous actions are not to be subjected to controlling constraints by others.* This principle provides the justificatory basis for the right to make autonomous decisions, which in turn takes the form of specific autonomy-related rights, such as liberty and privacy. The principle should be treated as a broad, abstract principle independent of restrictive or exceptive clauses such as "We must respect individuals' views and rights *so long as* their thoughts and actions do not seriously harm other persons." Like all moral principles, this principle has only prima facie standing. It asserts a right of noninterference and correlatively an obligation not to constrain autonomous actions. It is always an open question which restrictions may rightfully be placed on choices by patients or subjects when these choices conflict with other values. If choices endanger the public health, potentially harm a fetus, or involve a scarce resource for which a patient cannot pay, it may be justifiable to restrict exercises of autonomy severely, perhaps even by state intervention. If restriction is justified, the justification must rest on some competing moral principle such as beneficence or justice.

The principle of respect for autonomy does not determine what, on balance, a person ought to be free to know or do or what is to count as a valid justification for constraining autonomy. For example, in Case 6 a patient with an inoperable, incurable carcinoma asks, "I don't have cancer, do I?" The physician lies, saying, "You're as good as you were ten years ago." Because this lie denies the patient information he may need to determine his future course of action, it does override the principle of respect for autonomy. However, it may be (and here we state no opinion) that, on balance, the lie is justified by the principle of beneficence. (See Chapters 5 and 7.)

So far, our discussion of the moral requirements of the principle of respect for autonomy has focused primarily on a negative feature: avoidance of controlling constraints, including lying and coercion. However, the principle has clear positive implications when applied to certain relationships. For example, in research, medicine, and health care, it engenders a positive or affirmative obligation of respectful treatment in disclosing information and fostering autonomous decision making. There is no general obligation to disclose information to others, even if there is a general obligation not to lie to them (see the discussion of truthfulness in Chapter 7). But physicians and other health-care professionals and researchers do not have a right to do anything to patients or subjects without their consent, and the right to consent or refuse is grounded in the principle of respect for autonomy. In Justice Cardozo's famous statement, "Every human being of adult years and sound mind has a right to determine what shall be done with his own body."[10] For the patient's or subject's consent to be a valid authorization for the professional to proceed, it must be based on understanding and must be voluntary. Because of the unequal distribution of knowledge between professionals on the one hand and patients or subjects on the other, the principle of respect for autonomy entails that professionals have a prima facie obligation to disclose information, to ensure understanding and voluntariness, and to foster adequate decision making.

In addition, health-care professionals stand in special fiduciary relationships to their patients and thus have an affirmative obligation to disclose information:

The relationship between patient and physician is one known to the law as a "fiduciary relationship." Any person such as a physician, attorney, priest or other who enters into a relationship of trust and confidence with another has a positive obligation to disclose all relevant facts. If an individual wishes to buy a pig from a farmer, the farmer is not obliged to point out defects of the pig. If specifically questioned, the farmer commits fraud if he answers dishonestly, but he is not obliged to volunteer information which may be detrimental to the sale. However, since the essence of a professional relationship is that the professional knows more about his subject than the person who seeks his help . . . an affirmative duty of disclosure has always existed.[11]

The principle of respect for autonomy can easily be interpreted as too broad in scope. It does not apply to persons who are not in a position to act in a sufficiently autonomous manner—perhaps because they are immature, incapacitated, ignorant, coerced, or in a position in which they can be exploited by others. Infants, irrationally suicidal individuals, and drug-dependent patients are examples. The behavior of nonautonomous persons may be validly controlled on grounds of beneficence in order to protect them from harms that might result from their behavior. Those who defend rights of autonomy in biomedical ethics have never denied that some forms of intervention are justified if persons are either wholly or substantially nonautonomous and cannot be rendered autonomous for specific decisions—such as through the provision of information about proposed medical treatment.

We shall later discuss valid ways to override the principle of respect for autonomy, as well as how to handle those occasions in which a rational agent expresses an autonomous wish to waive consent, delegate authority to others, or take his or her own life. In particular, we will consider permissible paternalistic restraints in Chapter 5.

The meaning and justification of informed consent

The practice of obtaining informed consent developed in medicine and biomedical and behavioral research, where the disclosure and nondisclosure of information regularly occur in encounters between patients and physicians and between subjects and researchers. Since the Nuremburg trials, in which horrifying accounts of experimentation in concentration camps led to concern about the use of nonconsenting subjects in research, the issue of informed consent has probably received more attention than any other issue in biomedical ethics. Yet the term *informed consent* did not appear until a decade after these trials, and it did not receive serious examination until around 1972.

Increasingly the focus has changed from the physician's or researcher's obligation to *disclose* information to the quality of a patient's or subject's *understanding* and *consent*. The forces creating this shift of emphasis were largely, but not entirely, external to medicine and biomedical research and emerged primarily through the influence of law and ethics. Throughout this section we shall see how standards of informed consent have derived from the regulation of research, from case law regarding medical practice, and from changes in the patient-physician relationship.

Functions and justifications of rules of informed consent

Virtually all medical and research codes of ethics now hold that physicians and research investigators must obtain the informed consent of patients and subjects before undertaking procedures. These consent measures have been designed to enable autonomous choice by patients and subjects, but they serve other functions as well, including the protection of patients and subjects against harm and the encouragement of medical professionals to act responsibly in their interactions with patients and subjects.[12]

Although informed consent may serve each of these functions, two positions on the function and justification of informed consent requirements have permeated the literature. Throughout the early history of concern about research subjects, consent requirements were primarily viewed as a way to minimize risk to subjects. Reduction of risk and avoidance of unfairness and exploitation still function as the primary justifications for many professional, regulatory, and institutional controls and may be the driving *motive* behind the public and scholarly interest in the ethics of research and in guidelines on consent. Nonetheless, protection of autonomy has emerged in the last two decades as the primary *justification* of informed consent provisions, which are only one facet of the social rules and regulations that have been devised to protect research subjects. For example, in addition to evaluating proposed consent forms for research protocols, institutional review boards (IRBs), which are mandated for the evaluation of research involving human subjects in institutions receiving federal funds, must determine whether the proposed research has an acceptable risk-benefit ratio.

Enabling autonomous choice is a loosely defined goal that is often buried in vague discussions of the importance of protecting the welfare and rights of research subjects. Much the same can be said of the history of informed consent in clinical medicine. Enabling autonomous choice has thus been one of several imperfectly distinguished and poorly formulated goals in the quest for a satisfactory medical and research ethics. Historically we can claim little beyond the indisputable fact that a general, inchoate societal demand has developed for the protection of patients' and subjects' rights, most conspicuously their autonomy rights.

Throughout this chapter we accept the view that the primary function of informed consent is protecting and enabling individual autonomous choice. The alternative justification of protection from harm is based on the principles of nonmaleficence and beneficence (see Chapters 4 and 5). Second-party consent, or consent on behalf of a person given by another, is properly justified on this latter basis (unless the nonautonomous person's previous autonomous wishes are known), but a justification in terms of the principles of nonmaleficence and beneficence is not a sufficient justification of first-party consent. Autonomy deserves protection even if a person's choice would not maximize individual or social welfare.

The definition and elements of informed consent

Before we can fix the conditions under which we must obtain an informed consent—for example, when a procedure is intrusive, when there are significant risks, or when the purposes of the procedure need to be known—the concept of informed consent itself needs clarification. That is, we need to establish a meaning of informed consent, given the many different meanings that might be proposed. Unfortunately, the contexts in which practices of consent arose and have persisted often leave considerable vagueness around the term and thus create a need to sharpen the concept so that its meaning is clear and suitable.

Some recent commentators on informed consent in clinical medicine have reduced the idea to shared decision making between doctor and patient, so that informed consent and mutual decision making are identical ideas.[13] But despite the historical relationship in clinical medicine between decision making and informed consent, it is a confusion to treat informed consent and shared decision making as identical. Informed consent is not restricted to clinical medicine and is used no less frequently for research contexts, in which a model of shared decision making may or may not be appropriate, depending on the circumstances. Even in clinical contexts the informational interactions through which patients elect medical interventions should be distinguished from their act of permitting or approving the intervention.

TWO SENSES OF "INFORMED CONSENT."[14] The question "What is an informed consent?" is complicated because there are at least two entrenched meanings of *informed consent*. That is, the term is analyzable in different ways because of two different conceptions of informed consent.

In the first sense, informed consent is analyzable in terms of autonomous choice by patients and subjects: An informed consent is an *autonomous authorization* of a medical intervention or of involvement in research by individual persons. This first sense of informed consent requires that a patient or subject do more than express agreement with, yield to, or comply with an arrangement or a proposal. He or she must actively authorize the proposal in the act of consent. A patient does not authorize in this sense if he or she merely assents to a treatment plan by submission to a doctor's authoritative order; nor is there autonomous authorization if the treatment plan is not specific about what is authorized.

An example of the latter problem is found in the classic case of *Mohr* v. *Williams*, in which a physician obtained his patient Anna Mohr's consent to an operation on her right ear. In the course of the procedure he determined that the left ear was actually the one that needed surgery and operated on it instead. A court found that the physician should have obtained the patient's consent to the surgery on the left ear because express consent to a particular surgery is required:

If a physician advises a patient to submit to a particular operation, and the patient weighs the dangers and risks incident to its performance, and finally consents, the patient thereby, in effect, enters into a contract authorizing the physician to operate to the extent of the consent given, but no further.[15]

Accordingly, an informed consent in this first sense is an autonomous action by a subject or a patient that authorizes a professional either to involve the subject in research or to initiate a medical plan for the patient (or both). Following our analysis of autonomy, an informed consent occurs if a patient or subject with substantial *understanding* and in substantial *absence of control* by others *intentionally authorizes* a professional to do something. The authorization condition, then, is what distinguishes an act of informed consent from other forms of autonomous action. We note also that *disclosure* plays no role in this definition.

In the second sense, informed consent is analyzable in terms of *the social rules of informed consent* in those institutional contexts in which it is necessary to obtain legally valid consent from potential patients or subjects before proceeding with therapeutic procedures or research. Informed consents are not always autonomous acts in these settings and are not necessarily even meaningful authorizations. This second sense of consent may be understood in terms of institutional rules of consent, because informed consent here refers to an institutionally or legally effective authorization from a patient or a subject. An authorization is effective if obtained through procedures that satisfy the rules that govern specific institutional practices of consent. Any consent is informed if it satisfies the operative rules governing the practice.

The analysis of informed consent in terms of institutional rules of consent captures the current dominant conception in the regulatory rules of federal agencies and in health-care institutions. These documents derive from a conception of what the rules must be in order to enable effective authorizations in these institutions. A patient or subject can autonomously authorize an intervention and so give an informed consent in the first sense, but not effectively authorize that intervention and thus not give an informed consent in this second sense. For example, if a minor is not legally authorized to consent, he or she may autonomously authorize without giving an effective consent.

Because institutional rules of informed consent need not result in autonomous authorizations, some critics have argued that the courts have imposed on physicians a mere obligation to warn of risks of proposed interventions and treatments.[16] Jay Katz, for example, maintains that "This judicially imposed obligation must be distinguished from the idea of informed consent, namely, that patients have a decisive role to play in the medical decisionmaking process." By their actions and declarations, Katz believes, the courts as well as medical institutions have made informed consent a "cruel hoax" and have allowed "the idea of informed consent . . . to wither on the vine."[17] Katz's complaints can best be understood by utilizing the two senses of informed consent: A physician who obtains a consent under institutional criteria may still fail to meet the rigorous standards of an autonomy-based model, which alone Katz acknowledges as adequate.

Although it is easy to criticize institutional rules as superficial, there may be valid reasons why a court, an institution, or a physician cannot obtain a consent that satisfies the demands of strict rules protective of autonomy. Requirements to enable patients and subjects to make decisions about authorization must be evaluated not only in terms of respect for autonomy but also in terms of the fairness and the effects of imposing such requirements on various institutions. It is necessary to take account of what is fair and reasonable to require of health-care professionals and researchers, the effect of alternative consent requirements on efficiency and effectiveness in the delivery of health care and the advancement of science, and—particularly in medical care—the effect of consent requirements on the welfare of patients.

In conclusion, rules of informed consent need not conform to only one of the two classes of definitions we have discussed. They may conform to both. Many rules of informed consent in policy contexts reflect a strong and definite reliance on informed consent in the first sense. Furthermore, we take it as morally axiomatic that the first definition ought to serve—and sometimes has served—as the benchmark for the evaluation of the moral adequacy of rules framed for institutional purposes. This conclusion follows from an understanding of the primary goal of informed consent in medical care and in research as that of enabling potential subjects and patients to make autonomous decisions about whether to authorize medical and research interventions.

THE ELEMENTS OF INFORMED CONSENT. The most common approach to the definition of *informed consent* in literature on the subject has been to specify the elements of the concept, in particular the elements of the *information* component and the *consent* component. The information component refers to adequate disclosure of information and adequate comprehension by patients or subjects of what is disclosed. The consent component refers to a voluntary decision or agreement on the part of a competent person. Legal, philosophical, regulatory, medical, and psychological literatures have all tended to favor the following elements as the analytical components of informed consent:[18]

1. Disclosure
2. Understanding
3. Voluntariness
4. Competence
5. Consent[19]

These elements are often confusingly presented as the conditions of a definition of the term *informed consent*, such that one gives an informed consent to an intervention if (and perhaps only if) one receives a thorough disclosure about it, one comprehends the disclosure, one acts voluntarily, one is competent to act, and one consents to the intervention. Although this definition seems congruent with the uses of the term in such practical contexts as clinical medicine and law, this list of conditions is distorted by the specific orientations of medical convention and malpractice law. Conditions 1 through 5 are less suitable as conditions that express the meaning or character of informed consent than as a list of the elements of informed consent as they have emerged in institutional policies and social regulations that impose conditions for effective consent in medicine and research.

The above five-condition definition is, of course, superior to a one-condition definition in terms of disclosure, as courts and medical literature have some-times proposed.[20] But both approaches tend to distort informed consent by suggesting that *disclosure* is the key item in the act of giving an informed consent. Any definition that makes disclosure the chief condition incorporates dubious assumptions about medical authority, about physician responsibility, or about legal theories of liability, all of which delineate an *obligation* to make disclosures rather than a *meaning* of informed consent. The meaning of informed consent, as we saw, is better analyzed in terms of autonomous authorization.

However, in the remainder of this chapter we accept the idea of "elements" as explicating the basic topics about informed decision making that need analysis. We examine these standard elements in light of the goal of enabling autonomous choice by patients, but we do not propose that contemporary medicine and research should always be held to the standard of autonomous decision making. Our belief that this standard is the proper guidepost for framing conceptions of informed consent in institutional settings does not mean that everything about informed consent has to be measured in terms of whether an autonomous authorization has been achieved. Each of the following five elements is treated in this chapter, with an eye to possible improvements by using the model of autonomous authorization. (The importance of authorization in our analysis leads us to substitute element 5 below for "consent," which is listed above as condition 5.)

I. *Threshold Element*
  1. Competence
II. *Information Elements*
  2. Disclosure of Information
  3. Understanding of Information
III. *Consent Elements*
  4. Voluntariness
  5. Authorization

Because this chapter is about autonomy, and not merely informed consent, our treatment of these elements will extend beyond the context of consent and refusal into other regions of autonomous action and respect for autonomy.

Competence

Competence to consent—or decision-making capacity—might be more appropriately described as a presupposition of the practice of obtaining informed consent than as an element of informed consent, because *competence* is used to refer to a precondition of being able to authorize autonomously. The term is used in biomedical contexts in which both physical and mental conditions can render patients and subjects incapable—in psychological fact or in law—of adequate decision making. Here competence functions as a threshold concept to distinguish between persons from whom decisions should be solicited and those from whom they need not or should not be solicited.

However, the special commitments of medicine, law, psychiatry, philosophy, and other professions have led to competing theories of the abilities persons must have in order to be considered competent. The word *competence* has layers of meaning connected in diverse ways but with different purposes behind the different definitions. This situation has led some to observe that there is no standard definition of competence, consequently no accepted test of competence, and consequently no nonarbitrary line that can be drawn between those who are competent and those who are incompetent. But we need to keep definitions, tests, and boundary lines as distinct as possible, confining attention for the moment to the problem of definition.

A single core meaning of the word *competence* is present in all the varied contexts in which it is applied. That meaning is "the ability to perform a task."[21] By contrast to this core meaning, the criteria of particular competencies vary from context to context because the criteria are relative to specific tasks. For example, the criteria for someone's competence to stand trial, to raise dachshunds, to write checks, or to lecture to law students are starkly different. Moreover, a person should rarely be judged incompetent with respect to every sphere of life. We usually need to consider only some type of competence or incompetence, such as the competence to decide about treatment or participation in research. Judgments of competence and incompetence thus may affect only a limited range of decision making. For example, a person who is judged incompetent to drive an automobile may be competent to decide to participate in medical research and may be able to handle simple affairs easily while faltering before complex ones.

In Case 9, a woman who was involuntarily hospitalized because of periods of confusion and loss of memory was competent most of the time to perform ordinary tasks. Health professionals and a court were called upon to determine whether this legally incompetent patient could be provided with an alternative medical therapy suitable to her situation. The concept of "specific incompetence" has been invoked in such cases in law to prevent vague generalizations about competence from excluding persons from all decision making. When it proves difficult to determine the level of competence, it is appropriate to evaluate the patient over time—regarding understanding, deliberative capacity, and coherence—while supplying counseling and further support and information.

Some persons are incompetent to do something at one point in time and competent to perform that same task at another point in time. Judgments of competence about these persons can be complicated by the need to distinguish categories of illness that result in chronic changes of intellectual, language, or memory functioning from those that are characterized by rapid reversibility of these functions, as in the case of transient ischemic attack, transient global amnesia, and the like. In some of the latter cases patients may be competent even from hour to hour.

These conceptual points have practical significance. The law has traditionally presumed that a person incompetent to manage his or her estate is also incompetent to vote, make medical decisions, get married, and so on. Such laws were usually aimed at the protection of property rather than persons and so were ill suited to medical decision making. Their global sweep, based on a total judgment of the person, can and has at times been carried too far. To say that "person X is incompetent to do Y" should never carry the automatic implication that X is not competent to do Z—that is, not competent to perform an action other than Y. In one classic case a physician argued that a patient was incompetent to consent because she was epileptic.[22] Such judgments defy much that we know about the etiology of various forms of incompetence—even in the hard cases of the mentally retarded or in psychotic patients or patients with uncontrollably painful afflictions.

Sometimes a competent person who is generally able to select means appropriate to chosen goals will nonetheless act incompetently in a circumstance in which he or she is called on to act in accordance with these means and goals. Hospitals know these persons well. Consider the following patient who is hospitalized with an acute disc problem and whose goal is to control her back pain. The patient has decided to manage the problem by wearing a brace, a method she has used successfully in the past. She believes strongly that she should return to this treatment modality. This approach conflicts, however, with the advice of her physician, who unwaveringly and with conviction advocates surgery. When the physician—an eminent man who alone in her city is competent to treat her—asks her to sign the surgical permit, she is psychologically unable to refuse. The patient's hopes are vested in this assertive and, in her view, powerful physician; both her hopes and fears are exaggerated by her illness, and she has a passive personality. In the circumstance, it is psychologically impossible for her to act as she desires. She is a competent person and competent to choose in general but not competent in choosing on this occasion.

Competence is also a continuum concept. Persons are more or less competent to the extent that they possess a certain level or range of abilities. For example, an experienced and knowledgeable patient is likely to be more competent to consent to a procedure than a frightened, inexperienced patient in the emergency room. This continuum of competence runs from full competence through various levels of partial competence to full incompetence. For practical and policy reasons, we need cutoffs on this continuum, so that any person below a certain level of abilities will be treated as incompetent.[23] Not all competent individuals are equally competent and not all incompetent persons equally incompetent, but the function of competence determinations is to sort persons into these two basic classes, and thus to treat persons as either competent or incompetent in particular contexts. The validity of a consent or refusal will depend in complex ways on the nature of a patient's incompetence to consent and on the actual constraints of that person's circumstances.

Case 10 illustrates the difficulties often encountered in attempting to judge competence. In this case, a man who generally exhibits normal behavior patterns is involuntarily committed to a mental institution as the result of bizarre self-destructive behavior (pulling out an eye and cutting off a hand) that is influenced by his unorthodox religious beliefs. He is judged incompetent, despite his generally competent behavior and despite the fact that his peculiar actions follow "reasonably" from his religious beliefs. This troublesome case cannot be interpreted in terms of intermittent competence, but it might be argued that an analysis in terms of limited competence is justified. However, such an analysis would also suggest that persons with unorthodox (or even bizarre) religious beliefs are less than competent, even though they reason clearly in light of their beliefs. This criterion is morally perilous for policy purposes and thus is difficult to accept as a general guideline.

There should be a moral presumption in health care—parallel to the accepted legal presumption—of an adult's competence to make decisions. The burden of proof would then fall on those who believe that a particular adult is incompetent to decide, and it would be necessary for health-care professionals, often by appealing to the courts, to establish a patient's incompetence in order to disqualify him or her from decision making.

Standards of competence

Not surprisingly, the major question about competence in recent years has centered on standards for its determination. In both law and medicine, standards of competence to consent tend to feature mental skills or capacities—ones closely connected to the attributes of autonomous persons, such as cognitive skills and independence of judgment. However, properties of autonomy and psychological capacity are not the only criteria used in general standards. Many policies also use criteria of efficiency, feasibility, and social acceptability in order to determine whether a person has given a valid authorization. For example, age has conventionally been used as an operational criterion of valid authorization, with established thresholds of age varying in accordance with a community's standards, with the degree of risk involved, and with the importance of the prospective benefits.

Many believe that judgments of competence should be connected to judgments about experience, maturity, responsibility, and welfare. For example, they argue that as an intervention in medicine increases the risks for persons, the level of ability required for a judgment of competence to elect or refuse the intervention should be increased; and as the consequences for well-being become less substantial, the level of capacity required for competence should be decreased.[24] This proposal is generally sound. The welfare of patients and subjects, broad social interests in ensuring good outcomes, and cultural views about responsibility and authority appropriately contribute to the makeup of general standards of competence. These standards are our means of balancing benefit and harm to the patient or subject with the importance of autonomy. If the consequences for welfare are grave, the need increases to be able to certify that the patient possesses the requisite capacities; but if little in the way of welfare is at stake, the level of capacity required for competence may be reduced together with the means used to test for the capacity. Nevertheless, it is still reasonable to believe that the primary reference standard of competence is the autonomous person.

Some progress toward a useful set of standards for competence has come through criminal law and civil law. Legal standards cluster around various abilities to comprehend and process information and to reason about the consequences of one's actions. Although courts have disagreed about which properties are most crucial to a determination of general competence, the following diverse standards have all been proposed and implemented:[25] (1) capacity to reach a decision based on rational reasons, (2) capacity to reach a reasonable result through a decision, and (3) the capacity to make a decision at all. Without attempting to identify all the possible arguments for adopting one or more of these three standards, it seems promising to combine parts of these into a single standard: A person is competent if and only if that person can make reasonable decisions based on rational reasons. In biomedical contexts this standard suggests that a competent person is able to understand a therapy or research procedure, to deliberate regarding major risks and benefits, and to make a decision in light of this deliberation.[26]

These characteristics indicate how competence is closely tied to autonomy. Law, medicine, and to some extent philosophy presume a context in which the characteristics of the competent person are also the properties possessed by the autonomous person. Although *autonomy* and *competence* are very different in meaning (autonomy means self-governance; competence means the ability to perform a task), the criteria of the autonomous person and of the competent person are strikingly similar. It thus seems a plausible hypothesis that an autonomous person is necessarily a competent person. On this hypothesis, a person is generally competent to authorize or refuse to authorize an intervention if and perhaps only if the person is autonomous.

Value-laden judgments of competence

Professional judgments of competence or incompetence in medicine and law function to tell us whether X is the kind of person from whom it is appropriate to solicit a decision, whether a guardian should be appointed to look after X's interests, whether involuntary institutionalization is appropriate, and the like. Competence judgments thus have a distinctive normative role of qualifying or disqualifying the person, and the concept itself cannot be understood apart from this grading function. These normative judgments are sometimes highly contestable and yet are presented as empirical findings. For example, a person who appears irrational or unreasonable to others might be declared incompetent so that treatment can be provided against his or her wishes. Such a declaration, presented in the guise of an empirical determination of incompetence, may conceal a value judgment about what a rational person would do that harbors an unduly narrow conception of rationality. Virtually all theories of incompetence encounter difficulties about whether to promote the patient's autonomy or err on the side of safety by protecting the patient, a moral and not a medical problem.[27] If precise, nonevaluative criteria were available for making such determinations of competence, the gray area would vanish. But such criteria are not available, and moral judgments and policy choices about what to do with possibly incompetent persons cannot be avoided.[28]

Determining where the threshold of competence should be situated involves a judgment about the requisite abilities and also about how to establish thresholds for each of the abilities selected. There may also be a need to select a test of competence that establishes passing and failing grades. Thus, the following three ingredients all involve normative judgments about competence:

(1) the relevant abilities for competence;
(2) a threshold level of the abilities in item 1; and
(3) an empirical test for item 2.

In the tests under item 3, it is an empirical question whether someone possesses the requisite level of abilities, but this question can only be asked and answered if other criteria have already been fixed under items 1 and 2. Sometimes these criteria are fixed by an institution or by tradition, but at other times they are open to substantial development and modification. Generally, the criteria could have been different from what they are, and they still may shift over time.

The following schema expresses the range of *in*abilities currently required in various competing tests used to evaluate *in*competence.[29] These tests range from the test requiring the least ability (the test the largest number of persons likely will pass as a competence test) to the other end of the spectrum of difficulty:

1. Inability to evidence a preference or choice
2. Inability to understand one's situation or relevantly similar situations
3. Inability to understand disclosed information
4. Inability to give a reason

5. Inability to give a rational reason (although some supporting reasons may be given)
6. Inability to give risk/benefit-related reasons (although some rational supporting reasons may be given)
7. Inability to reach a reasonable decision (as judged, e.g., by a reasonable person standard)

These tests cluster around three kinds of abilities or skills. Test 1 looks for the simple ability to offer a preference. Tests 2 and 3 probe for abilities to understand information and to appreciate one's situation. Tests 4 through 7 relate to the ability to reason through a consequential life decision, although only test 7 restricts the range of acceptable outcomes of a process of reasoning. These tests could be used alone or in combination in order to determine incompetence.

A decision about which test or tests to use in order to determine whether a patient is competent to consent depends on a number of factors. In health-care institutions the selection of abilities, thresholds, and tests will depend on moral and policy questions related to the concerns that shape the selection of requirements for informed consent. A central issue concerns the number and weights of the moral principles to be balanced. The evaluative trade-off is usually between two principles: the principle of respect for autonomy on the one hand and that of beneficence on the other. For example, if one is especially concerned about preventing abuses of autonomy, one may accept test 1 as the only valid test of incompetence, or perhaps only tests 1, 2, and 3. But if one's primary concern is that sick persons receive the best medical treatment possible, one may require patients to pass all these tests, or at least tests 6 and 7. Those who accept a stringent test of incompetence (such as 6 and 7) will place the medical interests and safety of patients above their autonomy. By contrast, those committed broadly to autonomy rights, even for sick and psychiatric patients, will judge that these values have priority over values of health and safety and will therefore adopt one of the less stringent tests of incompetence.

Conflicts based on these different commitments should come as no surprise, because the conflicts are an instance of the most pervasive clash of principles in biomedical ethics, namely that between the principles of autonomy and beneficence. We will explore the full depth of this conflict in Chapter 5 (see pp. 209–15).

Disclosure of information

We have seen that from an institutional point of view informed consent is often understood primarily in terms of the obligation to inform patients. Disclosure has traditionally been portrayed as a necessary condition of valid informed consent, especially in the courts, which have spoken of a disclosure of facts as the staple ingredient in informed consent. The legal doctrine of informed consent has been primarily a law of disclosure based on a general obligation to exercise reasonable care by giving information. Litigation has erupted over the absence of informed consent because of an alleged civil injury to one's person or property that is intentionally or negligently inflicted by a physician's failure to disclose—an injury that is measured in terms of, and compensated by, money damages. This focus results from the legal system's need for a functional mechanism to assess injury and responsibility.

In theory the failure of a physician to obtain consent for medical treatment has always been remediable through appeal to the common law. However, physicians have traditionally regarded legal requirements as minimal and subject to discretion by physicians. When, at the beginning of the twentieth century, serious litigation over legal requirements of consent to medical treatment began to occur, courts progressively realized that standards for valid consent were more elusive than had traditionally been appreciated. A more complicated set of rules began to evolve, and some of the rules devised by courts, especially disclosure standards, came into conflict. In this context the term *informed consent* was born, and the doctrine of informed consent was conceived almost exclusively as a set of disclosure rules.

These disclosure requirements are vitally important in legal and regulatory contexts. However, from the moral point of view, informed consent has less to do with the liability of professionals as agents of disclosure and more to do with the autonomous choices of patients and subjects. Disclosure may be unimportant to a particular patient's or subject's decision. For example, the patient may already know the relevant information. From this perspective the focus on disclosure may be misleading, because it conveys the image of a physician having a body of information that needs to be transmitted, like disclosing a secret or issuing a warning. But in medicine, information transfer and decision making often do not fit this image. Both health-care professionals and patients need to ask and answer questions, which is less a matter of disclosing information than of discovering what information is relevant and how to frame and use it.

Nevertheless, disclosure is an important topic. Without an adequate transfer of information many patients and subjects will have insufficient information for decision making. The professional's own perspective, opinions, and recommendations are often essential for the patient's or subject's deliberation, as well as for mutual understanding. Even if not essential, they are generally worthwhile and material. Professionals, then, are generally obligated to disclose a core set of information, including (1) those facts or descriptions that patients or subjects usually consider material in deciding whether to refuse or consent to the proposed intervention or research, (2) information the professional believes to be material, (3) the professional's recommendation, and (4) the purpose of seeking consent and the nature of consent as an act of authorization.

Additional or supplementary types of disclosure have also been proposed—for example, statements of the purpose of the procedure and the persons in charge. Many related controversies surround what should be disclosed about a procedure's risks and negative consequences, as well as about the nature and purpose of the procedure, its benefits, and alternative procedures. If research is involved, disclosure may appropriately include a statement of the criteria used for the selection of subjects and a statement that the person has an opportunity to ask further questions and to withdraw at any time. Such lists could be expanded indefinitely, but the central moral issues turn more on the informational needs of particular patients and subjects than on lists of items.

Standards of disclosure

The main struggle in the courts has been to determine which standards should govern the disclosure of information. Two general standards of disclosure have emerged in these cases: the professional practice standard and the reasonable person standard. A third standard, the subjective standard, has also been proposed.

THE PROFESSIONAL PRACTICE STANDARD. The first standard holds that adequate disclosure is determined by the traditional practices of a professional community, such as a community of physicians or clinical psychologists. This standard was devised under the conviction that the doctor's proper role is to act in the patient's best medical interest. Medical care standards, rather than patients' rights, were deemed to determine the operative guidelines for disclosure. The custom in a profession, then, establishes the amount and kinds of information to be disclosed; and disclosure, like treatment, is a task that belongs to physicians because of their professional expertise, role, and commitment. As a result, only expert testimony from members of such professional groups could count as evidence that there has been a violation of a patient's right to information.[30]

Several difficulties afflict the professional practice standard. First, it is unclear that a customary standard exists regarding the communication of information in many situations in medicine. Moreover, if custom alone were conclusive, then pervasive negligence could be perpetuated. The majority of professionals could, in principle, offer the same inferior level of information. If there is no professional standard of disclosure or if the standard is set too low, then the patient's legal right to information is undermined by this legal standard. The goal of informed consent is undermined by the very standards of informed consent. Perhaps the chief objection to the professional practice standard is that it can undermine the patient's right of autonomous choice, which is the primary function and justification of rules of informed consent. Professional standards in medicine are fashioned for specifically medical judgments, but decisions for or against medical care, being nonmedical judgments, seem rightly the province of the patient. This has always been the point of the proscription against nonconsensual touching in law, however darkly it may have appeared in many court opinions.

It may also be questioned whether physicians have sufficient expertise to know what information is in the best interests of their patients. The assumption that they do have the expertise is largely an empirical assumption, but no reliable data substantiate the claim.[31] Moreover, the weighing of risks against a person's subjective beliefs, fears, and hopes is not reducible to an expert skill measured through a professional standard. Medical custom often expresses the presumptions, values, and goals of a medical orientation, but information provided to patients and subjects sometimes needs to be freed from the entrenched values and goals of medical professionals.

THE REASONABLE PERSON STANDARD. Although many legal jurisdictions in the United States have retained the more traditional professional practice standard, the reasonable person standard has gained acceptance in perhaps sixty percent of the states in the United States.[32] According to this standard, the kind and amount of information to be disclosed are determined by reference to a hypothetical reasonable person. The pertinence of a piece of information is measured by the significance a reasonable person would attach to it in deciding whether to undergo a procedure. By this standard the determination of informational needs is shifted from the physician to the patient, and physicians may be found guilty of negligent disclosures even if their behavior conforms to recognized and routine professional practice. The fundamental reason for this standard is the underlying belief that informed consent in law is a doctrine fashioned to permit patients to be the agents of decision making and authorization.

Most proponents of the reasonable person standard believe that considerations of autonomy generally outweigh those of beneficence and that, on balance, the reasonable person standard better serves autonomy than does the professional practice standard. This approach to the differences between these standards is found in Case 8. A patient was told in general terms about the risks of undergoing a general anesthetic and about the nature of ulcer surgery, but the physicians failed to disclose the inherent risks of the surgery itself. The operation appeared to be successful, but injuries to the spleen were subsequently discovered and a gastric ulcer developed—both events being risks inherent in the original surgery. The patient sued the physician, who had failed

to disclose these inherent risks. The physician argued that disclosures of outcomes of such low probability are uncommon in medicine and that he should
be held only to the standards of disclosure accepted by surgeons, a clear invocation of the professional practice standard. The court, however, concluded that
"the patient's right of self-decision is the measure of the physician's duty to
reveal." A physician is therefore required by the reasonable person standard to
disclose the "material information—that is, all information relevant to a meaningful decisional process," with respect to both the proposed therapy and its
inherent risks.

In a precedent case on which this court relied, medical obligations to disclose
were based on moral considerations of autonomy. The judge referred to these
considerations as "the patient's right of self-decision" and the patient's "prerogative to decide."[33] His point is that obligations of disclosure are at their
root moral rather than legal or medical and that these moral obligations inform
both law and medicine regarding appropriate standards. This conclusion of case
law, when combined with the moral standards of autonomy we have proposed,
suggests the following standard of disclosure: The patient or subject should be
provided with information that a reasonable person in the patient's or subject's
circumstances would find relevant and could reasonably be expected to assim-
ilate. In this way the moral requirement to respect autonomy is translated into
a reasonable person standard of disclosure.

Nevertheless, this reasonable person standard is still plagued by conceptual,
moral, and practical difficulties. First, "material information" and the central
concept of the reasonable person have never been carefully defined. Second,
there are questions about how the reasonable person standard can be employed
in practice. Its hypothetical structure is difficult for physicians to interpret,
because they have to project what a reasonable patient would need to know.

Another problem has emerged from empirical studies that examine whether
patients actually use information disclosed to them in reaching their decisions.
Data collected in one study indicate that although ninety-three percent of the
patients surveyed believed they benefited from the information disclosed, only
twelve percent actually used the information in their decisions to consent.[34]
This study, involving family-planning patients, reaches conclusions similar to
an earlier study of kidney donors.[35] In both studies the data indicate that patients generally make their decisions prior to and independent of the actual
process of receiving information. Other studies indicate that patients generally
accept a physician's recommendation without carefully weighing risks and
benefits[36] and that as many as eighty-six percent of patients would agree to a
procedure (upper gastrointestinal endoscopy in one study) without any discussion of risks.[37]

These data do not show that decisions by patients were uninformed or that
disclosed information was irrelevant. The patients may have believed only that

additional information did not alter their prior commitment to a particular course of action. For example, a kidney donor could reasonably decide that the eventual death of his brother outweighs the risks disclosed by a physician. Nonetheless, these empirical findings throw into question what should count as material information for the individual patient and whether the information is the same for the reasonable patient as for the individual patient. This problem invites discussion of the third standard of disclosure.

THE SUBJECTIVE STANDARD. In the reasonable person model, adequacy of information is judged by reference to the informational needs of the objective reasonable person, not by reference to the specific informational needs of the individual patient or subject, as proposed by the subjective standard. Individual informational needs can differ, because a person may have personal or unorthodox beliefs, unusual health problems, or unique family histories that require a different informational base than the reasonable person needs. For example, a female employee with a family history of reproductive problems might need information that other persons would not want before becoming involved in research on sexual and familial relations or accepting employment in certain industries. If a physician knows or has reason to believe that a person desires such information, then withholding it may deprive that patient of the opportunity to make an informed choice and thus undermine autonomy.

At issue is the extent to which the reasonable person standard should be tailored to the individual patient, made subjective. There is a continuum of possible interpretations. At one end, being ''in the patient's or subject's position'' could be taken to include only the person's medical condition and related physical characteristics. Under this interpretation, the health-care professional would be obligated to disclose only medical information that would be needed or wanted by the reasonable patient with these conditions and characteristics. At the other end of the continuum, the patient's position could be construed to include any factor particular to the patient's need or desire for information that a physician could reasonably be expected to know (or even to discover).

Under the latter construal, the reasonable person standard may be identical to the subjective standard. The physician is obligated to disclose information a particular patient desires or needs to know, so long as there is a reasonable connection between these desires and needs for information and what the physician should know about the patient's position. This construal suggests that the moral question is not whether the information necessarily, probably, or possibly would have led the patient to forgo therapy—a critical legal question—but rather whether the information was necessary for this patient's informed decision, regardless of the outcome.

Despite many problems that plague the subjective standard in law,[38] it is a preferable moral standard of disclosure from the standpoint of the principle of respect for autonomy, because it acknowledges the independent informational needs and desires of persons in the process of making difficult decisions. Nevertheless, exclusive use of a subjective standard is inappropriate for either law or ethics, because patients often do not know what information would be relevant for their deliberations, and a doctor cannot reasonably be expected to do an exhaustive background and character analysis of each patient to determine what information would be relevant. Again we note that the key question is not one of what quantum of information should be disclosed. It is rather the question of what professionals can do to facilitate decision making based on substantial understanding, if patients and subjects are ignorant or inexperienced.

The legal standards we have now examined may be appropriate for the needs of courts and even for some institutional policies, but these standards will contribute little to consent practices unless augmented by a broader conception of decision making by patients and subjects. The solution to the problem of disclosure is to be found in active participation by patients or subjects in the context of an informational exchange. What professionals customarily disclose and what an objective reasonable person needs may fail to contain some or even all of the information material to the person from whom a decision is being sought. Legal and professional rules of disclosure should, then, only serve to initiate the communication process necessary for good decision making. Unfortunately, when those rules are interpreted narrowly and minimalistically, professionals may be satisfied with a signed consent form, while paying little attention to the process of decision making.

Intentional nondisclosure

Several other problems about disclosure in clinical medicine center on justifications for a less complete disclosure than might have been made in the circumstances.

THE THERAPEUTIC PRIVILEGE. Legal exceptions to the rule of informed consent allow the health professional to proceed without consent in cases of emergency, incompetency, waiver, and the like. The most controversial exception is the therapeutic privilege, according to which a physician may intentionally and validly withhold information, based on a "sound medical judgment" that to divulge the information would be potentially harmful to a depressed, emotionally drained, or unstable patient.[39]

The precise formulation of this therapeutic privilege varies across legal jurisdictions. Some formulations permit physicians to withhold information if disclosure would cause any countertherapeutic deterioration in the physical, psychological, or emotional condition of the patient. But other formulations permit the physician to withhold information if and only if the patient's knowledge of the information would have serious health-related consequences—for example, by jeopardizing the success of the treatment or by critically impairing relevant decision-making processes through psychological harm. The narrowest formulation is analogous to a circumstance of incompetence; the therapeutic privilege can be validly invoked only if the physician reasonably believes that disclosure would render the patient incompetent to consent to or refuse the treatment. To invoke the therapeutic privilege under this last condition would not in principle conflict with respect for autonomy, because an autonomous decision could not be made.

Discretion by physicians must be permitted in many difficult cases, and courts have held, properly, that the patient's right to information may on occasion be validly qualified by a physician's judgment of the patient's welfare, based on the principles of beneficence and nonmaleficence. What may be doubted, as Jay Katz has argued, is that there can be "consistency" between physician discretion in disclosing information and the full disclosure of facts demanded by some courts. "Only in dreams or fairy tales," Katz suggests, "can 'discretion' to withhold crucial information so easily and magically be reconciled with 'full disclosure.' "[40]

There is no formal inconsistency between respecting autonomy and protecting from harm. Both purposes can be promoted through informed choice. However, the history of informed consent has left a legal and medical legacy in which demands for patient autonomy coexist with ill-defined exceptions recognized in both law and medicine. This complexity is understandable: Disclosures can harm some patients, and in many circumstances patients have a deep need for a health professional who assumes authority and, with reassuring confidence, issues orders that can aid the patient's recovery. Human needs for such authority pervade the medical context and complicate the process of reaching decisions with patients.

Problems of not harming or causing undue alarm to the patient by disclosures are further complicated by remote risks. In one case a woman had a fatal reaction during urography. The radiologist had intentionally not disclosed the slight chance of death (roughly one in ten thousand) because it might have upset the patient. The radiologist justified the nondisclosure on grounds of beneficence: The disclosure would be "dangerous" and "not in the best interest of the patient." This argument is plausible in some clinical contexts, but it may—and often does—serve as a rationalization. Hence the argument always requires careful scrutiny. One possible—and generally more acceptable—approach in anesthesia is "to tell all patients that there are serious, although remote, risks of anesthesia, but to allow the individual patient to decide how much additional information he or she wishes to obtain about these risks."[41]

This approach would also be applicable to other areas of medicine and health care.

THE THERAPEUTIC USE OF PLACEBOS. The therapeutic use of placebos merits special attention because it is common in medicine and usually involves deception or incomplete disclosure of information. A *placebo* (from the Latin for ''I shall please'') is a substance or procedure that the health-care professional believes to be pharmacologically or biomedically inert for the condition being treated. Studies indicate that placebos relieve some symptoms of approximately thirty-five percent of patients who suffer from such conditions as angina pectoris, cough, anxiety, depression, hypertension, headache, and the common cold.[42] Placebos are touted for speeding recovery but are probably most often used to relieve pain, a use that may cause a biochemical release of endorphins.[43] Fundamental moral questions appear in the use of placebos without the patient's knowledge or consent, where the physician engages in nondisclosure, incomplete disclosure, or deception.

One defense offered for such uses of placebos is that ''deception is completely moral when it is used for the welfare of the patient.''[44] But when beneficence trumps respect for autonomy (as in some cases of the beneficence model and paternalism discussed in Chapter 5), it is not enough to show that in the circumstances under consideration beneficence appears to be weightier. It is also necessary to meet the other conditions for justified infringements of prima facie principles, including effectiveness and necessity. Some available evidence suggests that the placebo effect—an improvement in the patient after the use of a placebo—can sometimes be produced without nondisclosure, incomplete disclosure, or deception. For example, the placebo effect can sometimes be produced even when patients have been informed that a substance is pharmacologically inert and have consented to its use.[45] And in many cases where placebos are effective, they appear to work because of the ''healing context,'' involving the professional's care, compassion, and skill in fostering hope and faith.[46] Thus, it may be possible to produce the placebo effect without administering actual placebos. Of course, such a practice may entail a different allocation of resources to enable physicians and other health-care professionals to spend more time in interaction with patients rather than dispensing pills.

Nevertheless, a placebo effect often does not appear to be likely unless an actual placebo is used without the patient's informed consent. The professionals involved in Case 5 thought that an undisclosed placebo offered the only hope of effective treatment of the patient's pain.[47] In that case, Mr. X, a sixty-five-year-old retired army officer who had been successful in the military and in teaching and research, had undergone several abdominal operations for gallstones, postoperative adhesions, and bowel obstructions. He subsequently experienced chronic pain. As a result he became somewhat depressed, lost weight, had poor personal hygiene, was unkempt, and withdrew socially because he assumed awkward or embarrassing postures trying to control his pain. After using Talwin six times a day for more than two years to control his pain, he had so much tissue and muscle damage that he had trouble finding injection sites for the Talwin, which has also been shown to be addictive. Mr. X sought therapeutic help ''to get more out of life in spite of [his] pain,'' and he voluntarily entered a psychiatric ward, which featured individual behavioral therapy programs, daily group therapy, and so on.

In this ward Mr. X reduced his Talwin usage to four times a day, but he insisted that this level was necessary to control his pain. After much discussion with their colleagues, his therapists decided to withdraw the Talwin over time without his knowledge by diluting it with increasing proportions of normal saline. Mr. X experienced nausea, diarrhea, and cramps, but he thought that these withdrawal symptoms were the result of Elavil (amitriptyline), which the therapists had introduced to relieve the withdrawal symptoms without informing the patient about its purpose. Mr. X continued practicing self-control techniques during this period, and the intervals between injections of the saline were increased. Mr. X was aware of the changes in intervals but not that the injections contained only saline.

After three weeks, his therapist informed him that he was receiving a placebo rather than this usual medication. After his initial incredulity and anger subsided, he asked that the saline be discontinued and that the self-control techniques be continued. When he was discharged three weeks later, he reported that he could control his abdominal pain more effectively with the self-control techniques than he could earlier with Talwin. Follow-up six months later indicated that he was still using the relaxation techniques and had resumed social activities and part-time teaching.

The therapists have defended their deceptive use of a placebo on the grounds that they ''felt ethically obliged to use a treatment that had a high probability of success'' for Mr. X, their patient. Not using the placebo would have ''protected some standard of openness'' but probably would not have been in Mr. X's best interests. The therapists maintained, ''We saw no option without ethical problems. Although it is precarious to justify the means by the end, we felt most obliged to use a procedure designed to help the patient achieve a personally and medically desirable goal.'' They argue in effect that the principle of beneficence outweighs or overrides respect for autonomy and truthfulness in this case.

However, the therapists also suggest that their actions did not infringe Mr. X's autonomy. It is possible that Mr. X's autonomy was so compromised by his addiction to Talwin (which he thought was nonaddictive) that it was not an infringement of his autonomy to provide a placebo without his consent. One goal was to restore Mr. X's autonomy, through relieving him of his pain, his addiction, and his false beliefs about withdrawal. (See our discussion of weak paternalism in Chapter 5.) The therapists also invoke the principle of respect for autonomy itself to justify their actions. According to this line of argument, they did not infringe Mr. X's autonomous choices and even acted in accord with his autonomous choices, when those choices are considered over time and in all their complexity. Such claims need careful examination in the context of this case.

One defense appeals to Mr. X's *implicit consent* when he voluntarily admitted himself to a psychiatric ward where adjustment in medication was a clear expectation. He accepted the goals of the therapy—"to get more out of life in spite of [his] pain." However, a fundamental question is what Mr. X implicitly consented to when he voluntarily entered the psychiatric ward. No appeal to implicit consent will succeed, because we know that he expressly refused to allow further reduction in his Talwin dosage level. It is not plausible to appeal to implicit consent to override current express refusals, unless the patient now has diminished autonomy—such as because of drug addiction—and thus cannot revoke previous consent, whether express or implied.

Another possible appeal to the principle of respect for autonomy to justify the undisclosed placebo appears in the therapists' apparent belief that Mr. X ratified their decision to use the placebo when he decided to continue the self-control techniques rather than returning to Talwin. However, actual or predicted *future consent* also does not satisfy the requirement to obtain informed consent, as an expression of the principle of respect for autonomy. The prediction of future consent can only provide evidence that the reasons for intervention against the patient's current wishes are important and perhaps sufficient. This predicted future ratification does not transform the current intervention without the patient's consent into respect for the patient's autonomy.[48]

The therapists note that they saw "no option without ethical problems." However, it is not clear that they had exhausted all moral options. One possibility would have been to obtain the patient's prior *general consent* to the administration of several drugs and placebos, as part of the effort to wean him from Talwin and to enable him to develop adequate self-control techniques to manage his pain. Such general consent might have been obtained at the outset and would have obviated the need for specific consent to the substitution of a placebo (saline) for the Talwin. In fact, when the placebo was administered, Mr. X was informed that his medication regimen would be modified, but he did not receive any specific details. He still insisted on maintaining the same Talwin dosage level (though not the same frequency). Another possibility, short of a deceptive use of a placebo, may have been inadequately considered because of the staff's therapeutic perspective. The staff defined the patient's therapeutic "problem" in terms of specific behaviors and devoted little attention to the "person responsible for those behaviors."[49] If the therapists had conceived Mr. X's problem in a broader way, they might have discovered alternative procedures with high probabilities of success and with fewer or no ethical problems.

We have examined this complex case in detail in order to discuss the use of placebos without the patient's informed consent. We have considered whether the use of an undisclosed placebo could be justified in this case by the principle of respect for autonomy, and we have concluded that this justification is deficient if it appeals to the patient's implicit consent against his explicit refusal or to his past or future consent against his current refusal. However, if the therapists had received the patient's prior general informed consent to the administration of several medications, including placebos, they would not have infringed his autonomy by not making a specific disclosure at the time of the placebo unless he had revoked his general consent. We also leave open the possibility that this paternalistic use of an undisclosed placebo could be justified by the principle of beneficence (see Chapter 5).

WITHHOLDING INFORMATION FROM RESEARCH SUBJECTS. Problems of intentional nondisclosure in clinical practice have parallels in research contexts, where investigators are sometimes unwilling to share some relevant information with subjects. In biomedical research, the prime example is the use of clinical trials involving randomization, placebos, blind experiments, and so on, all widely used to compensate for bias. Because we discuss clinical trials in a major section of Chapter 7, here we only make reference to them before discussing social-scientific research that involves nondisclosure or deception.

In randomized clinical trials, there is no justification for failure to disclose to potential subjects the full set of treatments and placebos that will be used, their risks and benefits, and their uncertainties. There is also no justification for failure to disclose the method of assignment in randomized clinical trials. But if these items of information are supplied, potential subjects may have an adequate understanding to be able to decide whether to participate in a clinical trial, even though they do not know which treatment or placebo they will receive.

Adequate disclosure does not always require complete disclosure, and in some cases there are ways of handling moral problems of incomplete disclosure. For example, subjects are sometimes informed that they cannot be told the purpose or the specific subject of the research, and in some cases they are asked to consent to studies after being informed that the research procedures will be intentionally deceptive. Here the question is whether potential subjects who understand that they are being kept partially ignorant about a particular intervention or research project can give an informed consent to that project or intervention.

A satisfactory answer to this question in any given case depends on a subject's ability to judge the materiality of the information being withheld. Subjects are not always in a good position to make such a judgment, and it is sometimes difficult to determine whether unknown information will prove to be important. At a minimum, the procedures involved should be carefully scrutinized—by investigators and review committees—to ensure that the risks to subjects are minimal and are outweighed by the anticipated benefits and to ensure that autonomy is protected by providing information that a subject would need in order to make a decision about participation. This recommendation is procedural rather than substantive. But it would be precipitous to maintain that patients and subjects can never give informed consents because they lack some facts. They may, in the end, have every material fact they need. In other cases, they may have inadequate information, and research investigators may need to resort to alternative research designs.

As substantial deception or substantial risk is added in a research project, justification becomes progressively more difficult. Stanley Milgram's well-known experiments on obedience raise these issues in a dramatic way. In these experiments, two people come to what appears to be a psychology laboratory to participate in what has been advertised as a study of memory and learning. One is designated as a "teacher" and the other as a "learner." The experimenter explains that the study is concerned with the effects of punishment on learning. The learner is conducted into a room and seated in a chair. His arms are strapped to prevent excessive movement, and an electrode is attached to his wrist. He is told that he is to learn a list of word pairs; whenever he makes an error, he will receive electric shocks of increasing intensity that will be administered by the other subject, the "teacher." The subject who is assigned the role of teacher is deliberately deceived by the experimenter. The learner is actually part of the research team, and the machine does not actually deliver shocks to the learner. The point of the experiment, as Milgram describes it, "is to see how far a person will proceed in a concrete and measurable situation in which he is ordered to inflict increasing pain on a protesting subject."[50]

Milgram contends that debate over his methods is biased if the research is described as "deception," and he proposes "morally neutral terms" such as "masking," "staging," or "technical illusions."[51] However, such morally neutral terms bias the debate even more by obscuring the moral issue that the experiment did involve deception without the subjects' consent to participate in deceptive practices.

In contrast to what consultants had predicted in advance, Milgram reports that as many as 62.5 percent of the subjects in some versions of the experiments continued to obey the experimenter's order to inflict shock up to the maximum of 450 volts, labeled on the machine "Danger—Severe Shock." Critics have questioned whether the research was necessary on the grounds that

historical evidence establishes the phenomenon of human obedience in inflicting pain; and others have proposed alternative nondeceptive research designs,
such as role-playing. The extensive ethical debate over this research during the
last twenty-five years has centered on the imposition of risks of harm to subjects without their informed consent.[52]

Through debriefing and friendly reconciliation with the "victim," Milgram
tried to minimize any harms that the subjects might experience through stress,
anxiety, guilt, and shame about their actions in the experiment. His primary
argument is that the subsequent responses of the participants ethically justify
the research: "To my mind, the central moral justification for allowing my
experiment is that it was judged acceptable by those who took part in it."[53]
Eighty-four percent said they were glad to have been in it, fifteen percent were
neutral, and one percent expressed negative opinions. These subsequent responses could be construed by defenders of the research as indicating that the
harms were minimal (and justified by the benefits) and as providing a form of
retroactive approval and consent.

We have already raised questions about the sufficiency of future or retroactive consent. The Milgram experiment itself may have created the conditions
for subsequent approval in the subjects' efforts to come to grips with what they
did. In any event, future or retroactive approval is not a substitute for the
exercise of autonomy in giving informed consent or refusal at the outset. In
considering alternatives to retrospective consent, Milgram is not satisfied with
presuming a subject's consent to deceptive research based on the responses of
a large number of informed people about the acceptability of the experiment.
This process, which has been called surrogate consent may help researchers
and review committees anticipate harms and reactions while deciding whether
to approve the research, but it does not constitute consent. A more promising
approach to consent, as Milgram recognizes, is obtaining subjects' prior general consent to participate in research involving deception or nondisclosure, as
long as certain conditions are met.[54]

In another problematic case, discussed in Chapter 2, a social scientist using
deception placed homosexual subjects at risk of public disclosure and embarrassment and invaded their privacy. Also, a revealing sociological study of the
practices of Italian priests in hearing confessions of sexual sins—published in
English as *Sex and the Confessional*[55]—involved the deception of priests and
the taping of their questions and advice. Although these cases, too, are behavioral rather than biomedical, they illustrate how deception and resulting risk
can and do occur during research.

Can such research be justified? We think not if (1) significant risk is involved, and (2) subjects are not informed that they are being placed at risk.
The critical question is whether subjects can voluntarily accept the risk with an
adequate understanding of the deceptive practices. It is a fundamental violation

of the principle of respect for autonomy to deceive subjects and also to place them at risk. This conclusion is far from innocuous, because much present-day research in the social sciences is deceptive and in many cases is approved by institutional review boards.

This conclusion does not imply that research involving deception can never justifiably be undertaken. Relatively risk-free and significant research—for example, in behavioral psychology and sociology—could not in some cases be undertaken without deception or incomplete disclosure. Simple examples include studies of visual and other perceptual responses. Cases in which disclosure would invalidate the research should be distinguished from cases in which disclosure would be inconvenient, time-consuming, or expensive, and from cases in which potential subjects would refuse to participate if adequately informed about the nature of the experiment. Generally, deception should be permitted in research only if it is essential to obtain important information, no substantial risk is attached, other moral principles are not violated, and subjects are informed that deception is part of the study and consent to participate. We return in Chapter 7 to some special problems and needed qualifications of this general conclusion, especially in the context of randomized clinical trials.

Understanding

If the analysis thus far is correct, we need to reconceive traditional problems of disclosure as follows: If patients and subjects are ignorant, sick, frightened, or inexperienced, what can professionals do to facilitate obtaining good decisions based on substantial understanding? That is, how can professionals enable patients and subjects to make autonomous choices? In this conception of the problem, understanding is a more important element than disclosure and may be the most important element in the process of obtaining an informed consent. The key to effective communication, understanding, and decision making is participation by patients or subjects in an exchange of information. Ordinarily, a professional has only limited insight into the distinct values, fears, hopes, and informational needs of others. Asking questions, eliciting the concerns and interests of the patient or subject, and establishing a climate that encourages the patient or subject to ask questions may be more important to the person's understanding than a whole corpus of disclosed information.[56]

Clinical experience and empirical testing indicate that patients and subjects exhibit wide variation in their understanding of information about diagnoses, procedures, risks, and prognoses. Although some patients and subjects are calm, attentive, and eager for dialogue, others are nervous or distracted in ways that impair or block understanding. Many conditions other than lack of sufficient information can limit their understanding—for example, illness, irrationality, and immaturity.[57] In Case 9, a woman suffering from chronic brain syndrome with arteriosclerosis has periods of confusion and mild loss of memory; she is sometimes but not always unable to understand her condition. Even if there were no concerns about general competence, problems about adequate understanding might remain, because information could be so distorted or unsuitable that communication fails.

The nature of understanding

There is no consensus about how to analyze understanding, but an analysis sufficient for our purposes is that one understands if one has justified beliefs about the nature and consequences of one's actions. This understanding need not be full or complete, because a substantial grasp of central facts and other descriptions will often be sufficient. Some facts are irrelevant or trivial; others are vital or even decisive. In many informed consent cases, the inadequacy of a person's understanding about a single risk or limitation is the reason why the person did not understand what he or she was consenting to. A single missing fact can thus deprive a person of adequate understanding.

Consider, for example, the actual case of *Bang* v. *Charles T. Miller Hospital,* in which patient Bang did not intend to consent to sterilization, which was an inevitable outcome of his prostate surgery.[58] Bang did, in fact, give his formal, intentional consent to prostate surgery but without having been apprised that sterilization was an inevitable outcome. (Sterilization is not necessarily an outcome of all prostate surgery, but it was an inevitable outcome of the specific procedure selected by Bang's surgeon.) Bang's failure to understand this one description of a consequence of the surgery substantially compromised what was otherwise an adequate understanding. It also invalidated what otherwise would have been an informed consent.

In the informed consent context it is usually of paramount significance that patients and subjects understand what a health-care professional believes a patient or subject needs to understand and should regard as material in order to authorize an intervention. Patient or subject and professional also need to share an understanding about the terms of the authorization. As in all contractual circumstances, unless there is agreement about the essential features of what is authorized, there can be no assurance that a patient or subject has made an autonomous decision. Even if both physician and patient use a word such as *stroke* or *hernia,* their interpretations may be vastly different inasmuch as standard medical definitions and conceptions may have no place in the patient's outlook. Effective communication thus may require the professional and the patient or subject first to come to terms with the other's conception.

It is sometimes argued that most patients and subjects cannot comprehend enough information or appreciate its relevance sufficiently to make decisions about medical care or participation in research. Franz Ingelfinger maintains, for example, that "the chances are remote that the subject really understands what he has consented to,"[59] and Robert Mulford similarly contends that "the subject is ordinarily not qualified to evaluate the true risks and expected benefits."[60] These statements are overgeneralizations based partially on unwarranted standards of full disclosure and full understanding. The ideal of complete disclosure of all possibly relevant knowledge promotes such claims about the limited capacity of subjects to comprehend. But if this ideal standard is replaced by a more acceptable account of the understanding of relevant information, such skepticism would be put to flight. Merely because our actions are never *fully* informed, voluntary, or autonomous, it does not follow that our actions are never *adequately* informed, free, or autonomous.

This is not to deny that some patients' knowledge base is so impoverished that communication about alien or novel situations is exceedingly difficult, especially if new theories and cognitive constructs are essential for making an appropriate interpretation. But even under such difficult situations there may be no grounds for foreclosing the possibility of making an adequate decision. Successful communication of novel, alien, and specialized information to laypersons can be accomplished by drawing analogies between such information and more ordinary events with which the patient or subject is familiar. Similarly, professionals can express probabilities in both numeric and nonnumeric terms, while helping the patient or subject to assign meanings to the probabilities through comparison with more familiar risks and prior experiences.

In this process of communication an adequate appreciation of some information can be as important as comprehending basic facts. However, to enable a patient not only to comprehend but also to appreciate risks and benefits can be a formidable task. For example, many patients confronted with coronary bypass surgery, orthopedic surgery, and many other forms of surgery understand that as a consequence of their consent to the surgery they will suffer postoperative pain. Nevertheless their projected expectations of the pain may be seriously inadequate. In some situations patients cannot, in advance, adequately appreciate the real nature of the pain, and many ill patients reach a point where they can no longer balance with clear judgment the threat of pain against the risks of surgery. At this point the benefits of surgery are overwhelmingly attractive, and the risks recede in their appraisals. In one respect these patients correctly understand basic facts about procedures that involve pain, but in other respects their understanding is less than adequate.

Many common situations in medicine require the physician to confront this problem. For example, in Case 24, a fourteen-year-old girl wishes to donate a kidney to her mother. Although she has exhibited a perceptive and relatively unemotional grasp of the situation, many doubt that a fourteen-year old child can either adequately appreciate the significance of future risks or carefully balance risks and benefits. Even the professional who is skillful and persistent

in giving patients a due appreciation of the situation may find this challenge
too much to meet.

Problems of information processing

With the exception of a few limited studies of the comprehension of patients,
most studies of informed consent have given little attention to information processing. Yet current knowledge about information processing raises many issues about adequate understanding. For example, information overload may be
an obstacle to adequate understanding and may be as likely as underdisclosure
to produce uninformed decisions. Although the implications of this phenomenon are not well understood, there are significant constraints on the amount of
information that can be meaningfully processed and retained by patients and
subjects. Information overload is exacerbated if unfamiliar terms are used or if
information cannot be meaningfully organized. Yet practical constraints generally require that disclosures occur in a compressed presentation. Patients and
potential subjects are likely to rely on some modes of selective perception, and
it will be difficult to determine when words have special meaning for them,
when preconceptions distort their processing of the information, and when other
biases intrude.

   Some revealing studies focus on difficulties in processing information about
risks. This literature indicates that risk disclosures often lead subjects to distort
information and may promote inferential errors and a disproportionate fear of
risks.[61] Some ways of framing information are so misleading and difficult to
eliminate that health professionals no less than patients find it almost impossible to interpret the information objectively. For example, choices between risky
alternatives can be heavily influenced by whether the same risk information is
presented as providing a gain or an opportunity for a patient, or as constituting
a loss or a reduction of opportunity.[62] In one study, radiologists, outpatients
with chronic medical problems, and graduate students in business were asked
to make a hypothetical choice between two alternative therapies for lung cancer: surgery and radiation therapy.[63] The preferences of all three groups were
affected by whether the information about outcomes was framed in terms of
probability of survival or probability of dying. When the outcomes were framed
in terms of probability of survival, only twenty-five percent chose radiation
over surgery. However, when the outcomes were framed in terms of probability
of death, forty-two percent preferred radiation. The mode of presenting the risk
of immediate death from surgical complications, which has no analogue in
radiation therapy, appears to have made the decisive difference.

   These framing effects reduce understanding of material information, with
direct implications for autonomous choice. If a misperception prevents a person
from understanding the risk of death and this risk is material to the person's

decision, then the person's choice of surgery is based on less than substantial understanding and would not qualify as an autonomous authorization. The lesson to be learned is not skepticism about information processing but the need for professionals to provide patients and subjects with both the positive and the negative sides of information—for example, both the mortality and the survival information.[64]

Other problems of information processing result from inappropriate contexts. Patients need to have time in which to make a decision and also need to know if there are alternatives deserving consideration. Yet health-care professionals frequently do not adequately address these needs. For example, they may disclose information in order to solicit consent immediately prior to treatment, when there is little time to make a decision. Without the proper climate, a request from a professional that the patient or subject ask for information is as likely to result in silence as to elicit a meaningful exchange.

Problems of nonacceptance and false belief

A person's ability to make decisions may be compromised by a refusal to accept information as true or untainted, even if he or she adequately comprehends the information. The distinction between comprehension of information and acceptance of information has often been obscured by reliance on recall tests. At best, "correct" answers on such tests provide evidence of a person's comprehension of what the physician or investigator has disclosed. These answers do not indicate whether the subject believed what was disclosed.

A false belief can invalidate a decision by a patient or subject. For example, a person might falsely and irrationally believe that a doctor will not fill out insurance forms unless the patient consents to a procedure the doctor has suggested, a sufficiently informed psychiatric patient capable of consent might agree to participate in nontherapeutic research under the false belief that it is therapeutic, or a seriously ill patient asked to make a treatment decision might refuse under the false belief that he or she is not ill.

Some false beliefs are more significant than others, and we also need to take account of the probabilities that may be involved in the belief. These problems are compounded by inconclusive evidence and failure to achieve agreement about the truth or falsity of beliefs. Many beliefs that are central and even decisive for a patient's decision may be regarded by others, including health-care professionals seeking consent, as highly questionable, poorly reasoned, or even absurd. Sometimes overwhelming medical evidence indicates that a patient is unjustified in holding a belief, while in other circumstances the patient's beliefs may be contestable but not refutable by hard counterevidence.

The probabilities and uncertainties that surround many beliefs indicate that truth claims should be judged by the available evidence, which itself can be

subject to different interpretations and even to outright dispute. There is often more than one standard of evidence, and all evidence must be gathered within some framework that determines what is to count as evidence. No evidence is independent of the framework that it presupposes, yet two or more frameworks may advance competing standards of evidence. If no agreement on the criteria for determining the justifiability of beliefs is available, there may be no adequate grounds for determining whether a given belief compromises understanding. This conclusion is not meant as a skeptical denial of the possibility of knowledge, but only as a warning that the evidence for believing that a belief is false may itself be rationally contestable.

However, if we assume that some beliefs are demonstrably false, the question arises whether patients and subjects should be forced to give up their false beliefs in order that they may reach an informed decision. Some have argued that when subjects specifically object to further information or persuasion, the information should not be imposed.[65] This position does not imply, however, that we should never coerce patients or subjects to change their beliefs or to process information differently. If a patient's or subject's autonomy is limited by his or her ignorance, as in the case of a false belief a patient has difficulty in surrendering, it may be legitimate and even obligatory to promote autonomy by attempting to impose the information on a patient who finds it unwelcome. And if this proves impossible, the principles of beneficence and nonmaleficence may still justify overriding the patient's nonautonomous choices (as we discuss in Chapter 5).

Consider the following case in which a false belief played a major role in a patient's refusal of treatment:[66]

A 57-year-old woman was admitted to hospital because of a fractured hip. . . . During the course of the hospitalization, a Papanicolaou test and biopsy revealed stage 1A carcinoma of the cervix. . . . Surgery was strongly recommended, since the cancer was almost certainly curable by a hysterectomy. . . . The patient refused the procedure.

The patient's treating physicians at this point felt that she was mentally incompetent. Psychiatric and neurological consultations were requested to determine the possibility of dementia and/or mental incompetency. The psychiatric consultant felt that the patient was demented and not mentally competent to make decisions regarding her own care. This determination was based in large measure on the patient's steadfast "unreasonable" refusal to undergo surgery. The neurologist disagreed, finding no evidence of dementia. On questioning, the patient stated that she was refusing the hysterectomy because she *did not believe* she had cancer. "Anyone knows," she said, "that people with cancer are sick, feel bad and lose weight," while she felt quite well. The patient continued to hold this view despite the results of the biopsy and her physicians' persistent arguments to the contrary.

In light of the medical evidence, this patient is unjustified in believing she does not have cancer. As long as the patient persists in holding this false belief, and if this belief is material to her decision, the patient cannot give an informed

refusal. In this case, the physician seriously considered overriding the refusal, but under intense scrutiny the patient was eventually persuaded of the falsity of her belief. This breakthrough is instructive about the complexities inherent in achieving effective communication in many situations. The patient was a poor white from Appalachia with a third-grade education. The fact that her treating physician was black was the major reason for her false belief that she had no cancer. Discussions with another physician (who was white) and with her daughter resulted in a change in belief and a consent to a successful hysterectomy.

The problem of waivers

A further problem about understanding is whether we ought to recognize waivers of informed consent. What are we to say about those individuals who choose to understand nothing about a circumstance or at least choose to have less information than a reasonable person would choose to have? In the exercise of a waiver, a patient voluntarily relinquishes the right to an informed consent; that is, the patient excuses the physician from the obligation to obtain informed consent. The patient may delegate decision-making authority to the physician or request not to be informed. In effect, the patient makes a decision not to make an informed decision.

At least two courts have held that "a medical doctor need not make disclosures of risks when the patient requests that he not be so informed."[67] Various studies purport to show that more than sixty percent of patients want to know virtually nothing about procedures or the risks of the procedures,[68] and other studies indicate that eighty-six percent would consent without disclosures of risk and that only about twelve percent use the information provided in reaching their decisions.[69] Some physicians claim that more uninformed patients defer to physicians than seek pertinent information, although one study also indicates that physicians underestimate patient preferences for information in twenty-nine percent of their interactions with patients.[70]

There are two major ways to respond to the problem of waivers. The contemplated medical procedure might be withheld until sufficient understanding is present, notwithstanding the person's autonomously expressed desire not to be informed. According to this approach, persons should be coerced into receiving undesired information. Alternatively, when a patient or subject adequately understands whether he or she wants further information and then waives the right to the information, the professional might proceed without insisting on any understanding beyond the person's understanding that he or she is waiving a right. In the second situation, the person's waiver is a valid consent to therapy or research, even if it is not an informed consent.[71]

Many circumstances can be imagined in which information waivers are justified. For example, if a committed Jehovah's Witness were to inform a doctor that he wished to have everything possible done for him but did not want to know if transfusions or similar procedures would be employed, it is hard to construct a moral argument to support the conclusion that he must be told. On the other hand, patients commonly have an inordinate trust in physicians, and the general recognition of waivers of consent in research and therapeutic settings could make patients more vulnerable to those who would use abbreviated consent procedures merely because of convenience. Even if a waiver does not in principle conflict with respect for a patient's autonomy, under what conditions can a patient make a voluntary and informed decision to waive the right to hear relevant disclosable information? How often would there be abuse of the waiver by physicians, and how difficult would it be to prevent such abuse?

No general solution to these problems about waivers is likely to emerge. Each case of consent and the possibility of waiver will have to be considered separately. There may, however, be procedural ways to contain the problem. There could be rules against allowing waivers, with provisions that these rules specify prima facie obligations that could be overridden after special consideration by deliberative bodies, such as institutional review committees and hospital ethics committees. Rules against waivers could be developed to protect patients and subjects, but if committees determined that the person's interest was adequately protected in a particular case despite a waiver of information, they could allow the waiver. This procedural solution is no mere evasion of the problem. It would be easy to violate autonomy and to fail to live up to our responsibilities by inflexible rules that either permit or prohibit waivers. This procedural suggestion at least provides a flexible arrangement for deliberation and decision.

Voluntariness

Being free to act is sometimes as important for autonomous action as being competent and being informed. Under the term *voluntariness,* we will concentrate on the condition of a person's being independent of manipulative and coercive influences exerted by others in order to control the person. As the law has long recognized, a consent coerced by threats or manipulated by clever misrepresentation is no consent at all. In our framework, such a consent fails to be an autonomous authorization, and those who solicit consent by these means fail to respect autonomy.

Our use of *voluntariness* is intentionally narrow, and we distinguish it from broader uses that make the word synonymous with *autonomy* itself. Some have analyzed voluntariness in terms of the presence of adequate knowledge, the absence of psychological compulsion, and the absence of external constraints.[72] Were we to adopt this broad meaning, the voluntariness condition would be the only condition—rather than one among other conditions—of autonomous action. We avoid this outcome by saying that a person acts voluntarily to the degree he or she wills the action without being under the control of another agent's influence. Voluntariness can also be affected by physical and psychological conditions such as compulsion and drug addiction, and we will return to these difficult issues in the section on paternalism in Chapter 5.

Although control entails an influence, not all influences are controlling. Many influences are resistible, and some are welcomed rather than resisted. The broad category of influence includes acts of love, threats, educational communications, lies, manipulative suggestion, and emotional appeals, all of which can vary dramatically in the impact they make on persons. If a physician orders a reluctant patient to undergo cardiac catheterization and coerces the patient into compliance through a treat of abandonment, then the patient is controlled by the will of the physician. If, by contrast, a physician persuades the patient to undergo the procedure when the patient is at first reluctant to do so, then the patient is not under the will of the doctor.

But there are degrees of influence, and many cases are difficult to categorize in health care. For example, a physician may express severe irritation if a patient does not make the "right" decision about taking the prescribed dosage of a drug, and the patient may be intimidated and fearful, ultimately changing his or her mind and accepting the physician's recommendation not because of reasoned arguments but rather because it appears that acceptance will meet the physician's approval and thus ensure better care. Here the patient agrees under a significant influence exerted by the physician's role, authority, and power. In other cases, the physician may allow the patient even less discretion by a subtle yet firm suggestion that the patient has no choice but to pursue a particular course.

The nature and types of influence

In our analysis, there are three primary categories of influence: coercion, manipulation, and persuasion. *Coercion* is the most frequently mentioned form of controlling influence in the literature on biomedical ethics.[73] This literature discusses, for example, interventions involving subtle threats of ill consequences if patients or subjects do not submit to a recommended course of action. Coercion, as we define it, occurs when one person intentionally uses a credible and severe threat of harm or force to control another. The threat of force used by police and hospitals in involuntary commitments is a typical example. For a threat to be credible, either both parties must know that the person making the threat can effect it or the one making the threat must successfully deceive the person threatened into so believing. Some threats will coerce virtually all persons, whereas others will coerce only a few persons. Whether coercion occurs therefore depends ultimately on the subjective responses of those at whom coercion is directed.

Coercion entirely compromises autonomy and so deserves to be placed at one end of a continuum of types of influence. At the other end of the continuum from coercion are weak forms of influence such as rational persuasion. In *persuasion,* as we use the term here, a person must be convinced to believe in something through the merit of reasons advanced by another person. The persuader must believe that his or her statements are warranted by the evidence but need not personally judge these statements to be sufficient reasons for a belief. It is enough if the person persuaded finds these reasons sufficient as the substantive basis for a belief. We thus do not recognize what Paul Appelbaum and Loren Roth label ''forceful persuasion'' as a form of persuasion. This form of influence requires that persistent and sometimes misleading language be used. They cite as an example the case of an intern who did not accept a patient's refusal of an X ray. The intern insisted that he ''absolutely must have the film and that he [the patient] could not refuse it.'' The patient then reluctantly agreed.[74] In our usage, neither nonrational nor forceful ''persuasion'' qualifies as a form of persuasion, because both are forms of manipulation.

Manipulation is not a single kind of social influence. The word is a label for a class of influence strategies whose common feature is that they are neither instances of persuasion nor instances of coercion. The essence of manipulation is getting people to do what the manipulator wants by means other than coercion or persuasion. For purposes of decision making in health care, the most important form of manipulation is informational manipulation, a deliberate act of managing information that successfully influences a person by nonpersuasively altering the person's understanding of a situation and thereby motivating the person to do what the agent of influence intends. Some forms of informational manipulation are incompatible with informed consent. For example, the most common form is deception that involves such strategies as lying, withholding information, true assertion that omits a vital qualification, and misleading exaggeration in order to cause persons to believe what is false.

A good example is found in a long-standing controversy in psychology about deception of human subjects and the role of informed consent.[75] In the classic case of Milgram's obedience experiments, discussed above, subjects were deceived about virtually every aspect of the research to which they were consenting. By our criteria, these consents are manipulated and therefore do not satisfy the conditions of informed consent.

Several problems encountered previously in discussing understanding reappear as issues of informational manipulation. For example, a recurrent concern in the relevant literature is that clinicians will use the therapeutic privilege to withhold information not in order to avert harm to patients but to manipulate patients into consenting to their recommendations.[76] The manner in which information is presented by tone of voice, by forceful gesture, and by framing information negatively rather than positively can also affect a patient's perception and response.

Nevertheless, it is easy to inflate the threat of control by influence beyond its proper significance. We almost always make decisions in a context of competing influences, such as wants, needs, familial interests, legal obligations, and persuasive arguments. Although significant, these influences may not be controlling to any substantial degree. From the perspective of decision making by patients and subjects, we need only establish general criteria for the point at which autonomy is imperiled, while retaining a due appreciation that no sharp boundary can be drawn in many cases between controlling and noncontrolling influences. We most need to know the point at which an influence becomes obstructive or controls the will of an agent. In each case the powers of an individual patient or subject must be assessed, because resistibility to influence varies from person to person. The health professional thus should consider the particular patient's capacities for autonomous choice and resistance to influence, not the yardstick of the reasonable person.

The obligation to abstain from controlling influence

Thus far we have primarily attempted to distinguish influences that are compatible with substantial autonomy from influences that are not. Now we can turn to questions about the justifiability of exerting these forms of influence.

Some influences are welcomed by patients and subjects and are compatible with autonomous decision making. For example, professionals are sometimes morally blameworthy if they do *not* attempt to persuade resistant patients to pursue treatments that are medically essential. Reasoned argument in defense of an option is a form of information giving and may be vital to ensuring understanding. It is never an unjustified form of influence. The primary challenge to the professional is often to restrict influence attempts to explanation and persuasion, in order to secure a nonmanipulated consent from the patient or subject.

We are here assuming that influence by appeal to reason—persuasion—is in theory and practice distinguishable from influence by appeal to emotion. As applied to professionals in health care, the challenge is to distinguish in particular cases which emotional and which cognitive responses are likely to be provoked and to take care not to overwhelm the person with frightening information, particularly if the person is in a psychologically vulnerable or compromised state. Disclosures or approaches that might rationally persuade one patient might overwhelm another patient with fear and panic, thereby bypassing reason.

Manipulation and coercion are at times justified, even if the occasions are infrequent. Generally we can say that the central moral issues about manipulation—the most intricate and elusive category—turn on how to differentiate those actions that are compatible with substantial autonomy from those that are not. In health care the concern is usually over which kinds of manipulation—threats, punishments, rewards, and offers—permit a patient or subject to make an autonomous choice and which kinds deprive the person of that opportunity.

The most difficult problems about autonomy and manipulation are not about punishment and threat, which are generally unjustified, but rather are about the effect of rewards and offers. For example, during the Tuskegee syphilis experiments, various methods were used to stimulate and sustain the interest of subjects in continued participation. They were offered free burial assistance and insurance, free transportation to and from the examinations, and a free stop in town on the return trip; they were rewarded with free medicines and free hot meals on the days of the examination. The socioeconomic deprivation of these subjects made them vulnerable to such manipulation.[77]

When an offer is made in a setting in which it is abnormally attractive—for example, money or freedom for deprived prisoners—it is always manipulative, never coercive. To maintain that irresistibly attractive offers coerce patients or subjects makes a mockery of the concept of coercion (unless, of course, the offer is a disguised threat), because then anyone who intentionally and successfully influenced another by presenting an offer so attractive that the person was unable to resist it—e.g., a large salary at a wonderful job—would have coerced the person.[78]

Nonetheless, some kinds of offers have long been viewed by numerous writers as inherently coercive instruments or circumstances. Among the best-known examples have been "irresistible offers" made to prisoners to become research subjects. Beecher was among the earliest to denounce such practices as coercive and as involving bribery inconsistent with obtaining informed consent:

> Whenever coercion could operate, however subtly, the consent of volunteers must be suspect. This applies especially to civil prisoners and other captive groups, such as medical students. . . .
> The prospect of an award of extreme benefit to the [prisoner] subject such as a great reduction in time of imprisonment or parole or pardon could constitute a bribe greater than the human spirit could be expected to support, with clear violation of the necessary requirements of the principle of consent.[79]

We agree that if a prison official said, "We will not allow you to leave when your time is up unless you become an experimental subject," this statement would constitute a threat and would be coercive. However, the offer described by Beecher is a genuine offer, not a veiled threat. We do not suggest that, because such offers are not instances of coercion, it is morally legitimate to use them to induce prisoners to be research subjects. The offer condemned by Beecher appears to be a morally impermissible manipulation, but, as described, it is not a threat and is not coercive.

The grounds for claiming that an influence is both controlling and morally unjustified seem clear in the abstract but unclear in many concrete cases. In Case 5, which was discussed at length earlier, a patient's medication was modified without his knowledge after he had refused to allow modification. This case of nondisclosure involved the intent to control choice and to manipulate the patient to the best medical outcome. The therapists clearly overrode the patient's autonomous wishes (unless one diagnoses the patient as addicted). However, such control may sometimes be justified on grounds of beneficence.

Some of the most difficult cases in health care involve manipulationlike situations involving patients or subjects in desperate need. To say that a person desperately needs something—such as a medication or a source of income—means that without it there is a strong probability that the person (or some loved one, etc.) will be seriously harmed. Very attractive offers such as free medication or extra money can leave such persons without any real choice other than to accept the offer. Here a person is controlled by a situation but not by the intentional manipulation of another person.

It might be thought that any such offer to a person already in desperate need is inherently exploitive. But this may not be the case. In 1722, several inmates of the Newgate Prison volunteered, as an alternative to hanging, to be subjects in an experiment on smallpox inoculation.[80] It might at first seem that they were controlled, but more plausibly this is a case of a manipulationlike circumstance in which a very welcome offer is made to persons in desperate need. The facts of the outcome indicate just how welcome and fortuitous: These condemned men all survived and were released.

But for patients who are abnormally weak, dependent, and surrender-prone, influences that might ordinarily be resisted can become controlling, and compliance may be induced by influencing or contributing to the desperation, anxiety, boredom, hope, or other human emotions pervasive in the lives of patients. Even the hope of more attention and better care can be a significant factor for a bedridden individual. Thus, what a health professional regards as an attempt at rational persuasion may irrationally influence the patient by tearing at his or her vulnerabilities. We are not implying that health professionals do routinely manipulate or exploit the patient's vulnerabilities, but only that many patients are vulnerable to such influence.[81]

It is especially important to ensure that autonomy rights are preserved in institutions whose populations are admitted involuntarily. There is no reason why prisoners, for example, could not validly consent to medical research if coercive tactics were not specifically involved and if there were no manipulative offers, such as unduly large amounts of money for high risk-taking. A coercive environment does not render a person incompetent or make all choices involuntary. The person may be vulnerable and may act involuntarily, but each individual case requires careful investigation.[82]

Conclusion

The intimate connection between autonomy and decision making in health care unifies the sections of this chapter. Although we have justified the obligation to solicit decisions for patients by the principle of respect for autonomy, we acknowledge that the principle's precise demands remain partially unsettled. For example, important issues concern how the principle is connected to rules of truthfulness, confidentiality, and privacy—three subjects discussed in Chapter 7. In other chapters, especially in Chapter 5 on beneficence, we will test the weight of this principle in competition with other principles. We have only argued thus far that making respect for autonomy a trump moral principle, rather than one moral principle in a system of principles, places an inappropriately high premium on autonomy.

Although respecting autonomy is more important than biomedical ethics had appreciated until the last two decades, it is not the only principle and should not be overvalued when it conflicts with other values. The human moral community—indeed morality itself—is founded no less on the other three principles that we discuss in subsequent chapters. In many clinical circumstances the weight of respect for autonomy is minimal, while the weight of nonmaleficence or beneficence is maximal. Similarly in public policy, the demands of justice can outweigh the demands of respect for autonomy.

Several conclusions in this chapter could be viewed as one-sided in deference to autonomy, on grounds that their implications for professional conduct exceed current legal and regulatory requirements of informed consent (in the social or institutional sense). For example, our proposed shift from a focus on disclosure to a focus on understanding and effective communication entails a different and more burdensome way of structuring the process of soliciting consent. Nevertheless, we have not argued that all our proposals ought to be, or could be, turned into enforceable legal requirements or into regulatory rules or hospital policies. The resources needed to provide a rich context of decision making in which professionals conduct themselves in accordance with the strategies suggested in this chapter will not always be justifiable. This problem invites judgments about justice and the allocation of resources (see Chapter 6) that compete with the obligation to obtain informed consent.

We have concentrated on informed decision making in health care in this chapter, but these issues are not the only ones raised by the principle of respect for autonomy. We will examine several other issues of autonomy in conjunction with other moral principles. Because moral dilemmas arise from conflicts of two or more principles, these issues could be treated in more than one chapter. For example, suicide could be treated as a problem of autonomy—that is, of determining when, if ever, suicide is autonomous and when, if ever, autonomous suicide may be forcibly prevented on grounds of beneficence. We will discuss these problems of suicide under paternalistic beneficence in Chapter 5. Questions of autonomy, in short, will be unavoidable as we test the limits and weights of the principles of nonmaleficence, beneficence, and justice in the next three chapters.

Notes

1. This core idea of autonomy has been helpfully treated by Isaiah Berlin, "Two Concepts of Liberty," in *Four Essays on Liberty* (Oxford: Oxford University Press, 1969), pp. 118–72; and Joel Feinberg, *Harm to Self*, Vol. III in *The Moral Limits of Criminal Law* (New York: Oxford University Press, 1986), chaps. 18 and 19.

2. See, for example, Stanley Benn, "Freedom, Autonomy and the Concept of a Person," *Proceedings of the Aristotelian Society* 76 (1976): 123f.

3. The theory of autonomy has undergone sustained investigation in recent years, and the three-condition analysis defended here is far from a consensus position. For influential treatments, see the articles cited below by Gerald Dworkin; and Harry Frankfurt, "Freedom of the Will and the Concept of a Person," *Journal of Philosophy* 68 (1971): 5–20.

4. Although it would not be appropriate here to defend the theses that the above three conditions are the basic conditions of autonomous action and that they need to be satisfied only to a substantial degree, that view has been defended elsewhere. See Ruth R. Faden and Tom L. Beauchamp, *A History and Theory of Informed Consent* (New York: Oxford University Press, 1986), chap. 7. Whether each condition is a necessary condition of autonomous action—as we believe—and whether they are jointly sufficient conditions—a more difficult thesis to sustain—are not matters on which we shall speculate in detail and not ones demonstrated in the above-cited work. Such claims would need extensive argument.

5. See Robert Paul Wolff, *In Defense of Anarchism* (New York: Harper and Row, 1970), pp. 4–6, 13f. See also Wolff's stronger claims in "On Violence," *Journal of Philosophy* 66 (October 1969): esp. 608. For an elaboration of the position argued below against Wolff, see Tom L. Beauchamp and Kenneth Witkowski, "Critique of Pure Anarchism," *Canadian Journal of Philosophy* 3 (1973): 533–39. For more recent developments in essentially the same controversy, see Joseph Raz, "Authority and Justification," *Philosophy and Public Affairs* 14 (1985): 3–29; and Christopher McMahon, "Autonomy and Authority," *Philosophy and Public Affairs* 16 (Fall 1987): 303–28.

6. See Gerald Dworkin, "Autonomy and Behavior Control," *Hastings Center Report* 6 (February 1976): 23.

7. These reflections are indebted to Gerald Dworkin, "Moral Autonomy," in *Morals, Science, and Sociality,* ed. H. Tristram Engelhardt, Jr., and Daniel Callahan (Hastings-on-Hudson, N.Y.: Hastings Center, 1978), pp. 156–71.

8. Immanuel Kant, *Groundwork of the Metaphysics of Morals,* trans. H. J. Paton (New York: Harper and Row, 1964); *The Doctrine of Virtue,* Part II of the "Metaphysics of Morals," trans. Mary Gregor (New York: Harper and Row, 1964).

9. John Stuart Mill, *Utilitarianism, On Liberty, and Essay on Mill,* ed. with intro. by Mary Warnock (New York: New American Library, 1974), pp. 136–38, 184–89.

10. *Schloendorff* v. *New York Hospital,* 211 N.Y. 125, 127, 129; 105 N.E., 92, 93 (1914). See also *Natanson* v. *Kline,* 186 Kan. 393, P.2d 1093 (1960), rehearing denied, 187 Kan. 186, 354 P.2d 670 (1960).

11. Angela Roddey Holder, *Medical Malpractice Law* (New York: John Wiley, 1975), p. 225.

12. See Alexander Capron, "Informed Consent in Catastrophic Disease and Treatment," *University of Pennsylvania Law Review* 123 (December 1974): 364–76.

13. See Jay Katz, *The Silent World of Doctor and Patient* (New York: Free Press, 1984), pp. 86–87; and President's Commission for the Study of Ethical Problems in Medicine and Biomedical and Behavioral Research, *Making Health Care Decisions* (Washington, D.C.: U.S. Government Printing Office, 1982), Vol. I, p. 15.

14. The analysis in this subsection is based on Faden and Beauchamp, *A History and Theory of Informed Consent,* chap. 8.

15. *Mohr* v. *Williams,* 95 Minn. 261, 104 N.W. 12 (1905), at 15.

16. This conclusion is thoroughly explored in Alan J. Weisbard, "Informed Consent: The Law's Uneasy Compromise with Ethical Theory," *Nebraska Law Review* 65 (1986): 749–67.

17. Jay Katz, "Disclosure and Consent," in *Genetics and the Law II,* ed. A. Milunsky and G. Annas (New York: Plenum Press, 1980), pp. 122, 128.

18. See, for example, Alan Meisel and Loren Roth, "What We Do and Do Not Know about Informed Consent," *Journal of the American Medical Association* 246 (1981): 2473–77; President's Commission, *Making Health Care Decisions,* Vol. II, pp. 317–410, esp. p. 318, and Vol. I, chap. 1, esp. pp. 38–39; National Commission for the Protection of Human Subjects of Biomedical and Behavioral Research, *The Belmont Report* (Washington, D.C.: DHEW Publication no. OS 78-0012, 1978), p. 10; Margaret A. Somerville, as prepared for the Law Reform Commission of Canada, *Consent to Medical Care* (Ottawa: Law Reform Commission, 1979), pp. 11ff, 24.

19. The fifth element has been alternatively depicted as the element of decision, shared decision making, authorization, and permission giving—all used, in effect, as substitute terms for the term *consent.* Whatever the precise formulation, the fifth element refers to the final stage in the act of giving an informed consent.

20. See U.S. Supreme Court, *Planned Parenthood of Central Missouri* v. *Danforth,* 428 U.S. 52, 67 n.8 (1976).

21. See the analysis and defense of this definition in Charles M. Culver and Bernard Gert, *Philosophy in Medicine* (New York: Oxford University Press, 1982), chap. 3.

22. *Pratt* v. *Davis,* 118 Ill. App. 161 (1905), aff'd, 224 Ill. 300, 79 N.E. 562 (1906).

23. See Daniel Wikler, "Paternalism and the Mildly Retarded," *Philosophy and Public Affairs* 8 (Summer 1979): 377–92; and Allen Buchanan and Dan W. Brock, "Deciding for Others," *Milbank Quarterly* 64, supp. 2 (1986): 22–28, 38–41.

24. See Willard Gaylin, "The Competence of Children: No Longer All or None," *Hastings Center Report* 12 (April 1982): 33–38, esp. 35; Buchanan and Brock, "Deciding for Others," pp. 31–37; President's Commission, *Making Health Care Decisions,* Vol. I, p. 60; *Lane* v. *Candura,* 376 N.E. 2d 1232 (Mass. App. 1978); and Virginia Abernathy, "Compassion, Control, and Decisions about Competency," *American Journal of Psychiatry* 141 (1984): 53–58, esp. 56.

25. We are indebted to Donald Bersoff for this tripartite approach.

26. See Paul S. Appelbaum, Charles W. Lidz, and Alan Meisel, *Informed Consent:*

Legal Theory and Clinical Practice (New York: Oxford University Press, 1987), chap. 5; Paul S. Appelbaum and Loren Roth, "Competency to Consent to Research: A Psychiatric Overview," *Archives of General Psychiatry* 39 (1982): 951–58; Roth and Meisel, "What We Do and Do Not Know"; Ruth Macklin, "Some Problems in Gaining Informed Consent from Psychiatric Patients," *Emory Law Journal* 31 (Spring 1982): 360–68; Paul S. Appelbaum, Stuart A. Mirkin, and Alan L. Bateman, "Empirical Assessment of Competency to Consent to Psychiatric Hospitalization," *American Journal of Psychiatry* 138 (1981): 1170–76.

27. See Jeffrie Murphy, "Incompetence and Paternalism," *Archiv für Rechts-und-Sozialphilosophie* 50 (1974): 465–86.

28. The analysis in the remainder of this section has profited from numerous discussions with Ruth R. Faden and Nancy King.

29. This schema is indebted to the above-mentioned articles by Appelbaum, Meisel, Lidz, and Roth.

30. See "Necessity and Sufficiency of Expert Evidence and Extent of Physician's Duty to Inform Patient of Risks of Proposed Treatment," *American Law Reports* 3d, 52 (1977): 1084; "Modern Status of Views as to General Measure of Physician's Duty to Inform Patient of Risks of Proposed Treatment," *American Law Reports* 3d, 88 (1978): 1008; David Seidelson, "Medical Malpractice: Informed Consent Cases in 'Full-Disclosure' Jurisdictions," *Duquesne Law Review* 14 (1976): 309–11; "Informed Consent and the Dying Patient," *Yale Law Journal* 83 (1974): 1637.

31. See, for example, Charles Keown, Paul Slovic, and Sarah Lichtenstein, "Attitudes of Physicians, Pharmacists, and Laypersons toward Seriousness and Need for Disclosure of Prescription Drug Side Effects," *Health Psychology* 3 (1984): 1–11; and Ruth R. Faden et al., "Disclosure of Information to Patients in Medical Care," *Medical Care* 19 (July 1981): 718–33.

32. See "Physician's Duty to Inform of Risks," *American Law Reports* 3d, 88 (1986): 1010–25 (and update, 50–60). Georgia appears to be the only state to have rejected the modern informed consent doctrine altogether. See *Spikes* v. *Health,* 332 S.E. 2d 889 (Ga. App. 1985), 889–93.

33. *Canterbury* v. *Spence,* 464 F.2d 772, at 785–87 (D.C. Cir. 1972). See the review and reaffirmation of these standards in *Crain* v. *Allison,* D.C. App., 443 A.2d 558 (1982), 558–66. In 1972, two other appellate decisions—*Cobbs* v. *Grant* (Case 8) and *Wilkinson* v. *Vesey*—joined *Canterbury* and established this reasonable person standard in the jurisdictions of Washington, D.C., California, and Rhode Island. *Wilkinson* v. *Vesey,* 295 A.2d 676 (R.E. 1972); *Cobbs* v. *Grant,* 8 Cal. 3d 229, 104 Cal. Rptr. 505, 502 P.2d 1 (1972). Other courts that subsequently addressed the problem of disclosure have, on occasion, switched to the reasonable person standard. For particularly instructive examples, see *Cross* v. *Trapp,* 294 S.E. 2d 446 (W.V. 1982), 446–61; and *Wheeldon* v. *Madison,* 374 N.W.2d 367 (S.D. 1985), 367–81. However, some courts that had already adopted the professional practice standard have declined to change their position. In addition, some later statutes have invalidated this new common-law standard in several jurisdictions. See Alan Meisel, "The Law of Informed Consent," in President's Commission, *Making Health Care Decisions,* Vol. III, pp. 206–45; and "Physician's Duty to Inform of Risks," pp. 1016–25.

34. Ruth R. Faden, "Disclosure and Informed Consent: Does It Matter How We Tell It?" *Health Education Monographs* 5 (1977): 198–215; Ruth R. Faden and Tom L. Beauchamp, "Decision-Making and Informed Consent: A Study of the Impact

of Disclosed Information,'' *Social Indicators Research* 7 (1980): 313–36; and, for an extension, Faden et al., ''Disclosure of Information.''

35. C. H. Fellner and J. R. Marshall, ''Kidney Donors—the Myth of Informed Consent,'' *American Journal of Psychiatry* 126 (1970): 1245; and idem, ''Twelve Kidney Donors,'' *Journal of the American Medical Association* 206 (1968): 2703–7.

36. See Meisel and Roth, ''What We Do and Do Not Know.''

37. Gerald T. Roling et al., ''An Appraisal of Patients' Reactions to 'Informed Consent,' '' *Gastrointestinal Endoscopy* 24 (1977): 69–70.

38. For two very different assessments of the viability of a subjective standard in law, see *Scott* v. *Bradford,* 606 P.2d 554 (Okl. 1979), 554–60; and *Barclay* v. *Campbell,* 704 S.W.2d 8 (Tex. 1986), 8–11.

39. *Canterbury* v. *Spence,* 464 F.2d at 789. For a broad formulation, see *Wilson* v. *Scott,* 412 S.W.2d 299, 301 (Tex. 1967). See also President's Commission, *Making Health Care Decisions,* Vol. I, pp. 95–96; M. J. Myers, ''Comment: Informed Consent in Medical Malpractice,'' *California Law Review* 55 (1967): 1396–1410; E. S. Glass, ''Restructuring Informed Consent: Legal Therapy for the Doctor-Patient Relationship,'' *Yale Law Journal* 79 (1970): 1533; ''Informed Consent—A Proposed Standard for Medical Disclosure,'' *New York University Law Review* 48 (1973): 548–63. For a fuller description pertinent to clinical medicine, including a survey of recent court cases, see Leslie J. Miller, ''Informed Consent: II,'' *Journal of the American Medical Association* 244 (1980): 2348–49.

40. Jay Katz, ''Informed Consent—A Fairy Tale? Law's Vision,'' *University of Pittsburgh Law Review* 39 (Winter 1977): 138 (see also p. 150); idem, *The Silent World,* pp. 60–65; and idem, ''Disclosure and Consent in Psychiatric Practice: Mission Impossible?'' in *Law and Ethics in the Practice of Psychiatry,* ed. Charles Hofling (New York: Brunner-Mazel, 1981), p. 93. Katz is quoting from *Salgo* v. *Stanford University Board of Trustees,* 154 Cal. App. 2d 560 (1957).

41. This proposal was actually based on a prospective randomized study of emotional responses to risk disclosure. See James W. Lankton, Barron M. Batehelder, and Alan J. Ominsky, ''Emotional Responses to Detailed Risk Disclosure for Anesthesia: A Prospective, Randomized Study,'' *Anesthesiology* 46 (April 1977): 294–96. This proposal can also be defended on grounds of the principle of respect for autonomy.

42. See the summary in Howard Brody, *Placebos and the Philosophy of Medicine: Clinical, Conceptual, and Ethical Issues* (Chicago: University of Chicago Press, 1980), pp. 10–11; and Herbert Benson and Mark Epstein, ''The Placebo Effect: A Neglected Aspect in the Care of Patients,'' *Journal of the American Medical Association* 232 (1975): 1225.

43. See J. D. Levine, N. C. Gordon, and H. L. Fields, ''The Mechanism of Placebo Analgesia,'' *Lancet* 2 (1978): 654–57.

44. Alan Leslie, ''Ethics and Practice of Placebo Therapy,'' in *Ethics in Medicine,* ed. Stanley Reiser, Arthur Dyck, and William Curran (Cambridge, Mass.: MIT Press, 1977), p. 242.

45. See L. C. Park et al., ''Effects of Informed Consent on Research Patients and Study Results,'' *Journal of Nervous and Mental Disease* 145 (1967): 349–57; and L. C. Park and L. Covi, ''Non-blind Placebo Trial: An Exploration of Neurotic Outpatients' Responses to Placebo When Its Inert Content Is Disclosed,'' *Archives of General Psychiatry* 12 (1965): 336–45.

46. Brody, *Placebos and the Philosophy of Medicine,* pp. 110, 113, et passim; Katz,

The Silent World, pp. 189–95. For a defense of placebos as a symbol of the physician's willingness to help the patient, see Howard Spiro, *Doctors, Patients, and Placebos* (New Haven: Yale University Press, 1986).

47. See Philip Levendusky and Loren Pankratz, "Self-Control Techniques as an Alternative to Pain Medication," *Journal of Abnormal Psychology* 84 (1975): 165–68. This case is discussed in several articles in that issue.

48. For a discussion of several kinds (e.g., implicit and presumed) and times (e.g., past and future) of consent, see James F. Childress, *Who Should Decide? Paternalism in Health Care* (New York: Oxford University Press, 1982), chap. 4.

49. See Herbert C. Kelman, "Was Deception Justified—And Was It Necessary?" *Journal of Abnormal Psychology* 84 (1975): 172–74.

50. Stanley Milgram, *Obedience to Authority* (New York: Harper and Row, 1974), pp. 3–4. See also Stanley Milgram, "Behavioral Study of Obedience," *Journal of Abnormal Psychology* 67 (1963): 371–78; and "Some Conditions of Obedience and Disobedience to Authority," *Human Relations* 18 (1965): 57–76.

51. Stanley Milgram, "Subject Reaction: The Neglected Factor in the Ethics of Experimentation," *Hastings Center Report* 7 (October 1977): 19.

52. For a sample of this debate, see Diana Baumrind, "Some Thoughts on Ethics of Research: After Reading Milgram's 'Behavioral Study of Obedience,' " *American Psychologist* 19 (1964): 421–23; Stanley Milgram, "Issues in the Study of Obedience: A Reply to Baumrind," *American Psychologist* 19 (1964): 848–52; and Steven C. Patten, "The Case That Milgram Makes," *Philosophical Review* 86 (July 1977): 350–64.

53. Milgram, "Subject Reaction," p. 21.

54. Ibid.

55. Norberto Valenti and Clara di Meglio, *Sex and the Confessional* (New York: Stein and Day, 1974).

56. For a powerful analysis applied to clinical medicine, see Katz, *The Silent World*.

57. A sensible approach to several problems of comprehension other than those mentioned here is found in Alan W. Cross and Larry R. Churchill, "Ethical and Cultural Dimensions of Informed Consent," *Annals of Internal Medicine* 96 (1982): 110–13.

58. *Bang v. Charles T. Miller Hospital*, 251 Minn. 427, 88 N.W. 2d 186 (1958).

59. Franz J. Ingelfinger, "Informed (But Uneducated) Consent," *New England Journal of Medicine* 287 (1972): 455–56; and idem, "Arrogance," *New England Journal of Medicine* 303 (1980): 1507–11.

60. Robert D. Mulford, "Experimentation on Human Beings," *Stanford Law Review* 20 (November 1967): 106.

61. The pioneering work has been done by Amos Tversky and Daniel Kahneman. See, for example, "Choices, Values and Frames," *American Psychologist* 39 (1984): 341–50; "Judgment under Certainty: Heuristics and Biases," *Science* 185 (1974): 1124–31; "The Framing of Decisions and the Psychology of Choice," *Science* 211 (1981): 453–58; and Daniel Kahneman and Amos Tversky, "Prospect Theory," *Econometrica* 47 (1979): 263–92. See also Daniel Kahneman, Paul Slovic and Amos Tversky, Baruch Fischoff, and Sarah Lichtenstein, "Behavioral Decision Theory," *Annual Review of Psychology* 28 (1977): 1–39; and Richard Nisbett and Lee Ross, *Human Inferences: Strategies and Shortcomings of Social Judgment* (Englewood Cliffs, N.J.: Prentice-Hall, 1980). We are indebted to Ruth Faden for directing us to much of this literature and for facilitating our understanding of it.

62. Kahneman and Tversky, ''Choices, Values and Frames,'' 344–46; and Tversky and Kahneman, ''The Framing of Decisions.''

63. S. E. Eraker and H. C. Sox, ''Assessment of Patients' Preferences for Therapeutic Outcome,'' *Medical Decision Making* 1 (1981): 29–39; Barbara McNeil et al., ''On the Elicitation of Preferences for Alternative Therapies,'' *New England Journal of Medicine* 306 (1982): 1259–62.

64. See, for example, Baruch Fischoff, Paul Slovic, and Sarah Lichtentstein, ''Knowing What You Want: Measuring Labile Values,'' in *Cognitive Processes in Choice and Decision Behavior*, ed. T. Wallston (Hillsdale, N.J.: Erlbaum, 1980), 117–41.

65. See H. Tristram Engelhardt, Jr., ''Basic Ethical Principles in the Conduct of Biomedical and Behavioral Research Involving Human Subjects,'' and Robert Veatch, ''Three Theories of Informed Consent,'' both in National Commission for the Protection of Human Subjects, appendix to *Belmont Report*, Vol. I.

66. The case and this analysis are presented in Faden and Beauchamp, *A History and Theory of Informed Consent*, p. 311. The case was reported in R. Faden and A. Faden, ''False Belief and the Refusal of Medical Treatment,'' *Journal of Medical Ethics* 3 (1977): 133–35.

67. *Cobbs* v. *Grant*, 502 P. 2d 1, p. 12 (Case 8 in the appendix); and *Sard* v. *Hardy*, 379 A. 2d, p. 1022.

68. See Ralph J. Alfidi, ''Controversy, Alternatives, and Decisions in Complying with the Legal Doctrine of Informed Consent,'' *Radiology* 114 (January 1975).

69. Cross and Churchill, ''Ethical and Cultural Dimensions,'' pp. 111–12.

70. William M. Strull, Bernard Lo, and Gerald Charles, ''Do Patients Want to Participate in Medical Decisionmaking?'' *Journal of the American Medical Association* 252 (1984): 2990–94.

71. For these issues turned in the direction of the patient's obligations to know and act autonomously, see Mark Strasser, ''Mill and the Right to Remain Uninformed,'' and David E. Ost, ''Information Waivers: Reply to Strasser,'' both in *Journal of Medicine and Philosophy* 11 (1986): 265–84.

72. This point, suitably modified for our purposes, derives from Joel Feinberg, *Social Philosophy* (Englewood Cliffs, N.J.: Prentice-Hall, 1973), p. 48.

73. See Henry K. Beecher, *Experimentation in Man* (Springfield, Ill.: Charles C. Thomas, 1959), pp. 18–20; idem, ''Editorial: Some Fallacies and Errors in the Application of the Principle of Consent in Experimentation,'' *Clinical Pharmacology and Therapeutics* 3 (March–April 1962): 144–45; American Psychological Association, ''Ethical Standards for Psychological Research,'' *APA Monitor* 2 (1971): 14; Carl Cohen, ''Medical Experimentation in Prisoners,'' *Perspectives in Biology and Medicine* (Spring 1979): 357–72; Richard Singer, ''Consent of the Unfree: Medical Experimentation and Behavior Modification in the Closed Institution, Part II,'' *Law and Human Behavior* 1 (1977): 105–22; Willard Gaylin, ''On the Borders of Persuasion: A Psychoanalytic Look at Coercion,'' *Psychiatry* 37 (1974): 1–8; Ingelfinger, ''Informed (But Uneducated) Consent,'' p. 466.

74. Paul S. Appelbaum and Loren H. Roth, ''Treatment Refusal in Medical Hospitals,'' in President's Commission, *Making Health Care Decisions*, Vol. II, p. 443, also pp. 452, 462, 466.

75. See Alan C. Elms, ''Keeping Deception Honest: Justifying Conditions for Social Scientific Research Stratagems,'' in *Ethical Issues in Social Science Research*, ed. Tom L. Beauchamp et al. (Baltimore: Johns Hopkins Press, 1982), pp. 232–45.

76. See, for example, Charles W. Lidz and Alan Meisel, ''Informed Consent and the

Structure of Medical Care," in President's Commission, *Making Health Care Decisions*, Vol. II; Alan Meisel, "The Exceptions to the Informed Consent Doctrine," *Wisconsin Law Review* 1979 (1979): 413–88.

77. See James H. Jones, *Bad Blood* (New York: Free Press, 1981); Thomas G. Benedek, "The 'Tuskegee Study' of Syphilis: Analysis of Moral Versus Methodologic Aspects," *Journal of Chronic Diseases* 31 (1978): 35–50, esp. 37–38; A. M. Brandt, "Racism and Research: The Case of the Tuskegee Syphilis Study," *Hastings Center Report* 8 (December 1978): 21–29; David J. Rothman, "Were Tuskegee & Willowbrook 'Studies in Nature'?" *Hastings Center Report* 12 (April 1982): 5–7, esp. 7.

78. The dominant position in the philosophical literature conceives coercion exclusively in terms of threats of severe negative sanctions. For example, Bernard Gert takes the firm position that if a person acts to secure an offered good, no matter how attractive or overwhelming the offer, coercion is not involved. Robert Nozick's pioneering analysis of coercion similarly implies that only threats can be coercive, in part because he believes that people shun threats but welcome offers. We accept this analysis. The essence of coercion is control of a person's behavior by the presenting a threat of a negative sanction. See Bernard Gert, "Coercion and Freedom," in *Coercion: Nomos XIV*, ed. J. Roland Pennock and John W. Chapman (New York: Aldine, 1972), pp. 36–37; Robert Nozick, "Coercion," in *Philosophy, Science and Method: Essays in Honor of Ernest Nagel*, ed. Sidney Morgenbesser, Patrick Suppes, and Morton White (New York: St. Martin's Press, 1969), pp. 440–72.

79. Beecher, "Editorial," pp. 144–45.

80. Henry K. Beecher, *Research and the Individual: Human Studies* (Boston: Little, Brown, 1970), p. 6.

81. See Charles W. Lidz et al., *Informed Consent: A Study of Decisionmaking in Psychiatry* (New York: Guilford Press, 1984), chap. 7, esp. pp. 110–11, 117–23.

82. The problems mentioned in this paragraph were under intense examination in *Kaimowitz v. Department of Mental Health*, Civil No. 73-19434-AW (Circuit Court, Wayne County, Mich., July 10, 1973), pp. 31–32. Summarized at *U.S.L.W.* 42 (July 31, 1973), 3062. See also Cohen, "Medical Experimentation in Prisoners"; Appelbaum and Roth, "Competency to Consent to Research"; and Jeffrie G. Murphy, "Therapy and the Problem of Autonomous Consent," *International Journal of Law and Psychiatry* 2 (1970): 415–30.

4

The Principle of Nonmaleficence

The concept of nonmaleficence or not inflicting harm has been associated with the maxim *Primum non nocere,* "Above all [or first] do no harm." This maxim has wide currency in discussions of the responsibilities of health-care professionals; yet its origins are obscure. Often proclaimed the fundamental principle in the Hippocratic tradition in medical ethics, it is not found in the Hippocratic corpus, and a venerable statement often confused with it—"At least, do no harm"—is not the most accurate translation of a passage that does appear in Hippocrates.[1] Nonetheless, the Hippocratic oath does express a duty of nonmaleficence together with a duty of beneficence: "I will use treatment to help the sick according to my ability and judgment, but I will never use it to injure or wrong them."

In this chapter we examine the nature and implications of the principle of nonmaleficence. We apply the principle to several major issues in biomedical ethics, including the distinction between killing and letting die, the difference between withholding and withdrawing life-sustaining treatments, the role of judgments of quality of life, the treatment of seriously ill newborns, and the duties of proxy decision makers for incompetent patients. These issues often concern our obligations to avoid harm when these obligations conflict with other obligations, such as respect for autonomy, justice, and beneficence.

120

The concept and obligation of nonmaleficence

The distinction between nonmaleficence and beneficence

A principle of nonmaleficence is recognized in many rule-deontological and rule-utilitarian theories, some of which regard this obligation as the foundation of social morality. For example, H. L. A. Hart presents a utilitarian argument that a minimum content for moral and legal systems can be formulated by examining characteristics of the human condition, one of which is ''human vulnerability'':

> The common requirements of law and morality consist for the most part not of active services to be rendered but of forbearances, which are usually formulated in negative form as prohibitions. Of these the most important for social life are those that restrict the use of violence in killing or inflicting bodily harm. The basic character of such rules may be brought out in a question: If there were not these rules what point could there be for beings such as ourselves in having rules of any other kind? The force of this rhetorical question rests on the fact that men are both occasionally prone to, and normally vulnerable to, bodily attack.[2]

Other formulations of the obligation of nonmaleficence appear in deontological writings by W. D. Ross, where it is distinguished from the obligation of beneficence, and by John Rawls, where it is distinguished from an obligation of ''mutual aid.''[3]

Not all philosophers view nonmaleficence and beneficence as distinct and separate obligations. For example, William Frankena holds that a single principle of beneficence includes four elements:

1. One ought not to inflict evil or harm (what is bad).
2. One ought to prevent evil or harm.
3. One ought to remove evil or harm.
4. One ought to do or promote good.[4]

He acknowledges that the fourth obligation may not, strictly speaking, be a moral obligation, and he arranges these elements serially so that—other things being equal in a case of conflict—the first takes moral precedence over the second, the second over the third, and the third over the fourth. When these elements conflict, he appeals—somewhat inconsistently—to the principle of utility as a mediating or heuristic maxim: Maximize good and minimize evil.

Nonmaleficence and beneficence are not easily separable, because many issues, especially in biomedical ethics, present the need to balance them together, as we discuss in the next chapter. However, to conflate them into one principle is to obscure distinctions that we make in ordinary moral discourse, which incorporates the defensible conviction that certain obligations not to injure others are not only distinct from but often (though not always) more stringent than obligations to take positive steps to benefit others. For example, the obligation not to push someone who cannot swim into deep water seems stronger than the obligation to rescue someone who has accidentally strayed into deep water. It is also morally imperative to accept substantial risks to personal safety in some cases in order not to endanger others, but acceptance of even moderate risks is not generally required to benefit others. If we try to encompass the ideas of benefiting others and not injuring them under the single principle of beneficence, we will still be forced to distinguish, as Frankena does, among the various elements of this principle that correspond roughly to what we call nonmaleficence and beneficence. Therefore, we treat the two principles as distinct, prima facie principles that may on occasion come into conflict.

In cases of conflict we can expect nonmaleficence to be overriding on many occasions, but not on all occasions. For example, a harm we inflict such as a surgical wound may be negligible or trivial yet necessary to prevent a major harm such as death. Whenever we are in a circumstance in which we must either avoid a harm or provide a benefit, we need a decision rule for choosing one course over the other. However, because the weights of these moral principles—like all moral principles—can vary in the circumstances, there can be no general mediating rule that always favors avoiding harm over providing benefit.

The moral relevance of the distinctions among elements 1 through 4 in the scheme above is more difficult to sustain than has often been appreciated. Refraining from aiding another person (by not providing a good or by not preventing or removing harm) can be as devastating in its consequences and as morally wrong as inflicting a harm. Suppose the same harm occurs to X either by your not assisting X and allowing the harm to occur or by your inflicting the harm on X. And suppose the harm that is either inflicted or allowed is equally intentional, equally sure to occur, and equally avoidable; and suppose you are equally at low risk in the two scenarios. For example, the harm of death can be inflicted by killing a person or can be caused by failing to put a person on a respirator. There is no moral relevance to the only difference in these cases, which is inflicting harm and refraining from assistance so as to allow harm. This shows that there is no moral difference between these two (or the above four) categories as categories. Moral differences occur in such cases only at the level of the kind and magnitude of the harms inflicted on or allowed to occur to X.

Nonetheless, it is preferable to distinguish the principles of nonmaleficence and beneficence in the following way:

Nonmaleficence
1. One ought not to inflict evil or harm.

Beneficence
2. One ought to prevent evil or harm.
3. One ought to remove evil or harm.
4. One ought to do or promote good.

All three forms of beneficence involve positive acts—preventing harm, removing harm, and promoting good—whereas nonmaleficence involves noninfliction of harm.

There are disputes about how to classify or characterize particular actions under categories 1 through 4 and also about which obligations are involved in various circumstances. For example, in Case 25, Robert McFall was dying of aplastic anemia, and his physicians thought that a bone marrow transplant from a genetically compatible donor could increase his chances of surviving for one year from twenty-five percent to forty to sixty percent. The patient's cousin, David Shimp, agreed to undergo the tests to determine his suitability to be a donor, but after completing the test for tissue compatibility he refused to undergo the test for genetic compatibility. He had changed his mind. McFall's lawyer asked a court to compel Shimp to undergo the second test and to donate his bone marrow if the test indicated a good match. Public discussion focused on whether Shimp had an obligation of beneficence toward McFall in the form of an obligation to prevent or remove harm or to promote McFall's welfare. McFall's lawyer also contended (unsuccessfully) that even if Shimp did not have a legal duty of beneficence to try to rescue McFall, he had a legal duty of nonmaleficence, which required that he not make McFall's situation worse. Thus, the lawyer argued, when Shimp agreed to undergo the first test and then backed out, he created a "delay of critical proportions" and violated the duty of nonmaleficence. The judge ruled that Shimp did not violate any legal duties but held nonetheless that Shimp's actions were "morally indefensible." [5] This case shows both the difficulties inherent in applying the principles of beneficence and nonmaleficence and the different approaches law and ethics may take to the same sequence of events. Other important issues in the distinction between the principles of nonmaleficence and beneficence will be considered in Chapter 5. In the remainder of this chapter we will concentrate on nonmaleficence.

Albert Jonsen has constructed a typology of uses of the principle "Do no harm" in biomedical ethics. [6] The typology includes (1) the moral requirement that medical practitioners strive to serve the well-being of their patients, (2) standards of due care, (3) risk-benefit assessments, and (4) detriment-benefit assessments. Item 1 is general and is implicit throughout this volume (especially in our discussion of professional-patient relationships in Chapters 5, 7, and 8); items 2 and 4 are analyzed below; and 3 and 4 are both treated in Chapter 5.

The distinction between risk-benefit analysis and detriment-benefit analysis is uncomplicated: The former focuses on risks of harm, whereas the latter focuses on the harms that occur at the time of the procedure or benefit. For example, an amputation is subject not only to risk-benefit analysis in view of possible infection but also to detriment-benefit analysis, because the loss of the limb is a certain detriment not subject to the probabilistic language of risk. The detriment-benefit analysis figures prominently in determining when actions that cause or permit death can be viewed either as nonviolations or as justified infringements of the principle of nonmaleficence (and its derivative rules, such as the prohibition of killing). Because death can be a major harm, causing death is at least prima facie prohibited by the principle of nonmaleficence. Much of this chapter is devoted to questions of the justification, if any, for actions that have a causal connection to another's death.

The concept of harm

The concept of nonmaleficence is frequently explicated by the terms *harm* and *injury*, both of which need analysis. *Injury* may refer to harm, disability, or death on the one hand, or to injustice or wrong on the other. Ross, for example, regards "not injuring others" as a synonym of "nonmaleficence" and includes under the duty of nonmaleficence several of the Decalogue's prohibitions of harmful actions, such as killing, stealing, committing adultery, and bearing false witness.[7]

The term *harm* has a similar ambiguity. As Joel Feinberg notes, to say that X harmed Y may mean that X wronged Y or treated Y unjustly, or that X invaded and thus thwarted, defeated, or set back Y's interests.[8] We cannot here dispose of the intricate conceptual problems that surround analysis of the notion of harm, but in order to explicate the principle of nonmaleficence, we will construe harm in the latter sense: the thwarting, defeating, or setting back of the interests of one party by the invasive actions of another party. Not every invasion of another's interests is wrong—or wrong on balance—merely because it is harmful. Some harmful actions are justifiable and excusable setbacks to another's interests. For example, all justified criminal punishments satisfy this description. It is important not to confuse statements about the justification of a harm with statements about the nature of a harm.

Some definitions of harm are broad enough to include setbacks to reputation, property, privacy, or liberty—all viewed as interests of persons. Within this broad definition trivial harms can be distinguished from serious harms by the order and magnitude of the interests affected. Other definitions have a narrower focus and view harms exclusively as setbacks to physical and perhaps mental interests (e.g., health and survival), thus disallowing setbacks to other interests, such as property and liberty. Whether the broad or the narrow definition of harm is preferable is not critical for our discussion. We will concentrate on physical harms, including pain, disability, and death, without denying the importance of mental harms and setbacks to other interests. In particular, we will emphasize intending, causing, and permitting death and the risks of death.

Because of the wide range of types of harms, the principle of nonmaleficence supports several moral rules. Rules prohibiting harmful actions are at the core of morality—for example, "Don't kill," "Don't cause pain," "Don't disable," "Don't deprive of freedom of opportunity," and "Don't deprive of pleasure."[9] Neither the principle of nonmaleficence nor any of these derivative moral rules is absolute; they are all prima facie binding. For instance, it is often appropriate—with the patient's consent—to inflict a harm in order to prevent death. Furthermore, it is sometimes justifiable to inflict harm on one person in order to protect another. For example, a policeman sometimes justifiably shoots a criminal in order to protect the criminal's intended victims or hostages. However, these prima facie principles and rules of nonmaleficence identify actions that always stand in need of moral justification *because* they inflict harm. Some philosophers, including Ross, assign a priority in their system to principles and rules that prohibit infliction of harm.[10] We will not, however, follow this ordering principle or any other hierarchical arrangement of principles.

The standard of due care

Duties of nonmaleficence include not imposing risks of harm as well as not inflicting actual harms. It is possible to violate the obligation of nonmaleficence without acting maliciously and without being aware of or intending the harm or risk of harm. Such a violation may involve omission as well as commission. In cases of risk imposition, law and morality recognize a standard of due care. This standard can be met when the goals sought are weighty and important enough to justify the imposition of risks on others. Grave risks require commensurately important goals for their justification, and emergencies may justify risks that calculations of good and evil in nonemergency situations will not justify. For example, saving lives after a major accident may justify the dangers created by speeding emergency vehicles. (We will return to these themes when we discuss the weight of beneficence and risk-benefit analysis in Chapter 5, where we will also provide a fuller analysis of risk.)

Negligence—that is, a departure from the standard of due care toward others—includes not only deliberately imposed risks that are unreasonable but also carelessly imposed risks. The moral requirement to act carefully is not separate from other moral duties such as nonmaleficence, and there is no moral rule against negligence as such. Rather, the term *negligence* applies to various forms of failure to meet moral obligations, including the failure to guard against risks of harm to others.[11] Under negligence we will concentrate on conduct that falls

below a standard of due care, established by law or by morality, for the protection of others from the careless or unreasonable imposition of risks.[12]

The standard of due care is commonly applied in legal cases. Courts determine responsibility and liability for harm, often because a patient, client, or
customer seeks compensation for setbacks or punishment of the responsible
party, or both. Legal liability or compensation need not be considered here,
but the legal model of responsibility for harmful action does suggest a general
framework that can be adapted to express the idea of moral responsibility for
harm caused by health-care professionals. With regard to due care, legal standards and moral standards should be reasonably similar, although there are
good reasons why the law cannot always follow moral standards. (See our
discussion of the law of informed consent in Chapter 3 and our general discussion of law and morality in Chapter 1.)

In the due care model, to be morally blameworthy a harm must be caused
by negligence, that is, by a failure to discharge a socially, legally, or morally
imposed duty to take care or to act reasonably toward others. Therefore, the
following are essential elements in a professional model of due care:

(1) the professional must have a duty to the affected party;
(2) the professional must breach that duty;
(3) the affected party must experience a harm; and
(4) this harm must be caused by the breach of duty.[13]

Professional malpractice is an instance of negligence in which professional
standards of care have not been followed—for example, when a physician fails
to follow a standard therapy that any competent physician should follow.

For health-care professionals, the legal and moral standards of due care include proper training, skills, and diligence. In making services available, physicians create the expectation that they will observe these standards. If their
conduct falls below these standards, they act negligently. Even if the therapeutic relationship proves to be harmful or unhelpful, the patient cannot successfully charge malpractice unless the physician failed to meet professional standards of care. For example, in *Adkins* v. *Ropp,* the supreme court of Indiana
considered a patient's claim that a physician had been negligent in removing
foreign matter from the patient's eye and that, as a result, the eye became
infected and blinded. The court held as follows:

When a physician and surgeon assumes to treat and care for a patient, in the absence of
a special agreement, he is held in law to have impliedly contracted that he possesses
the reasonable and ordinary qualifications of his profession and that he will exercise at
least reasonable skill, care and diligence in his treatment of him. This implied contract
on the part of the physician does not include a promise to effect a cure and negligence
cannot be imputed because a cure is not effected, but he does impliedly promise that he

will use due diligence and ordinary skill in his treatment of the patient so that a cure may follow such care and skill, and this degree of care and skill is required of him, not only in performing an operation or administering first treatments, but he is held to the like degree of care and skill in the necessary subsequent treatments unless he is excused from further service by the patient himself, or the physician or surgeon upon due notice refuses to further treat the case. In determining whether the physician or surgeon has exercised the degree of skill and care which the law requires, regard must be had to the advanced state of the profession at the time of treatment and in the locality in which the physician or surgeon practices.[14]

What constitutes due care will vary from context to context. The customs, practices, and policies of the medical profession—and specializations within the profession—will in part contribute to establishing some applicable standards. For example, the Principles of Medical Ethics of the American Medical Association require physicians to provide "competent medical service" and to "continue to study, apply and advance scientific knowledge." Furthermore, in some circumstances, "a physician shall . . . obtain consultation, and use the talents of other health professionals when indicated." These dicta establish standards, although they must allow for the inherent fallibility of clinical judgment. Due care requirements cannot eliminate mistakes or prevent all harms; they can only reduce the probability of things going badly in diagnosis and treatment.

The principle of double effect

Through a long history, primarily but not exclusively in the Roman Catholic tradition, the principle of double effect has been invoked to support claims that an act having a harmful effect such as death does not always fall under moral prohibitions such as the rule against killing.[15] This principle has been widely used in certain deontological writings, especially those holding that some actions are wrong in themselves regardless of their consequences.

Conditions and applications of the principle

According to this principle there is a morally relevant difference between the intended effects of a person's action and the nonintended though foreseen effects of the action. An act of killing the innocent is wrong in itself, but it may nevertheless be permissible to allow the bad effect of a person's death to occur if this effect is a nonintended consequence of an action performed for the sake of a good (and overriding) effect. The good effect is seen as direct and intended; the harmful effect is seen as indirect, unintended, or merely foreseen. The principle, then, allows an agent to bring about a bad effect indirectly that it is not permissible to bring about directly. To say that the effect is indirect is to say that it is not intended either as a means to another end or as an end in itself.

The Roman Catholic position on abortion provides an instructive example of the use of the principle of double effect. Catholic opposition to abortion is based on an acceptance of the prohibition against killing innocent human beings and the conviction that human life begins at conception. Here a moral principle is combined with a claim about the beginning of human life. Despite the prohibition of abortion, which is viewed as the moral equivalent of murder, Catholic teaching acknowledges at least two situations in which the death of the fetus—as a result of a physician's actions—does not lead to a judgment that the physician performed an abortion or committed a moral wrong. Both situations involve conditions that threaten the pregnant woman: cancerous uterus and ectopic pregnancy. In both, the death of the fetus is held to be the indirect, unintended effect of a morally legitimate medical procedure. The argument is not that abortion is justified in these cases but that these deaths do not count as abortions because they are indirect and unintended.[16]

The principle of double effect specifies four conditions that must be satisfied for an act with both a good and a bad effect to be justified. (1) The action itself (independent of its consequences) must not be intrinsically wrong (it must be morally good or at least morally neutral). (2) The agent must intend only the good effect and not the bad effect. The bad effect can be foreseen, tolerated, and permitted but must not be intended; it is therefore allowed but not sought. (Some philosophers prefer to use Jeremy Bentham's language of "obliquely intentional" for these "merely foreseen" effects.) (3) The bad effect must not be a means to the end of bringing about the good effect; that is, the good effect must be achieved directly by the action and not by way of the bad effect. (4) The good result must outweigh the evil permitted; that is, there must be proportionality or a favorable balance between the good and bad effects of the action.[17]

Although traditional formulations require that all four conditions be satisfied, some recent formulations have highlighted one or more conditions while downplaying others. Some theologians now emphasize the fourth element of the principle—proportionality between good and bad effects—almost to the exclusion of other elements. As a result, it is difficult to distinguish their position as a mode of reasoning from utilitarianism, despite the differences in their more general conceptions of values and disvalues. By contrast, some theologians and philosophers focus primarily on the agent's intention rather than on the effects caused by the agent.[18] Traditionalists, however, insist on all four conditions, each strictly formulated.[19]

Catholic moralists have traditionally applied these four conditions to a range of moral problems. The removal of a cancerous uterus that results in the foreseen but not intended death of the fetus is a widely used test case. The action of removing the cancerous uterus in this situation is a permissible obstetrical procedure that has good and bad effects. The physician intends only the good effect (saving the mother's life), not the bad effect (the death of the fetus). This claim about the acceptability of the agent's intention is made, in part, because the fetus's death is not a means to the end of saving the mother's life. If the fetus's death were a means, it would be intended along with the end. But saving the mother's life is only contingent upon the fetus's removal, not upon its death. Its death is an unintended though foreseen effect and is neither an end nor a means to an end. Finally, saving the mother's life is a sufficient reason for performing the medical procedure and for allowing the death of the fetus, because the good effect outweighs the evil one.

Suppose, by contrast, that a physician determines that it is necessary to perform a fetal craniotomy—now rare—in order to save a woman in labor. Here the woman will die if the fetus's head is not crushed. This procedure is disqualified by the principle of double effect, because killing the fetus is the means to the good end of saving the mother's life. Whereas the woman's death is not intended by the decision not to operate (she is permitted to die), the fetus's death would be directly, even if regrettably, willed and brought about (an act of murder). Since a papal decree in 1884, this procedure has been condemned in the Roman Catholic tradition for failing to meet the conditions of the principle of double effect.

Sometimes the principle of double effect is also invoked to justify the deaths of civilians in wartime as the indirect result of an attack on a legitimate military target or to justify an agent's acceptance of the risk of death for a good cause. If the conditions of the principle of double effect are met, the former is not considered murder and the latter is not considered suicide. In traditions that condemn suicide, intentional risk-taking can be justified in life-threatening circumstances, so long as one does not intend to cause one's death either as a means or as an end. Heroes, martyrs, and the like presumably fit this description.

More generally, appeals to the principle of double effect have been prominent when obligations or values conflict and not all can be realized simultaneously. These obligations are often to different parties, such as the pregnant woman and the fetus, but two obligations to the same party also may conflict. The latter conflict may occur in the care of terminally ill patients when there is an obligation of nonmaleficence, including an obligation not to kill, and also an obligation of beneficence to make the patient comfortable by inducing sleep and alleviating pain. If these obligations conflict, it may be possible to make the patient comfortable only by using medications that may hasten and thus cause the patient's death. If the four conditions of the principle of double effect are met and thus a physician intends only relief of pain and not death, its adherents agree that hastening the patient's death does not qualify as homicide and is justified.

For example, according to the Ethical and Religious Directives for Catholic Health Facilities, "it is not euthanasia to give a dying person sedatives and analgesics for the alleviation of pain, when such a measure is judged necessary, even though they may deprive the patient of the use of reason, or shorten his life."[20] Similarly, the statement on euthanasia by the Vatican accepts the use of painkillers that may hasten and thus cause death: "In this case, of course, death is no way intended or sought, even if the risk of it is reasonably taken; the intention is simply to relieve pain effectively, using for this purpose pain-killers available in medicine."[21] However, if an agent using the same medication intends the same death, the action would not be acceptable.

Critique of the principle

Despite its intuitive plausibility, the principle of double effect has several problems that cannot be overcome short of transforming the principle into a different principle. We shall examine two types of problems with the principle: (1) conceptual and theoretical issues about the nature of acting (or omitting) intentionally and about what counts as an intended effect, and (2) moral problems about whether the principle of double effect correctly locates a morally relevant difference between actions or effects of action.

Adherents of double effect need an account of intentional actions and intended effects of action that allows them to be distinguished in just the right way from nonintentional actions and unintended effects. But the literature on intentional action is filled with diverse accounts that analyze the notion in terms of actions variously described as volitional, deliberate, self-controlled, willed, reasoned, planned, or instrumental. One of the few widely shared views in this literature is that intentional acts require an agent's plan—a blueprint, map, or representation of the means and ends proposed for the execution of an action.[22] Thus, for an act to be intentional, it must correspond to the agent's conception of how it was planned to be performed. Intentional actions also do not merely happen to people, and they are not accidental, inadvertent, or performed by mistake. Instead, the actor must make the act happen or, in the case of omission, control the outcome.

A critical question for theories of double effect is whether unwanted effects of actions that are willed in accordance with a plan are intended effects. Adherents of the principle accept the view that foreseen effects that the actor does not want or desire are not intentional. Alvin Goldman uses the following example in an attempt to prove that merely foreseen effects are unintentional.[23] Imagine that Mr. G is taking a driver's test to prove competence, he comes to an intersection that requires a right turn, and he extends his arm to signal for a turn, although he knows it is raining and his hand will get wet. According to Goldman, Mr. G's signaling for a turn is an intentional act. By contrast, his getting a wet hand is an unintended effect or "incidental by-product."

Such effects in double-effect theory are viewed as merely foreseen. They are wanted only in the distant sense that the actor wants to perform an act that entails them more than he or she wants not to perform the act. Here, we suggest, it is better to discard the language of wanting altogether and to say, as Hector Castañeda puts it, that they are "tolerated" effects.[24] They are not so undesirable as to cause the actor to choose against performing the desired act that entails them. The undesired effect is entailed in the plan of an intentional action, but adherents of double effect insist that not all effects entailed in intentional action are intended effects. To a defender of the principle, the physician who foresees a patient's death because of heavy administration of sedatives does not intend to bring about the patient's death when he or she administers medication to relieve pain.

In order to avoid the conclusion that an agent intentionally brings about all the consequences of an action that the agent foresees, the defender of double effect elects a narrow conception of what is intended. The defender distinguishes between acts and effects and then between effects that are desired or wanted and effects that are foreseen but not desired or wanted. This narrow zone of what is intended is a vital element in the theory because it is the moral basis on which foreseen harmful outcomes can be permitted; without this narrowed conception of what is intended, a physician, for example, could never intentionally do anything that would allow a harmful or otherwise bad outcome and thus would often be suspended in action while avoiding doing good for patients. But with this account of what is intended, there is no need to absolutely prohibit any particular outcome such as death, because prohibitions apply only to certain kinds of intentional acts.

However, if we use a broader model of intentionality based on what is willed rather than what is wanted, intentional actions and intentional effects can be interpreted to include any action and any effect willed in accordance with a plan, including tolerated as well as wanted effects.[25] In this conception a physician can want not to do what he intends to do, in the same way that we can be willing to do something but at the same time be reluctant to do it. Undesirable effects or risks of harm that attend particular procedures almost always fall into this category. In this connection of intentional acts and intentional effects, then, the distinction between what is intended and what is foreseen is not viable.[26]

This account of intended effects can be developed as follows. If a person knowingly and voluntarily acts to bring about an effect, the person brings about the effect intentionally. The effect is intended even if the person did not desire it, did not will it for its own sake, or did not intend it as the goal of the action. This is not to say (as the defender of double effect steadfastly resists, and rightly so) that a person intends all the consequences of any action that is intentional, for that is manifestly false. The man who intentionally pulls a trigger in the effort to kill a snake but instead shoots himself in the foot does not intend to shoot himself in the foot. But if the snake were on his foot and he voluntarily and knowingly shot through the snake's head and into his foot, then he intentionally shot himself in the foot (and intended the consequence of a bullet-impacted foot). To say that he did not intentionally shoot himself in the foot would be similar to saying that when one enters a room and flips a switch that one knows turns on both a light and a fan, and one desires only to activate the light, one therefore turns on the fan unintentionally. If the fan makes an obnoxious whirring that the person wishes to avoid, it seems conceptually mistaken to say that the person unintentionally brought about this obnoxious sound by flipping the switch.

A person is also morally responsible for any effect of an action of this description. Clearly it is not true that because someone does not want a particular effect of a voluntary action the person is relieved of moral responsibility for causing the effect. But no proponent of double effect would say this, either; double-effect theory is not an attempt to absolve persons of responsibility for what they bring about but only to determine what it is permissible to bring about.

The moral relevance of the distinction between direct willing of a good effect and indirect willing of a bad effect can now be further considered. First, is it plausible to distinguish morally between intentionally causing the death of a fetus by craniotomy and intentionally removing a cancerous uterus that causes the death of a fetus? In both actions, the intention is to save a woman's life with knowledge that the fetus will be lost. In these cases, no agent desires a bad result (the fetus's death) for its own sake, and none would have tolerated the bad result if its avoidance were morally preferable. Each party wants the bad effect only because it cannot be eliminated without losing the good effect. Thus, the agents in our various examples above do not appear to want, will, or intend in ways that make a moral difference. None of these agents is in a position that is morally more favorable than that of the contrasting agents in these examples.

In the standard interpretation of double effect, the vital difference is that the fetus's death is a means to saving a woman's life in the unacceptable case but is merely a side effect in the acceptable case. A means must be intended, whereas a side effect need not be. The problem with this reply, as we have seen, is that it is questionable as an account of what is intended. Worse, the account would permit too much because it would justify all deaths that are the side effects of agents' plans (if the other conditions of double effect are satisfied). This approach seems to allow that almost anything can be foreseen as a side effect rather than intended as a means. For example, in the craniotomy case, why not say that the surgeon does not intend the death of the fetus but only intends to change its spatial location so that the woman will not die? The child will die, but can we not say this is an unwanted and (on this theory) unintended consequence?[27]

There may be a way out of these puzzles for defenders of double effect, but it is doubtful that any way has been found as yet.[28] Meanwhile, other complaints have been heard that need to be answered. For example, those who accept a broadly consequentialist rather than deontological account of ethical theory have also complained that there are unacceptable moral consequences that are deemed acceptable in double-effect theory. For example, processes of starvation or slowly causing death by pain medication may involve painful days or weeks of a life that a patient wishes to end, whereas a more active means to death such as a larger and lethal dose of the same painkiller would end the matter more quickly and with less pain. The claim is that double effect drives its exponents to less humane methods of ending human life than can and should be provided.

One effort to retain an emphasis on intention without entirely abandoning or neglecting the point of the principle of double effect focuses on the way actions display a person's motives and character—a theme that will be developed at greater length in Chapter 8.[29] From this perspective, the question is whether a person's conduct flows from a proper motivational structure or a good character. Thus, performing a craniotomy to save a pregnant woman's life need not display a disregard for human life or a positive desire to end it. While it seems implausible to distinguish the above two cases of fetal death in terms of the physician's intention, the physician may not want or desire the death of the fetus and may regret it in removing a cancerous uterus or in performing a craniotomy. These facts about the physician's motivation and perhaps character may make a decisive moral difference. But the principle of double effect seems unable to reach this conclusion on its own. In effect, the principle has been transformed into another moral framework about motivation and character.

Although the principle of double effect is fashioned for the discussion of actions and the effects of actions, it would perhaps be a better principle if it were reconstructed as an account of the motives of agents. We would, on this account, rightly evaluate the following two physicians quite differently. (1) Physician A lets a chronically ill, debilitated patient die out of frustration with the patient and the patient's family. (2) Physician B lets an identically situated chronically ill, debilitated patient die out of mercy and at the request of the patient and the family. Both physician A and physician B intend to let the patient die and use the same merciful means. Still, the different desires, goals, and motives of the two agents entail different evaluations of them. In the final analysis, the moral theory proposed by adherents of double effect seems to us sound in spirit but misplaced. One's motives in bringing about a consequence do make a significant difference in moral evaluation, but this is not because one either intends or does not intend the outcome.

Regarding the care of patients, few would dispute the conclusions reached by adherents of double effect about the justifiability of hastening death by relieving pain and inducing sleep in some circumstances. But the principle fails to resolve many of the difficult cases and cannot do all the moral work that must be done. As we argue below, some actions that intentionally and directly result in death are justifiable. For example, removing a respirator with the intention of terminating life is justified under some conditions. When the Council on Ethical and Judicial Affairs of the American Medical Association holds that the physician "should not intentionally cause death," this pronouncement comes immediately after the statement that it is ethical to "cease or omit treatment to permit a terminally ill patient whose death is imminent to die."[30]

Because omissions and cessations may involve the intentional causation of death, it is misleading and ill considered to say that physicians morally should not intend to cause death. The double-effect account seems to place us in the untenable position of saying that physician X is morally better than physician Y if X is able to keep away from consciousness the idea that X's action has an intended goal or consequence of a certain sort such as death. That is, if physician Y simply cannot avoid thinking that his or her act is undertaken to bring about the death of a patient, then Y must be judged morally defective by comparison to X, who does successfully avoid framing the same act as being undertaken to bring about the patient's death. There is also a further related defect in the case of hastening the death of terminal patients: If a physician called upon to alleviate a patient's pain so as to risk death cannot avoid the mental act of intending the patient's death in the act of administering the pain relief, then the physician morally cannot administer the additional medication. This does seem an unsatisfactory outcome of a moral theory.

In many cases, especially those of patients who wish to die, the proper moral question is not whether a patient's death is intended as an end or as a means but whether the conditions are sufficient to justify an intentional act of causing death—an answer that cannot be forthcoming from the principle of double effect alone. To obtain appropriate answers, we need first to consider the distinction between killing and letting die and its use in moral arguments.

Killing and letting die

In a well-known case, a sixty-eight-year-old doctor who suffered severely from terminal carcinoma of the stomach collapsed with a massive pulmonary embolism. He survived because one of his young colleagues performed a pulmonary embolectomy. Upon recovery, the doctor-patient requested that no steps be taken to prolong his life if he suffered another cardiovascular collapse. He wrote an authorization to this effect for the hospital records. Viewing his pain as too much to bear given his dismal prospects, he asked to be allowed to die, under specified conditions. However, he did not ask to be killed.[31]

In Case 20, a newborn with Down syndrome needed an operation to correct a tracheoesophageal fistula. The parents and physicians determined that survival was not in this infant's best interests and decided to allow the infant to die rather than to perform an operation. In these and other cases, we need to ask whether certain actions, such as intentionally not attempting to save the patient after a cardiovascular collapse and not performing an operation, can legitimately be described as ''allowing to die'' or ''letting die'' rather than ''killing,'' and whether such actions are justifiable.

For many people, it is important both to distinguish between killing and letting die and to prohibit the former while authorizing the latter in some cases. After prohibiting ''mercy killing'' or the ''intentional termination of the life of one human being by another,'' the American Medical Association House of Delegates in 1973 held that cessation of treatment is morally justified when the patient or the patient's immediate family, with the advice and judgment of the physician, decides to withhold or withdraw ''extraordinary means to prolong the life of the body when there is irrefutable evidence that biological death is imminent.''[32] Although several terms in this statement, including *extraordinary, irrefutable,* and *imminent,* need careful examination, the statement clearly permits some instances of intentional allowing to die by withholding or stopping treatment, but it excludes killing. Whether letting particular patients die is morally acceptable depends in this policy on several factors. But if their deaths in identical circumstances were to involve killing rather than being merely allowed to die, they are never justifiable, according to the guidelines.

Attacks on the distinction between killing and letting die

In recent years, the distinction between killing and letting die has come under frequent attack. Some critics focus on developments in biomedical technology that appear to make it conceptually difficult to classify acts as instances either of killing or of letting die. Stopping a respirator is a standard example of this problem. Other critics dismiss the distinction as a conceptual quibble without moral significance.

Before we explore and assess the arguments for and against this distinction, we note that acceptance or rejection of the conceptual distinction does not by itself determine moral conclusions about particular cases. For instance, one might deny that there is a clear conceptual difference between killing and letting die, while at the same time holding either that some cases of so-called killing and letting die are morally permissible or that all cases are morally impermissible. It is also possible to affirm the distinction and yet to hold that many cases of letting die and all cases of killing are morally wrong. Even if the distinction is morally significant, the labels "killing" and "letting die" should not be used to dictate moral conclusions about particular cases. For example, it would be absurd to affirm the moral significance of the distinction and then to accept all cases of letting die as morally fitting. Even instances of letting die must meet other criteria such as the balance of benefits over burdens to the patient, and some cases of allowed death involve egregious negligence.

In a widely discussed argument for rejecting both the distinction between active and passive euthanasia and the AMA policy statement, James Rachels contends that killing is not, in itself, worse than letting die.[33] That is, the "bare difference" between acts of killing and acts of letting die is not in itself a morally relevant difference. Rachels argues that if it is morally permissible to act intentionally so that a person dies, then the only morally significant question about how death may occur concerns which method will minimize the person's suffering. Part of Rachels's strategy is to sketch two cases that differ only in that one involves killing while the other involves allowing to die. He contends that if there is no morally relevant difference between these cases, the bare difference between acts of killing and allowing to die cannot be morally relevant. In his two cases, two young men, Smith and Jones, want their six-year-old cousins dead so that they can gain inheritances. Smith drowns his cousin while the boy is taking a bath. Jones plans to drown his cousin, but as he enters the bathroom he sees the boy slip and hit his head. Jones stands by, doing nothing, while the boy drowns. Thus, Smith killed his cousin, but Jones merely allowed his cousin to die.

While we agree with Rachels that these acts are equally reprehensible because of the agents' motives and actions, we do not accept his conclusion that these examples show that the distinction between killing and letting die is morally irrelevant. Several rejoinders to Rachels are in order. First, Rachels's cases and the cessations of treatment envisioned by the AMA are so markedly disanalogous that Rachels's argument is misdirected. In some cases of unjustified acts, including both of Rachels's examples, we are not interested in moral distinctions per se. As Richard Trammell points out, some examples have a "masking" or "sledgehammer" effect; the fact that "one cannot distinguish the taste of two wines when both are mixed with green persimmon juice, does not imply that there is no distinction between the wines."[34] Because Rachels's examples involve two morally unjustified acts by agents whose motives and intentions are despicable, it is not surprising that some other features of their situations, such as killing and letting die, do not seem morally compelling considerations in the circumstances.

Second, in Rachels's cases Smith and Jones are morally responsible and morally blameworthy for the deaths of their respective cousins, even if Jones, who allowed his cousin to drown, is not causally responsible. The law might find only Smith, who killed his cousin, guilty of homicide (because of the law's theory of proximate cause), but morality condemns both actions alike because of the agents' commissions and omissions. We find Jones's actions reprehensible because he could and morally should have rescued the child. Even if he had no other special duties to the child, the obligation of beneficence requires affirmative action in such a case.

Third, the point of the cases envisioned by the AMA is not inconsistent with Rachels's points. The AMA's central claim is that the physician is always morally prohibited from killing patients but is not morally bound to preserve life in all cases. According to the AMA, the physician has a right and perhaps a duty to stop treatment if and only if three conditions are met: (1) the life of the body is being preserved by extraordinary means, (2) there is irrefutable evidence that biological death is imminent, and (3) the patient or the family consents. While Rachels's cases involve two unjustified actions, one of killing and the other of letting die, the AMA statement distinguishes cases of unjustified killing from cases of justified letting die. The AMA statement does not claim that the moral difference is entirely predicated on the distinction between killing and letting die. It also does not imply that the bare difference between (passive) letting die and (active) killing is the major difference or a morally sufficient difference to distinguish the justified from the unjustified cases. The point is rather that the justified actions in medicine are confined to (passive) letting die.

The AMA statement holds that "mercy killing" in medicine is unjustified in all circumstances, but it holds neither that letting die is right in all circumstances nor that killing outside medicine is always wrong. For an act that results in an earlier death for the patient to be justified, it is necessary that it be an act of letting die, but this condition is not sufficient to justify the act; nor is the bare fact of an act's being a killing sufficient to make the act wrong. This AMA declaration is meant to control conduct exclusively in the context of the physician-patient relationship.

Even if the distinction between killing and letting die is morally irrelevant in some contexts, it does not follow that it is morally irrelevant in all contexts. Although Rachels does effectively undermine all attempts to rest moral judgments about ending life on the "bare difference" between killing and letting die, his target may nonetheless be made of straw. Many philosophers and theologians have argued that there are independent moral, religious, and other reasons both for defending the distinction and for prohibiting killing while authorizing allowing to die in some circumstances or based on some motives.

One theologian has argued, for example, that we can discern the moral significance of the distinction between killing and letting die by "placing it in the religious context out of which it grew."[35] That context is the biblical story of

God's actions toward his creatures. In that context it makes sense to talk about "placing patients in God's hands," just as it is important not to usurp God's prerogatives by desperately struggling to prolong life when the patient is irreversibly dying. But even if the distinction between killing and letting die originated within a religious context, and even if it makes more sense in that context than in some others, it can be defended on nontheological grounds without being reduced to a claim about a "bare difference." We turn next to this defense of the distinction.

A defense of the distinction between killing and letting die

Even if there are sufficient reasons in some cases to warrant mercy killing, there may also be good reasons to retain the distinction between killing and letting die and to maintain our current practices against killing *in medicine*, albeit with some clarifications and modifications. We defend this perspective in this section.

ACTS AND PRACTICES. The most important arguments for the distinction between killing and letting die depend on a distinction between acts and practices.[36] It is one thing to justify an act; it is another to justify a general practice. As we saw in our examination of rule utilitarianism and rule deontology, many beliefs about principles and consequences are applied to rules rather than directly to acts. For example, we might justify a rule of confidentiality because it encourages people to seek therapy and because it promotes respect for persons and their privacy, although such rule might lead to undesirable results in particular cases. Likewise, a rule that prohibits "active killing" while permitting some "allowed deaths" may be justifiable, even if it excludes some particular acts of killing that in themselves are justifiable. For example, the rule would not permit us to kill a patient who suffers from terrible pain, who will probably die within three weeks, and who rationally asks for a merciful assisted death. In order to maintain a viable practice that expresses our principles and avoids seriously undesirable consequences, it may be necessary to prohibit some acts that would not otherwise be wrong. Thus, although particular acts of killing may not violate the obligation of nonmaleficence and may be humane and compassionate, a policy that authorizes killing in medicine—in even a few cases—stands to violate the obligation of nonmaleficence by creating a grave risk of harm in many cases.

The prohibition of killing even for "mercy" expresses principles and supports practices that provide a basis of trust between patients and health-care professionals. When we trust such professionals, we expect them to promote our welfare and to do us no harm without a prospect of benefit as well as our consent. Trust, or the attitude of confidence and reliance placed in persons and institutions, can exist with little actual evidence of real trustworthiness (the quality or character trait of reliability, which is closely associated with fidelity and loyalty). The prohibition of killing is an attempt to promote a solid basis for trust in the role of caring for patients and protecting them from harm. This prohibition is both instrumentally and symbolically important, and its removal could weaken a set of practices and restraints that we cannot easily replace.[37]

WEDGE OR SLIPPERY SLOPE ARGUMENTS. This last argument—a wedge or slippery slope argument—is plausible but needs to be stated carefully. Because of the widespread misuses of such arguments in biomedical ethics (and perhaps because of their heavily metaphorical character—"the leading, entering, or thin edge of the wedge," "the first step on the slippery slope," "the foot in the door," and "the camel's nose under the tent"), there is a tendency to dismiss them whenever they are offered. However, as expressions of the principle of nonmaleficence, they are defensible in some cases.[38] They also force us to consider whether unacceptable harms may result from attractive and apparently innocent first steps. All of the metaphors invoked in this connection are used to express the conviction that legitimation of some forms of action, such as active voluntary euthanasia, will lead to other acts or practices that are morally objectionable even if some individual acts of this type are acceptable in themselves. The claim is that accepting the act in question would cross a line that has already been drawn against killing; and once that line has been crossed, it will not be possible to draw it again to preclude unacceptable acts or practices.

Wedge or slippery slope arguments appear in two versions: *logical-conceptual* and *psychological-sociological*. The first version maintains that there is no defensible line between acts leading to legitimate deaths and those leading to illegitimate deaths, unless there is a clear distinction sustained by moral reasons. A justification offered for one sort of act that strikes us as right may logically support another sort of act that strikes us as wrong. For example, some justifications offered for abortion logically imply a justification of infanticide under relevantly similar circumstances, and yet the act of infanticide seems wrong (to defenders of the similar act of abortion).

This first version of the wedge argument derives its power from the principle of universalizability discussed in Chapter 1. That principle commits us to ethical consistency and thus to judging relevantly similar cases in a similar way. If we judge X to be right, and we can point to no morally relevant dissimilarities between X and Y, then we logically cannot judge Y to be wrong. This first version of the wedge argument focuses on how support for one sort of action that seems acceptable logically implies support for another unacceptable action, where it is not possible in principle to identify morally relevant differences.[39]

Defenders of the prohibition of mercy killing sometimes appeal to this version of the wedge argument in the following way. Whereas we morally justify killing aggressors in self-defense and war, these killings do not threaten the following rule, which is derived from the principle of nonmaleficence: Do not directly kill innocent persons. Killing in self-defense or war is justified because the persons killed are not innocent. By contrast, if we once support the killing of innocent persons in medical settings, there is no clear way to limit the killing to legitimate cases of mercy directed at appropriate parties, because there will be no way to distinguish these parties from the vulnerable, the defenseless, the socially nonproductive, and the like.

Wedge arguments of this type may not be as damaging as they may seem at first. As Rachels correctly contends, "there obviously are good reasons for objecting to killing patients in order to get away for the weekend—or for even more respectable purposes, such as securing organs for transplantation—which do not apply to killing in order to put the patient out of extreme agony."[40] In other words, the counterreply is that relevant distinctions can be drawn, and we are not subject to uncontrollable implications from general principles. This first version of the wedge argument thus does not assist supporters of the distinction between killing and letting die as much as they might suppose. Indeed, it can be used against them: If it is rational and morally defensible to allow patients to die under conditions X, Y, and Z, it is rational and morally defensible to kill them under those same conditions. If it is in their best interests to die, it is (prima facie) irrelevant how death is brought about. Rachels makes a similar point when he argues that reliance on the distinction between killing and letting die may lead to decisions about life and death made on irrelevant grounds—such as whether the patient will or will not die without certain forms of treatment—instead of being made in terms of the patient's best interests.[41]

For example, in Case 20, a baby suffering from several defects needs an operation to correct a tracheoesophageal fistula; otherwise the baby will die. A baby suffering from those same defects but without the fistula may be kept alive, while the baby who needs the operation may be allowed to die. It is possible to argue that we need to determine the conditions under which death is in the baby's best interests and then choose to kill or to let die by determining which means would be more humane and compassionate in the circumstances. In the now famous Johns Hopkins Hospital case, an infant with Down syndrome and duodenal atresia was placed in a back room and died eleven days later of dehydration and starvation. This process of dying, which senior physicians had recommended against, was extremely difficult for all the parties involved, particularly the nurses. If the decision makers legitimately determine that a patient would be better off dead (we think the parties mistakenly came to this conclusion in these two cases), how could an act of killing violate the patient's interests if the patient will not die when artificial treatment is discontinued? A morally irrelevant factor would be allowed to dictate the outcome, and this would violate the rule of universalizability. This first version of the wedge or slippery slope argument, then, does not offer a clear and compelling reason to oppose mercy killing.

By contrast, the causal-empirical version does offer a strong reason for maintaining the distinction between killing and letting die. This psychological-sociological version focuses on what the wedge is driven into by examining the society and culture in order to determine the probable impact of making exceptions to rules or changing rules in a more permissive direction. If certain restraints against killing are removed, a moral decline might result, because various psychological or social forces make it unlikely that people will draw distinctions that are, in principle, clear and defensible. For example, in some settings it is plausible to argue that (1) to authorize killing patients for their own benefit when they are suffering excruciating pain or have a bleak future could open the door to a policy of killing patients for the sake of social benefits such as reducing financial burdens, and that (2) voluntary euthanasia might open the door to nonvoluntary and perhaps involuntary euthanasia.

These arguments do not depend on the conceptual version of the wedge or slippery slope arguments, because there are clear and defensible distinctions, rooted in moral principles, between voluntary and involuntary euthanasia and between killing patients at their request for their own benefit and killing them without their request for social benefits. Nevertheless, if there are psychological and social forces such as racism, an increasing number of handicapped newborns who survive at large expense to the public, or a growing number of aging persons with medical problems that require larger and larger proportions of a society's financial resources, this wedge argument becomes more compelling. We acknowledge that the success or failure of the argument depends on admittedly speculative predictions of a progressive erosion of moral restraints because of psychological or sociological forces; those, including the present authors, who accept this causal version of the wedge argument need a premise on the order of "better safe than sorry."

The main reservation expressed in this argument is the following. If rules permitting mercy killing were once introduced, society might gradually move in the direction of nonvoluntary and perhaps involuntary euthanasia—for example, in the form of killing handicapped newborns to avoid social and familial burdens. There could be a general reduction of respect for human life as a result of the official removal of barriers to killing. Rules against killing in a moral code are not isolated fragments; they are threads in a fabric of rules, drawn in part from nonmaleficence, that support respect for human life. The more threads we remove, the weaker the fabric becomes. If we focus on attitudes and not merely rules, the general attitude of respect for life may be eroded by shifts in particular areas. Determination of the likelihood of such an erosion depends not only on the connectedness of rules and attitudes but also on operative forces in the society.

THE NAZI ANALOGY. In debates about euthanasia, the holocaust under Nazi rule continues to serve as a powerful vision of the bottom of the slippery slope for a society that adopts mercy killing. Although the analogies are sometimes overplayed, this period left a string of inadequately answered questions about euthanasia. After the Nuremberg trial of German physicians, an American physician, Leo Alexander, argued that the Nazis started by accepting euthanasia for the incurably ill and then moved on to their policies of genocide:

Whatever proportions [the Nazi] crimes finally assumed, it became evident to all who investigated them that they had started from small beginnings. The beginnings at first were merely a subtle shift in emphasis in the basic attitude of the physicians. It started with the acceptance of the attitude, basic in the euthanasia movement, that there is such a thing as life not worthy to be lived. This attitude in its early stages concerned itself merely with the severely and chronically sick. Gradually the sphere of those to be included in this category was enlarged to encompass the socially unproductive, the ideologically unwanted, the racially unwanted and finally all non-Germans. But it is important to realize that the infinitely small wedged-in lever from which this entire trend of mind received its impetus was the attitude toward the nonrehabilitable sick.[42]

This image of "small beginnings" also appears in Robert Lifton's study of Nazi physicians, which describes the first steps as well as the final horror of implementing the general principle of "life unworthy of life" in an effort to "uncover psychological conditions conducive to evil."[43] Lifton notes that "prior to Auschwitz and the other death camps, the Nazis established a policy of direct medical killing: that is, killing arranged within medical channels, by means of medical decisions, and carried out by doctors and their assistants." Crucial to the program was the removal of a social and psychological barrier against killing through the "medicalization of killing," where killing was justified in the name of healing the society, a "therapeutic imperative." Lifton argues that although this program was called euthanasia, the term simply "camouflaged mass murder."

Contemporary proponents of mercy killing often properly insist that the rationale of the Nazi program was racist ideology, not respect for personal wishes and interests. They dispute the appropriateness of the Nazi analogy, because the Nazis concentrated on nonvoluntary and especially involuntary killing against the wishes of the victims—a program inappropriately labeled euthanasia, or good death. Thus, many argue, it is not the case that the Nazis took one step on the slippery slope and then could not stop. Rather, their ideology drove them to extremes.[44] Even if they had not changed their social and legal rules against killing innocent persons, their ideology encouraged redefining the "innocent" to exclude people they viewed as social threats. Hence, critics of the Nazi analogy contend, rules against mercy killing are neither necessary nor sufficient to prevent such a horrible state of affairs.

We accept this argument, but we also maintain that rules against killing, including mercy killing, are important in order to protect vital social practices and to maintain attitudes of respect for life, even if it is difficult to determine the degree of risk. This argument is not meant to suggest that mercy killing is always wrong. Rules against killing, like all moral rules, are prima facie, not absolute. We are now concentrating on rules at the level of social policy, professional ethics, and institutional directives. At this level, traditional restraints against killing are justifiable and appropriate.[45] In a particular case, the prima facie duty to refrain from killing may be outweighed by the prima facie duties to relieve suffering or to respect patients' autonomous wishes. Nevertheless, the empirical version of the wedge argument, in combination with some elements of the conceptual version and with other considerations of consequences, supports a strong rule of practice against mercy killing, backed by legal, social, and professional sanctions designed to caution health professionals and family members against expedient or ill-considered resort to killing.

An example of mercy killing that prohibitory rules should help deter was reported in the *Journal of the American Medical Association* in January 1988 under the provocative title "It's Over, Debbie."[46] A gynecology resident rotating through a large private hospital was awakened by a telephone call from a nurse who told him that a patient on the gynecologic-oncology unit, not the resident's usual duty station, was having difficulty getting rest. The chart at the nurses' station provided some details. A twenty-year-old woman named Debbie who was dying of ovarian cancer was experiencing unrelenting vomiting, apparently as a result of the alcohol drip administered for sedation (a procedure that some have criticized). The woman was emaciated, weighed eighty pounds, had an intravenous line, was receiving nasal oxygen, and was sitting in bed suffering from severe air hunger. She had not eaten or slept in two days, and she was receiving only supportive care because she had not responded to chemotherapy. The patient's only words to the resident were, "Let's get this over with." It was not reported whether the middle-aged female visitor in the room made any comments. After having the nurse draw twenty milligrams of morphine sulfate into a syringe, the resident took it into the room and injected it intravenously into the patient after telling the two women that it "would let her rest" and "to say good-bye." The patient died within a few minutes.

If this is an actual case—and doubts have been voiced about its authenticity—the resident acted rashly. Other medications could perhaps have relieved the patient's pain and suffering and enabled her to rest comfortably. The resident's intention was to kill the patient out of "mercy," not simply to provide comfort at the risk of hastening her death. But in the absence of any previous contact with the patient, the resident had no basis for interpreting her words as a request to be killed, and he or she (the gender of the resident was not reported) did not consult with anyone else before making a quick, momentous, and irreversible decision.

MERCY KILLING AND THE PRACTICE OF MEDICINE. In addition to fears of abuse of individuals such as the mentally disabled who cannot consent, there are other legitimate fears. Consider the following two types of wrongly diagnosed patients:[47]

1. Patients who are wrongly diagnosed as hopeless and who will survive if a treatment is ceased (in order to allow a natural death)
2. Patients who are wrongly diagnosed as hopeless and who will survive only if the treatment is *not* ceased (in order to allow a natural death)

If a social rule that allows some patients to die were in effect, doctors and families who followed it would only lose patients in the second category. But if killings were permitted, at least some of the patients in the first category would be needlessly lost. Thus, a rule prohibiting killing would save some lives that would be lost if both killing and allowing to die were permitted. Such a consequence is not a decisive reason for a policy of (only) allowing to die, because the numbers in categories 1 and 2 are likely to be small, and other reasons for killing, such as extreme pain and autonomous choice, might be weighty. But it is a morally relevant reason for the policy.

Proponents of the practice of killing certain patients sometimes appeal to a range of exceptional cases that override normal constraints against killing. Among the strongest reasons for killing some patients is to relieve unbearable and uncontrollable pain and suffering. No one would deny that pain and suffering can so ravage and dehumanize patients that death appears to be in their best interests. Prolonging life and refusing to kill in such circumstances may appear to be cruel and to violate the obligation of nonmaleficence. Often proponents of mercy killing appeal to nonmedical situations to show that killing may be more humane and compassionate than letting die—as, for example, in the case of a soldier mortally wounded on the battlefield or an accident victim inextricably trapped in a burning vehicle who cries out for a merciful death. In such tragic situations the present authors are reluctant to say that those who kill at the behest of the victim act wrongly. At least some such persons act justifiably and commendably.

There are, nevertheless, serious objections to building into medical practice an explicit exception that licenses physicians to kill their patients in order to relieve uncontrollable pain and suffering. It is not clear that many, if any, cases in medical practice are relevantly similar to the person trapped in a burning wreck. In medical practice the physician can usually relieve pain and make a patient comfortable without killing, or intending to kill, the patient, even if the medications may hasten death. We agree that clinicians have a moral obligation, based on nonmaleficence, beneficence, and autonomy, to relieve patients' pain in accord with their wishes and interests. However, it is important to preserve the distinction between the intention to relieve pain at the risk of hastening death and the intention to kill in order to relieve pain, however difficult it will be in borderline cases to apply the distinction. In the case of Debbie presented above, the medical resident intended to kill Debbie through the large dose of morphine sulfate in order to relieve her pain and give her rest. He or she failed to pursue other available measures that could have relieved Debbie's pain and enabled her to rest with the risk of hastened death.

Clinicians also have a moral obligation to inform patients of alternative approaches, such as a hospice, which assign a high priority to the relief of pain and suffering. The increased risk of addiction has often been overestimated and unduly feared in the care of terminally ill patients.[48] However, public policymakers in the United States have resisted legalizing heroin, a powerful painkiller, even in the care of terminally ill cancer patients, because of their fear of the harmful consequences that might flow from such an act, including not only addiction of surviving patients but also the legitimation of heroin and the possibility of abuses. Yet heroin has been used for terminally ill cancer patients for several years in Great Britain without evidence of uncontrollable problems. We thus see no merit in the societal prohibition of the use of heroin to relieve pain in terminally ill cancer patients. However, the main point is that clinicians already have under their control measures of pain relief that are both legal and generally effective. If clinicians took more seriously their obligation to relieve pain, the arguments for mercy killing from unbearable pain would be less powerful.[49]

Another reason for not giving physicians a license to kill is that we should be reluctant to construct a social or professional ethic on borderline situations and emergency cases, even if medical practititoners do confront some cases of unmanageable pain and suffering. It is dangerous to generalize from emergencies, because hard cases may make bad social and professional ethics as well as bad law. As Charles Fried writes,

The concept of emergency is only a tolerable moral concept if somehow we can truly think of it as exceptional, if we can truly think of it as a circumstance that, far from defying our usual moral universe, suspends it for a limited time and thus suspends usual moral principles. It is when emergencies become usual that we are threatened with moral disintegration, dehumanization.[50]

EXCEPTIONAL CASES. There are, we believe, ways to accept acts of killing in exceptional circumstances without altering the rules of practice in order to accommodate them. Juries often find those who kill their suffering relatives not guilty by reason of temporary insanity. Consider a famous case in New Jersey.[51] In June 1973, George Zygmaniak was in a motorcycle accident that left him paralyzed from the neck down. The paralysis was considered to be irreversible, and Zygmaniak begged his brother to kill him. Three days later, his brother brought a sawed-off shotgun to the hospital and shot Zygmaniak in the head, after having said, "Close your eyes now, I'm going to shoot you." A judgment of temporary insanity in this case springs from the lack of a legal channel to say the act was, under the circumstances, justifiable. Verdicts such as "not guilty by reason of temporary insanity" function under law to excuse the agent by finding (somewhat implausibly) that he or she lacked the conditions of responsibility necessary to be legally guilty.

The legal rule against killing can be maintained even if physicians and others sometimes find that it is morally permissible to engage in justified conscientious or civil disobedience against those rules. This is another way of acknowledging that there can be justified exceptions to enforceable rules against killing.[52] The conditions that justify conscientious refusals to follow the rule against killing patients are too complex and diverse to be considered here, but the important point is that if pain and suffering of a certain magnitude can in principle justify active killing, then only acts of conscientious refusal to follow the rule of practice will be justified (as long as certain other conditions are met), not fundamental changes in the rule itself. We do not invoke the language of "conscientious refusal" to evade acceptance of the justifiability of active killing in the difficult cases. In Chapter 8 (pp. 377–78), we present an actual case of nonvoluntary active killing by a physician that we believe was justified. We also do not believe that our position commits us to side primarily with utilitarians against deontological constraints on killing. Nothing in deontological rules of prima facie obligation prohibits killing under all possible circumstances, even for health-care professionals.

Finally, we need to ask which side in the debate has the burden of proof— the proponents or the opponents of a practice of selective killing. One prominent view is that supporters of the current practice of prohibiting killing bear the burden of proof because the prohibition of voluntary euthanasia infringes liberty and autonomy.[53] However, a policy of voluntary euthanasia, based on either a negative right to die (a right to noninterference) or a positive right to die (a right to be killed), would involve such a change in society's vision of the medical profession and in medical attitudes that a shift in the burden of proof to the proponents of change seems to us essential. We have argued that the prohibition of killing expresses important moral principles and attitudes whose loss, or serious alteration, could have major negative consequences. Because the current practice of prohibiting killing while accepting some "allowed deaths" has served us well, if not perfectly, it should be altered only with the utmost caution. Lines are not easy to draw and maintain, but in general we have been able to respect the line between killing and letting die in medical practice. Before we undertake any major changes, we need more evidence than we now have that the changes are needed in order to avoid important harms or secure important benefits and that the good effects will outweigh the bad effects.

PROBLEMS IN THE ACTIVE/PASSIVE DISTINCTION. Plaguing discussions of killing and allowing to die is the unclear status of the distinction between active measures (as in active euthanasia or killing) and passive measures (as in passive euthanasia or allowing to die). This distinction raises difficult questions about intentionality and causation that parallel the issues we encountered in our discussion of the principle of double effect and that we shall encounter later in this chapter when discussing the withholding of hydration and nutrition in order to let a patient die. Some say that this act is one of starving the patient and therefore is active killing, not passive allowing to die at all. No one has, as yet, succeeded in clearly formulating this distinction so that the active and the passive fall neatly into two different classes, just as no one has succeeded in theories of double effect in distinguishing the intentional and the nonintentional in the critical cases.

This conceptual problem provides another reason why we should be cautious about relaxing rules against killing. If it is conceptually difficult to distinguish killing from allowing to die,[54] it is an imprudent risk to relax our present constraints against killing. But the following must also be admitted: If it is permissible to unplug respirators and detach intravenous lines knowing that death will eventuate, we are already on a moderately slippery slope. If these are acts of killing (and it is doubtful that we have a sufficiently powerful theory of causation to decide that they are not acts of killing in many pertinent cases), the real logic of our present situation is that we are struggling to preserve as many traditional restraints against killing as we can, consistent with taking a humane approach toward seriously suffering patients and respecting their autonomy. The present authors are content to frame the issue in just this way, although we recognize that it leaves us short of clear and distinct principles and categories. We also acknowledge that those who have attacked the killing/letting die and active/passive distinctions have provided profound insights into the fragility of some of our restraints against killing and taking life.

Withholding and withdrawing life-prolonging treatments

Part of the debate about the distinctions between killing and letting die and active and passive steps focuses on acts of omission in contrast to acts of commission. Because of our views on killing and letting die, we do not hold that it is absolutely wrong to kill innocent persons when it is in accord with their wishes and interests, just as we do not hold that it is always right to omit treatment and let patients die. We cannot, then, use the omission/commission distinction without all the same reservations we have just noted. However, confusion persists about the distinction between withholding (not starting) and withdrawing (stopping) treatments. Many professionals and family members are more comfortable withholding treatments they have never started than withdrawing treatments they have started.[55] But does this psychological fact have moral significance, and should acts of withdrawing (stopping) be viewed as killing rather than letting die?

Some of these issues appear in the following case. An elderly man suffered from several major medical problems, including terminal cancer, with no reasonable chance of recovery. He was comatose and could not communicate with others. He had not expressed his wishes while competent, and he had no family to serve as proxy decision makers. The members of the staff quickly agreed on a no code or do not resuscitate (DNR) order. If the patient suffered a cardiac arrest, he would not be resuscitated but would be allowed to die. The staff was comfortable with this decision because of the patient's overall condition and prognosis and because not resuscitating the patient in the event of cardiac arrest could be viewed as withholding rather than withdrawing treatment. The patient was being kept alive by antibiotics to fight infection and by an intravenous line (IV) to provide nutrition and hydration.

Some members of the health-care team thought that all medical treatments, including artificial nutrition and hydration and antibiotics, should be stopped, because they were "extraordinary" or "heroic" treatments in this case. (We will return later to the question whether artificial nutrition and hydration may be considered extraordinary medical treatments in some cases; at present we are focusing on the distinction between withholding and withdrawing treatments). Others, perhaps a majority, thought it was wrong to stop these treatments once they had been started. A major disagreement erupted about whether it would be permissible not to insert the IV line again if it became infiltrated—that is, if it broke through the blood vessel and was leaking fluid into surrounding tissue. Some who argued against stopping treatment felt comfortable about not inserting the IV line again, because they viewed the action as one of omission rather than commission, of not starting rather than stopping, of withholding rather than withdrawing. They were still more emphatic about not inserting the IV line again if it required a cutdown (an incision to gain access to the deep large blood vessels) or a central line into the heart. Others viewed the provision of artificial nutrition and hydration as a single process and felt that inserting the IV line again was simply restarting or continuing what had been interrupted. For them, not restarting was equivalent to withdrawing and thus morally wrong.[56]

Although it is easy to understand these feelings of reluctance to withdraw treatments, the distinction between withdrawing and withholding treatments is morally indefensible and dangerous. The discomfort about withdrawing treatments appears to reflect the view of many care-givers that the action renders them more responsible for a patient's death than not starting a treatment to sustain life. However, withdrawing may be an omission in some cases, such as not recharging batteries for respirators or not putting the infusion into the feeding tube. Even if withdrawing were exclusively an act of commission rather than omission, it might still be justifiable, because some acts of commission such as disconnecting respirators may be viewed as instances of justifiable allowing to die.

A second source of care-giver discomfort about withdrawing treatments is the conviction that starting a treatment often creates expectations that it will be continued, and stopping it appears to breach faithfulness and contractual obligations to the patient and family. (See the discussion of rules of fidelity in Chapter 7.) However, wrong expectations and misleading promises should be avoided from the outset. The only appropriate expectation or promise is that care-givers will act in accord with the patient's interests and wishes, as limited by defensible systems for the allocation of health care and defensible social rules such as the prohibition of killing. Withdrawing a particular treatment, including life support, does not always amount to abandonment of the patient. It can follow the patient's directives, and it is appropriate in many cases to consider other modes of care that may or should be provided after a life-sustaining treatment is stopped.

The courts recognize that a crime can be committed by omission if a duty to act is present. Judgments turn on whether a physician has a duty to act in cases of either withholding or withdrawal of treatment. The court in the *Spring* case (Case 17), raised the primary legal problem about continuing dialysis as follows: "The question presented by . . . modern technology is, once undertaken, at what point does it cease to perform its intended function?" This court argued that "a physician has no duty to continue treatment, once it has proven to be ineffective." The court viewed this determination as "essentially medical," but the court also suggested that there should be a balancing of benefits and burdens to determine overall effectiveness and that the patient should, if possible, be the primary decision maker.[57] Although legal responsibility cannot be equated with moral responsibility in these cases, this conclusion is consistent with the moral conclusions for which we are arguing at present.

We believe that the moral burden of proof should generally be heavier when the decision is to withhold rather than to withdraw treatments.[58] In many cases, only after starting treatments will it be possible to make a proper diagnosis and prognosis as well as to determine what might be done for a patient and then to balance prospective benefits and burdens. The distinction between withholding and withdrawing treatment also may lead to overtreatment in some cases, that is, to continuation of a treatment that has been started although it would have been permissible never to have started it in the first place. Less obviously, but importantly, the distinction may lead to undertreatment. In one case, a seriously ill newborn died after several months of treatment, much of it against the parents' wishes, because one physician was unwilling to stop the respirator once it had been connected. Later it was reported that as a result of this experience, this physician was "less eager to attach babies to respirators now."[59] A sharp distinction between not starting and stopping treatments, combined with a reluctance to stop treatments, creates a dangerous situation for patients. Their wishes and interests may be violated if care-givers are afraid to commence treatments on the grounds that it is somehow wrong to withdraw a treatment even when it has become clear that its continuation is unwarranted.

Finally, the felt distinction between not starting and stopping may also account for—even though it does not adequately justify—the ease with which hospitals and health-care professionals have accepted no code or DNR. Policies regarding cardiopulmonary resuscitation (CPR) in the hospital setting (and we do not deal with CPR outside that setting) are particularly important, because cardiac arrest inevitably occurs in the dying process regardless of the underlying cause of death.[60] Hence, it would be possible to use CPR in an attempt to prolong, at least briefly, the lives of many patients who die in hospitals. Although death is often certain unless CPR is administered promptly, there is debate about whether the success of CPR should be measured by immediate or long-term results and whether the long-term results warrant CPR in as many cases as it is currently used, such as on terminally ill cancer patients.[61]

Policies regarding CPR have emerged with some measure of independence from other policies about life-sustaining technologies, such as respirators, in part because health-care professionals view not providing CPR as withholding rather than withdrawing treatment. Their decisions to provide or not provide CPR are especially problematic when made without advance consultation with patients or their families.[62] Futhermore, it is often unclear to hospital staffs, as well as to patients or their families, what orders not to resuscitate imply, if anything, about other levels of care and other technologies. For example, some patients with DNR orders still receive chemotherapy, surgery, and admission to the intensive care unit, while others do not.

No adequate justification has been given for viewing decisions about CPR in hospitals as different from decisions about other life-sustaining technologies, and a justification is not found in the distinction between withholding and withdrawing treatments. The identical substantive and procedural standards should apply to CPR as to other life-sustaining treatments. These standards have often been discussed under the distinction between ordinary and extraordinary means of treatment, a topic to which we turn next.

Optional and obligatory means of treatment

Ordinary and extraordinary means

The distinction between ordinary and extraordinary means of treatment has a prominent history, especially in the Roman Catholic tradition, in medical practice, and in judicial decisions. The previously cited 1973 statement by the AMA House of Delegates holds that the patient or the patient's immediate family can decide about the "cessation of extraordinary means to prolong the life of the body when there is irrefutable evidence that biological death is imminent." Like the distinctions between direct and indirect effects and between killing and letting die, this distinction has been employed to determine whether an act that results in death counts as killing, and especially as culpable killing in violation of the obligation of nonmaleficence. As developed by Roman Catholics to deal with problems of surgery (prior to the development of antisepsis and anesthesia), it was used to determine whether a patient's refusal of treatment should be classified as suicide. Refusal of ordinary means was considered suicide; refusal of extraordinary means was not considered suicide. Likewise, families and physicians did not commit homicide if they only withheld or withdrew extraordinary means of treatment from patients.

Unfortunately, a long history does not guarantee clarity or acceptability, and the distinction between ordinary and extraordinary means of treatment is both vague and unacceptable in the forms it has been presented. Several recent commentators have urged that the distinction be replaced by other categories, and we shall do so as well, adopting instead the terms *optional* and *obligatory*. *Ordinary* can then be reconstructed to mean morally obligatory, mandatory, required, or imperative; *extraordinary* can be reconstructed to mean morally optional, elective, or expendable.[63]

Here overtly moral categories replace what were often confusingly presented as medical practice categories. *Ordinary* has often been wrongly taken to mean "usual" or "customary," while *extraordinary* has often been taken to mean "unusual" or a departure from custom. The ordinary has then been interpreted as the customary in medical practice, in connection with the professional practice standard discussed in Chapter 3 or with the due care standards discussed earlier in this chapter. Treatments have been considered extraordinary and sometimes heroic if unusual or uncustomary for physicians to use in the relevant contexts. The terms have also become attached to technologies used in those contexts.

Although what is customary or usual in medical practice can be relevant to a moral judgment, it cannot always be morally decisive. It may be customary medical practice to treat disease X by means of technology Y, but whether this practice should be repeated for a particular patient depends on the patient's wishes and condition as a whole, not merely on what is customary treatment for X.[64] An example is treating pneumonia with antibiotics. This treatment is usual but may be morally optional for a patient irreversibly and imminently dying from cancer or AIDS. Ethics is not reducible to custom or professional consensus or traditional codes and oaths, as useful and indispensable as these may be in many professional contexts.

Criteria other than usual and unusual medical practice have also been proposed for determining which treatments are ordinary (obligatory) and extraordinary or heroic (optional). Some practitioners and commentators have proposed criteria such as whether the treatment is simple or complex, natural or artificial, noninvasive or invasive, inexpensive or costly. If a treatment is simple, natural, noninvasive, or inexpensive, it is more likely to be viewed as ordinary or obligatory than if it is complex, artificial, invasive, or costly. But these criteria are relevant only because they rely on deeper moral principles. For example, if a complex treatment is available and in accord with the patient's wishes and interests, it is difficult to see why morally it should be handled differently from a simple treatment that is also in accord with the patient's wishes and interests.

Several oddities emerge if the criteria of natural and artificial are invoked. According to one study conducted after the Natural Death Act was implemented in California, physicians in that state generally viewed respirators, dialyzers, and resuscitators as artificial, but they split evenly on intravenous feeding, while two-thirds viewed insulin, antibiotics, and chemotherapy as natural.[65] In general, they viewed mechanical systems as more artificial than drugs and other treatments. Nevertheless, physicians' construals of some treatments as artificial and others as natural are not morally relevant to judgments about whether and when those treatments may be withheld or withdrawn, unless these judgements are connected with the moral considerations that should govern these decisions. Criteria such as the degree of invasiveness and cost have the same limitations.

The misleading language of *ordinary* and *extraordinary* can be used if the substance of the distinction is explicated in ways similar to our use of *optional* and *obligatory*. According to Gerald Kelly, S.J., the distinction should be understood in the following way:

Ordinary means are all medicines, treatments, and operations, which offer a reasonable hope of benefit and which can be obtained and used without excessive expense, pain, or other inconvenience. Extraordinary means are all medicines, treatments, and operations, which cannot be obtained or used without excessive expense, pain, or other inconvenience, or which, if used, would not offer a reasonable hope of benefit.[66]

If we assume that excessiveness is to be determined by the probability and magnitude of the benefit, the substance of Kelly's distinction follows the lines of our distinction between the obligatory and the optional. If there is no reasonable hope of benefit, then any expense, pain, or other inconvenience is excessive. But if there is a reasonable hope of benefit, the amount of expense, pain, or other inconvenience may be significant without being excessive. Therefore, the point of the distinction and its application turn on a balance between benefits and burdens, including immediate detriment, inconvenience, risk of harm, and other costs. So understood, we have no substantial objection to the distinction.

However, neither the traditional distinction between ordinary and extraordinary means of treatment nor the distinction we recommend between obligatory and optional treatments is sufficient for the work that needs to be done on these subjects, because neither clearly envisions circumstances in which it may be wrong to treat and thus obligatory not to treat. Accordingly, as the following chart indicates, the range of pertinent distinctions and moral judgments that we propose as substitutes for the more traditional categories is threefold:

I. Obligatory	II. Optional	III. Wrong (Obligatory Not
	A. Neutral	to Provide)
	B. Heroic	

Most ethical discussions have focused on I and II, but with little attention paid to the two different possible interpretations of *optional*. A treatment might be optional in the sense that it is morally neutral whether an agent provides it. However, it could be optional because providing it would be heroic and praiseworthy, while not providing it would not be morally blameworthy. (For a discussion of heroic and praiseworthy acts, see Chapter 8.) Often the terms *heroic* and *extraordinary* are used to indicate that agents are expending additional time, effort, energy, and resources when there is a very limited chance of success.

To turn to category III, is it ever wrong to provide some treatments and even obligatory not to provide them? If the moral principles of nonmaleficence and beneficence establish a presumption in favor of providing life-sustaining treatments, as they do, they also indicate some of the conditions for rebutting that presumption. Even for an incompetent person, life-sustaining treatment may sometimes violate that person's interests. For example, the pain may be so severe and the physical restraints so burdensome as to outweigh the limited anticipated benefits, such as brief prolongation of life. In these circumstances, providing the treatment may be inhumane or cruel in violation of the principle of nonmaleficence. It will often, perhaps usually, be difficult to determine the balance of benefits and burdens to the incompetent patient, particularly when he or she has never had a life as a competent person expressing values; but, in principle, the burdens can so outweigh the benefits to the patient that the treatment is wrong rather than optional.

We reserve a systematic treatment of cost-benefit and risk-benefit judgments for the next chapter. Our concern at present is with substantive standards that distinguish obligatory and optional treatments. These standards may vary for competent patients making choices about treatments and for other parties making decisions for incompetent patients. Competent patients who can make informed and voluntary choices should have more latitude than other parties in balancing benefits and burdens and in accepting and refusing treatment. As noted throughout this chapter, the incompetent patient's vulnerability to harm may require actions, based on the principle of nonmaleficence, that would violate respect for a competent patient's autonomy unless authorized by the patient.

We concentrated on competent patients in our discussion of autonomy in Chapter 3, and we shall return to this class of patients in our discussion of paternalism in Chapter 5. We concentrate in this chapter primarily on substantive criteria of optional and obligatory treatments for incompetent patients. These criteria specify the conditions under which it is possible to rebut the presumption, based on the principles of nonmaleficence and beneficence, that the means to prolong life are obligatory and should be provided.

Conditions for overriding the prima facie obligation to treat

POINTLESS TREATMENT. Treatment is not obligatory when it offers no prospect of benefit to the patient because it is pointless. Several forms of treatment are pointless. First, if a patient is dead, he or she can no longer be harmed by the cessation of treatment, and a standard of best interests does not dictate treatment. Refined criteria for determining death will not alter this generalization, because it is irrelevant to the present point which criteria of death turn out to be the most acceptable.[67]

Second, there are patients who are irreversibly dying. The AMA standard indicates that some treatments may be discontinued when death is imminent. It is not clear whether this statement holds that all means of prolonging life can be considered extraordinary when death is imminent, except those that are palliative, or that only extraordinary means can be discontinued when death is imminent. Whatever the intention of the AMA statement, the first interpretation is more defensible. If it can be determined that a patient is irreversibly dying and that his or her death is imminent, modes of treatment such as resuscitation and respiration become optional. Because anything that we ought to do implies that we can do it (*ought* implies *can*), there is no medical indication for a curative treatment. Optimal care does not entail maximal treatment, and respect for life does not entail actions that prolong dying. Our paradigms of care for the dying should be fashioned so that technological interventions do not overwhelm human responses of care.

In cases involving either those who are dead or those who are irreversibly dying, objective medical factors are primary, and the role of expert judgment is central. The possibility of judgmental error should lead to efforts to prolong life in cases of serious doubt about whether patients are irretrievably in these categories unless certain conditions discussed below are met. Another problem involves specifying central terms such as an imminent death. The term *imminent* allows physicians latitude of judgment but suffers from vagueness. It could mean, for example, "any second now" or "in less than a year." A similar lack of specificity plagues attempts to classify patients as terminally ill and as dying.

As important as medical judgments are in decisions about the treatment of dying patients, they should not always be decisive. The values of patients and families are no less important and can be decisive. For example, in one case, two elderly women were severely burned in an accident, and the burn team agreed that survival was unprecedented in their cases. They were told that they were irreversibly dying. According to the burn team, both women were competent and rational after the accident before they began to experience serious problems from the burns. The burn team asked both if they wanted to choose between maximal treatment, which had never been efficacious in such cases at their burn center, and palliative care. Both chose palliative care.[68]

By contrast, in one case, Mr. C., a patient irreversibly dying from emphysema, insisted on having his life prolonged as long as possible by all available means. He demanded aggressive treatment, although the staff considered his condition hopeless. When Mr. C. became unconscious, his family and the staff had to decide whether to respect their earlier agreement with him or let him die. If this case did not involve a clear prior statement of Mr. C.'s wishes, there would be no moral difficulty in terminating treatment on the grounds that it was only prolonging his dying. But even with the prior agreement, following Mr. C.'s previous wishes might not be justified because of limited health-care resources—for instance, if other patients who were not irreversibly dying could not otherwise gain access to the ventilator and space in the intensive care unit.

BURDENS OUTWEIGHING BENEFITS. If the patient is not dead or dying, medical treatment is not obligatory if its burdens outweigh its benefits to the patient. When patients are not irreversibly dying and their deaths are not imminent, medical treatment may be optional even if it could prolong life for an indefinite period. The principle of nonmaleficence does not imply the sanctity of biological life without regard to the patient's pain, suffering, discomfort, and other problems. Nor does the principle mandate beginning or continuing maximum treatment for all nondying patients. For example, in Case 17, seventy-eight-year-old Earle Spring developed numerous medical problems, including chronic organic brain syndrome and kidney failure. The latter problem was controlled by hemodialysis. Although several aspects of the case are in dispute—such as whether Spring was conscious, aware, and able to express his own wishes—there is at least a plausible argument (although far from a definitive one) that the family and health-care professionals were not morally obligated to continue hemodialysis, which was necessary to sustain his life, because of the balance of benefits and burdens to the patient himself. However, this case, like many others, is complicated by the fact that the family was in a position of potential conflict of interest (because of their obligations to pay mounting health-care costs) in specifying the patient's interests.

Few decisions are more important than those to withhold or stop a medical procedure that sustains life. But in some cases it is unjustified to begin or to continue therapy knowing that it will produce a greater balance of suffering for someone incapable of choosing for or against such therapy. As the supreme judicial court of Massachusetts held in the *Saikewicz* case (16), ''the 'best interests' of an incompetent person are not necessarily served by imposing on such persons results not mandated as to competent persons similarly situated.''[69]

Quality of life

Judgments that treatments are optional often presuppose or otherwise rely on standards of the quality of life. In the Saikewicz case (Case 16), a sixty-year-old man with an IQ of 10 and a mental age of approximately two years and eight months suffered from acute myeloblastic monocytic leukemia. Chemotherapy would have produced extensive suffering and possibly serious side effects. Remission under chemotherapy occurs in only thirty to fifty percent of such cases and typically only for between two and thirteen months. If not given chemotherapy, Saikewicz could expect to live for several weeks or perhaps several months, during which he would not experience major pain or suffering. In not ordering treatment, the lower court considered ''the quality of life available to him [Saikewicz] even if the treatment does bring about remission.'' The supreme judicial court of Massachusetts, however, rejected this formulation if construed to equate the value of life with a measure of the quality of life—in particular, with Saikewicz's lower quality of life because of mental retardation. The court construed ''the vague, and perhaps ill-chosen, term 'quality of life' . . . as a reference to the continuing state of pain and disorientation precipitated by the chemotherapy treatment.''[70] It thus balanced prospective benefit against pain and suffering, finally determining that the patient's actual interests supported a decision not to provide chemotherapy. From a moral as well as a legal standpoint, we would agree with the conclusion reached in this opinion. However, we will object to its procedural requirements and standards in the last section of this chapter.

Such slogans as ''quality of life'' may mislead as often as they illuminate, and they thus need careful analysis. One proposal, defended by Paul Ramsey, is to reject all judgments about quality of life and to rely instead on medical indications. We need only to determine which treatment is medically indicated in order to know which treatment is obligatory and which is optional for incompetent patients. For dying patients, the relevant choices are between further palliative treatments and no treatments. For unconscious or incompetent nondying patients, there is an obligation to use the treatment medically indicated. Ramsey worries that we are gradually moving toward a policy of active, involuntary euthanasia for unconscious or incompetent nondying patients, and he resists this trend by asserting an "undiminished obligation first of all to save life and in the second instance, to use palliative treatments where possible."[71] Above all, quality-of-life judgments are to be avoided, he argues, because they violate the principle of equality of human lives.

It is doubtful, however, that objective medical factors—such as medical criteria used in the classification of patients as dying and nondying and in the determination of medical indications for treatment—can carry the weight Ramsey intends. These factors themselves reflect values that inspire, control, and limit medical interventions. It seems impossible to determine what will benefit a patient without presupposing some quality-of-life standard and judgments about the kind of life the patient will have after a medical intervention. Any attempt to make life—understood as a set of vital logical processes—unconditionally good in itself is a "vitalism" that should be rejected in favor of a view that life is only conditionally good.[72] The maintenance of biological life thus should not automatically be considered a (net) benefit to the person.

A good example is a patient, such as Karen Ann Quinlan, in a condition of permanent unconsciousness. Accurate medical diagnosis and prognosis are indispensable, but the judgment about whether to use life-prolonging measures hinges on the anticipated quality of life. The benefits of life-prolonging treatment to a permanently unconscious patient appear to be so limited as to render the treatment pointless.[73] Any benefit to the patient would appear to rest in the slight possibility of a diagnostic or prognostic error or of a medical breakthrough, rather than in the quality of the life that is prolonged.

Ramsey has objected that a quality-of-life approach wrongly shifts from the question of whether treatments are beneficial to patients to the question of whether patients' lives are beneficial to them. The latter question, he insists, opens the door to active, involuntary euthanasia.[74] He appeals to the wedge argument and contends that quality-of-life criteria commit us to active, involuntary euthanasia. The critical question is whether the criteria for quality of life—or, as we prefer, the criteria for determining the patient's best interests—can be stated with sufficient precision and cogency to avoid the dangers envisioned by wedge arguments. We think they can, but the vagueness surrounding terms such as *dignity* and *meaningful life* is a cause for concern, and cases in which seriously ill or handicapped newborn infants have been "allowed to die" under questionable justifications provide a reason for caution. A good example of an unjustified allowed death is Case 20, in which Infant Doe died six days after he was born with Down syndrome and respiratory and digestive complications requiring major surgery, which his parents refused to authorize.

Several conditions of patients should be excluded from consideration in these cases. For example, just as the supreme judicial court in Massachusetts found it inappropriate in the *Saikewicz* case to include mental retardation in a determination of the quality of life, we concur that this factor is irrelevant in determining whether treatment is in the patient's best interest.

It is also important not to confuse quality of life for the patient with the quality or the value of life for others. Quality of life is not tantamount to social worth or to group preferences. We have concentrated exclusively on the balance of benefits and burdens to the patient. Competent patients may autonomously choose to refuse life-sustaining treatment in part or primarily because of their unwillingness to burden their families or society with the costs of their care. However, proxies should not refuse treatment against the incompetent patient's interests in order to avoid burdens to the family or costs to society. The incompetent patient's best medical interests generally should be the decisive criterion for a proxy, even if these interests conflict with familial interests.

The President's Commission recognized a broader conception of best interests that includes the welfare of the family: "The impact of a decision on an incapacitated patient's loved ones may be taken into account in determining someone's best interests, for most people do have an important interest in the well-being of their families or close associates."[75] A patient may have an interest in the family's welfare, but it is a long step from this premise to a conclusion about whose interests should be overriding. When the incompetent patient has never been competent or never previously expressed his or her wishes while competent, it is not proper to impute altruism—a desire to relieve the family of its burdens—to that patient against his or her medical best interests.[76] If, however, the treatment is optional because it offers no reasonable chance of benefit or because the burdens to the patient outweigh the benefits to the patient, then the family's interests may become a legitimate factor in the calculus of interests.

Further questions about burdens to society arise in the context of the allocation of scarce resources for and within health care. We will treat this subject in Chapter 6.

Applications to seriously ill newborns

Some of the most difficult questions about the treatment of incompetents involve the other end of the continuum of age: seriously ill newborns. Some societies have circumvented the obligation of nonmaleficence in these cases by definitional ploys. To take an extreme example, the Nuer tribe viewed seriously handicapped newborns as nonhuman ''hippopotamuses'' who were mistakenly born to human parents and who should be returned to their natural habitat, the river. Although such conceptual maneuvers about human life are generally excluded in our society as far as newborns are concerned, some have argued that newborns are not persons and thus lack the rights of persons. We will return to this dispute about personhood later, but first we will consider the applications of our framework to newborns in order to determine appropriate treatment or nontreatment decisions in neonatal care.

Although neonatal intensive care can now salvage the lives of many newborns with physical conditions that would have been fatal a decade or so ago, the resultant quality of life is sometimes so low as to raise questions about whether the intensive care has produced more harm than benefit for the patient. Some commentators have argued that avoidance of harm is the best guide to decisions on behalf of infants in neonatal nurseries,[77] whereas others have argued that intensive care for neonates may violate the obligation of nonmaleficence if one or more of three conditions is present: ''inability to survive infancy, inability to live without severe pain, and inability to participate, at least minimally, in human experience.''[78]

H. Tristram Engelhardt, Jr., draws on the obligation of nonmaleficence to develop a concept of the ''injury of continued existence.'' Although he rejects active euthanasia for infants (on prudential grounds), he argues that nonmaleficence may morally require that death be allowed under some conditions: ''The concept of injury for continuance of existence, the proposed analogue of the concept of tort for wrongful life, presupposes that life can be of a negative value such that the medical maxim *primum non nocere* ('first do no harm') *would require not sustaining life.*''[79] Engelhardt makes a plausible case for the claim that there is sometimes a moral obligation not to sustain life in circumstances in which the burdens seriously outweigh the benefits to the patient. However, our goal here is the narrower one of showing that under some conditions allowing seriously handicapped newborns to die is morally permissible, because it does not violate the obligation of nonmaleficence (and satisfies other relevant justifying conditions).

Although moral controversy often focuses on newborns with neural tube defects or with Down syndrome, the most common cases—approximately seven percent of all live births in the United States each year—involve infants with low birth weight, often as a result of prematurity. In these cases, the primary problem is respiratory distress syndrome caused by hyaline membrane disease, a result of inadequate lung development. Judgments about reasonable chance of success and the balance of benefits and burdens vary widely in these circumstances.

Among the congenital anomalies, it would be justifiable under the conditions mentioned thus far to withhold or to withdraw treatment from newborns or infants who have Tay-Sachs disease, which involves increasing spasticity and dementia and usually results in death by age three or four. It would also be justifiable to withhold or to withdraw treatment from those who have Lesch-Nyhan disease, which involves uncontrollable spasms, mental retardation, compulsive self-mutilation, and early death.

Neural tube defects constitute another major type of congenital anomaly. In severe cases newborns lack all or most of the brain; death is inevitable for these anencephalic newborns, and there is general agreement that life-sustaining treatments are futile. More problematic is meningomyelocele (protrusion of part of the covering and substance of the spinal cord because of a defect in the vertebral column). The wide range of possible outcomes makes it difficult to know whether to treat vigorously all cases or only selected cases. The difficulty stems from the fact that some children with meningomyelocele can have a meaningful life, while the chances are slim for others. Dr. John Lorber argued at one point for vigorous and comprehensive treatment for all spina bifida babies (babies who have a defective closure of the bony encasement of the spinal cord), but he later concluded that such treatment results in only a marginal gain in survival rates and often preserves lives with severe disabilities and handicaps. He then proposed specific criteria, such as the site of the spinal lesion and the degree of paralysis, for determining the level of treatment on the first day after birth. When the decision is made to omit treatment for this disorder, normal custodial care and feeding are provided. Some of the babies who are not treated for spina bifida survive; however, their overall condition is not as good as it would have been had they been vigorously treated from the outset.[80]

Lorber's approach has the following merit: It is difficult to generalize over classes of infants (usually classified by disease categories), and it is usually necessary to examine the particulars of the case, such as the lesions and degree of paralysis, in order to make a defensible decision. However, these decisions are not reducible to technical medical criteria, because they presuppose judgments of value about probable outcomes.[81]

A final type of congenital abnormality involves newborns with a life-threatening problem that can be corrected and a permanent, uncorrectable handicap, such as Down syndrome, which causes mental retardation (and which occurs in one out of every seven hundred live births). The presence of a life-threatening condition provides the occasion for a decision about treatment or nontreatment, as in the well-known Johns Hopkins Hospital case in which a newborn with Down syndrome starved to death over several days after his parents refused permission for surgery to correct a duodenal atresia (obstruction of the upper part of the small intestine).[82] We suggested in our discussion of quality of life that Down syndrome, with resulting mental retardation, is not a sufficient reason to allow a newborn to die, even if the newborn suffers from other life-threatening conditions that require treatment. However, we also accept the restrictive standard offered by the President's Commission: "Permanent handicaps justify a decision not to provide life-sustaining treatment only when they are so severe that continued existence would not be a net benefit to the infant."[83]

In the United States the debate about treatment or nontreatment of seriously ill newborns was stimulated by a 1973 article in which Raymond S. Duff and A. G. M. Campbell reported that 43 of 299 consecutive deaths in the intensive care nursery at the Yale–New Haven Hospital had occurred following a decision for nontreatment based on the infant's extremely poor or hopeless prognosis for meaningful life.[84] This and similar reports led to a public debate in the United States that went unaccompanied by government intervention for almost a decade. But in April 1982, the Reagan administration took vigorous action in response to the Infant Doe case (Case 20). In this case, parents refused permission for surgery to correct a tracheoesophageal fistula (an opening between the breathing and the swallowing tubes that prevents passage of food to the stomach) in their newborn infant with Down syndrome, and the infant soon died from starvation. The regulations proposed by the Reagan administration were based on laws prohibiting discrimination because of handicaps and appeared to require maximal treatment in all cases except those in which treatment would be futile because the newborn was irreversibly and imminently dying. These regulations were overturned by the U.S. Supreme Court, but, as a result of the controversy, Congress passed amendments to the Child Abuse and Treatment Act that defined as child abuse the "withholding of medically indicated treatment" from newborns.[85]

The law and regulations define "medically indicated treatment" as all treatment that is likely to ameliorate life-threatening conditions. However, some conditions under which life-sustaining treatment is optional are recognized. Treatment is optional if, in the attending physician's medical judgment:

(1) the infant is chronically and irreversibly comatose;
(2) the provision of such treatment would either merely prolong dying, not be effective in ameliorating or correcting all of the infant's life-threatening conditions, or otherwise be futile in terms of the survival of the infant; or
(3) the provision of such treatment would be virtually futile in terms of the survival of the infant, and the treatment itself under such circumstances would be inhumane.

This approach is problematic, or at least misleading, on several grounds. We have already argued that medical indications themselves presuppose values and often standards of quality of life. Clearly conditions 1 through 3 do not amount as a unit to a definition of *medically* indicated treatment; rather, these conditions express Congress's view of *ethically* indicated treatment.[86] For instance, the judgment in condition 1 that a human life in an irreversible coma is not worth prolonging is based on a standard of quality of life, and the judgment in condition 3 depends on considering the inhumaneness of treatment in relation to the limited prospects of success ("virtually futile"). Even in these circumstances, the physician is obligated to provide "appropriate nutrition, hydration, or medication." It is unclear whether these elements of care are always deemed to be appropriate—particularly artificial nutrition and hydration (see the discussion below)—or whether they are appropriate only if they are necessary for the patient's comfort.[87] Although it is too early to determine the long-term impact of this legislation, some critics contend that this debate about neonatal intensive care has led to neglect of other modes of care, such as prenatal care, that are essential to protect infants.

In cases of incompetent patients, including seriously ill newborns, we should begin with the normal presumption in favor of the prolongation of life. Decision makers should then work diligently to determine the patient's actual interests. Judgments about the best interests of seriously ill newborns must be made by considering the prospective benefits and burdens as objectively as possible, in light of the patient's condition, without benefit of their previous declarations or meaningful inferences from their actions. Although the possibility of error is substantial, it is no greater than in many other judgments in medicine. Because of potential error in diagnosis, prognosis, and judgments about the patient's interests, the normal obligation to preserve life dictates erring on the side of sustaining life, at least in cases of serious doubt about the available evidence.

However, there is an important reason why this argument from nonmaleficence—and no doubt other similar ones in this chapter—remains incomplete. In the case of seriously ill newborns, the irreversibly comatose, the fetus, and others, we need to determine not only the applicable rules and their priority when they conflict but also to whom these rules apply. If we are certain that a particular being is a person, then we can usually be confident that the full complement of moral principles applies. But if, for example, we make a judgment that fetuses or certain neonates are not persons or are not properly the objects of rules about sustaining life (as the Nuer tribe example illustrates), this verdict would dramatically alter the requirements of newborn care. In short, moral analysis of these difficult cases involves inquiry into the proper objects of moral principles and not simply into the implications of the principles themselves. This controversy about human life and personhood is impossible to decide on the basis of the moral principles that form the core principles in this book. Rather, we need supplementary principles (perhaps nonmoral principles) that will allow us to distinguish persons from nonpersons, the dead from the alive, and the like.

On the one hand, if the fetus, for example, does not qualify as a human being—or a person, depending on which category is held to be relevant—then causing its death may not violate the principle of nonmaleficence. On the other hand, if a being is not a human being or a person, it may still be protected by principles such as nonmaleficence. For example, there is general agreement that it is wrong to inflict gratuitous pain on animals (although there is less agreement about when such pain has been inflicted) and that there are some harms that researchers should not inflict on animals even to generate scientific knowledge to benefit humans (although society is divided about which prospective benefits to humans, if any, can justify which harms to animals in experiments).[88] These problems cannot be resolved without an integrated theory of the nature and moral relevance of categories such as human being, person, animal, mammal, and the like. Unfortunately, this immense task is more than we can undertake in the present volume.

The omission of artificial nutrition and hydration

If our analysis of optional and obligatory means of treatment is correct, no medical treatment as such is always obligatory for care-givers to provide. The justifiability of any medical treatment's use is contingent on the circumstances. In recent years, however, there has been widespread debate about whether medical technologies for nutrition and hydration are ever optional.

In one case a seventy-nine-year-old widow had been a resident of a nursing home for several years. In the past she had experienced repeated transient ischemic attacks (stoppages of blood flow). Because of progressive organic brain syndrome, she had lost most of her mental abilities and had become disoriented. She also had episodes of thrombophlebitis as well as congestive heart failure. Her daughter and grandchildren visited her frequently and obviously loved her deeply. One day she was found unconscious on the bathroom floor of the nursing home. She was hospitalized and diagnosed as having suffered a "massive stroke." She made no recovery, remaining obtunded and nonverbal, but she continued to manifest a withdrawal reaction to painful stimuli and exhibited some purposeful behaviors. She strongly resisted a nasogastric tube being placed in her stomach; at each attempt she thrashed about violently and pushed the tube away. After the tube was finally placed, she pulled out of her restraints and managed to remove it. After several days on intravenous lines, her sites for IV lines were exhausted. The question for the staff was whether to take further "extraordinary" or "heroic" measures to maintain fluid and nutritional intake for an elderly patient who had made no recovery from a massive stroke and who was largely unaware and unresponsive. After much discussion with nurses on the floor and with the patient's family, the physicians in charge reached the conclusion that they should not provide further IVs, cutdowns, or a feeding tube. The patient had minimal oral intake and died quietly the following week.[89]

In a ground-breaking case in 1976, the New Jersey supreme court held that it was permissible for a guardian to disconnect Karen Ann Quinlan's respirator and allow her to die.[90] After the respirator was removed she lived for almost ten years, protected by antibiotics and sustained by nutrition and hydration provided through a nasogastric tube. Unable to communicate with anyone, she lay comatose in a fetal position, with increasing respiratory problems and bed-sores and her weight dropping from 115 pounds to 70 pounds. A moral issue developed over those ten years: If it is permissible to remove the respirator, is it also permissible for the same reasons to remove the feeding tube? Several Catholic moral theologians advised the parents that they were not morally re-quired to continue medical nutrition and hydration (MN&H) or antibiotics to fight infections. However, the Quinlans believed both that the feeding tube did not cause pain and that the respirator did.

While Karen Ann Quinlan lingered, the New Jersey supreme court faced another case that involved artificial nutrition and hydration. In *Conroy* the court considered the request of a guardian to withdraw MN&H for an eighty-four-year-old nursing-home resident and held that the provision of nutrition and hydration through nasogastric tubes and other medical means is not always legally required.[91] A similar decision was reached in the Brophy case (see Case 18) in Massachusetts, involving a forty-nine-year-old man who had been in a persistent vegetative state for more than three years following surgery for a ruptured brain artery.[92] The debate about MN&H has also surfaced in treatment decisions about handicapped newborns.[93]

A major issue is whether all medical treatments, depending on the circum-stances, can be construed as optional rather than obligatory. In particular, are MN&H by peripheral or central intravenous lines, nasogastric tubes, or gas-trostomies relevantly similar to other medical and surgical procedures that are sometimes construed as optional? Is it appropriate to view the provision of nutrition and hydration as medical treatment when it involves medical proce-dures or surgery and requires medical and health-care professionals? Are arti-ficial nutrition and hydration more similar to other medical treatments—and thus subject to the same standards of evaluation—than to the normal provision of food and water?[94]

Society is divided over these questions. One prominent view was advanced by the aforementioned President's Commission, which maintained in 1983 that no medical intervention, including a feeding procedure, is required if it merely delays the moment of death. It also suggested that "only rarely should a dying patient be fed by tube or intravenously." In the instance of permanently unconscious patients, the commission held that the sole conceivable "benefit" is sustaining the body, which it viewed as no real benefit at all. Not only can costs be burdensome to the family and society, but, in the commission's view, a policy of MN&H violates the autonomy of the patient if the patient formerly expressed a preference not to be treated.[95]

The American Medical Association has also made two influential pronouncements on this general subject. In 1982, the AMA's Council on Ethical and Judicial Affairs stated that in cases of well-confirmed irreversible coma, "all means of life support may be discontinued."[96] In 1986, the council clarified the earlier statement by specific reference to MN&H, holding that "life-prolonging medical treatment includes medication and artificially or technologically supplied respiration, nutrition, or hydration."[97] Although most pronouncements by professional organizations have been limited to terminally ill and irreversibly dying patients or to permanently unconscious patients, some commentators have gone farther by accepting the withdrawal of fluids from some patients who are seriously but not terminally ill.[98]

In sharp disagreement with these views, philosopher G. E. M. Anscombe contends that "for willful starvation there can be no excuse. The same can't be said quite without qualification about failing to operate or to adopt some courses of treatment."[99] Others have joined her with arguments to exempt MN&H from the general claim that any medical treatment is optional under some circumstances. These arguments try to establish that MN&H are not relevantly similar to other medical treatments and that the principle of universalizability (treat similar cases in a similar way) does not require or even permit the same judgments about MN&H that we make about other medical procedures. We will now consider several of these arguments.

The first argument holds that MN&H are always required because they are always necessary for patient comfort and dignity. Such a view may have been held by the nurse whose whistle-blowing led to an indictment against two California physicians who had discontinued intravenous nutrition to a patient who had suffered severe brain damage after the loss of oxygen following routine surgery. She insisted that "food is an ordinary means. And everyone has a right to ordinary treatment."[100] This view also underlies the rule proposed by the Department of Health and Human Services (July 5, 1983) for treatment of handicapped newborns: "The basic provision of nourishment, fluids, and routine nursing care is a fundamental matter of human dignity, not an option for medical judgment."[101] This rule includes medical as well as nonmedical means of providing nutrition and hydration. A similar conviction about patient comfort and dignity supports the exclusionary clause in several natural death acts that do not allow advance directives about artificial nutrition and hydration, although they permit advance directives about other medical procedures that prolong life.[102]

Whether the rationale is life prolongation or patient comfort and dignity, an absolute requirement to provide nutrition and hydration is not defensible. The procedures themselves may involve risks—such as, from a central IV—and discomfort and indignity—such as, from physical constraints to prevent patients from removing the lines or tubes. There is also some evidence that patients who are allowed to die without artificial hydration may die more comfortably than patients who receive such hydration.[103] It may be misleading to project the common experience of hunger and thirst on the dying patient who is malnourished and dehydrated. Whenever MN&H are required for an incompetent patient's comfort and dignity, they should always be provided. However, caring for patients by meeting their needs for comfort—such as by relieving their parched lips—may not entail the provision of medically adequate nutrition and hydration. Competent patients have an autonomy right to decline measures intended for comfort as well as measures intended to prolong life.

A second argument that MN&H are never optional focuses on their symbolic significance. Medical professionals generally find it intuitively devastating to starve someone. Denying food and water to anyone for any reason seems the antithesis of expressing care and compassion; provision of nutrition and hydration symbolizes the essence of care and compassion in medical as well as nonmedical contexts. Some reasons for the symbolic significance of food and water are obvious. We respond with care to the newborn by providing food and water. Feeding the hungry has been viewed as a fundamental human relationship and "the perfect symbol of the fact that human life is inescapably social and communal."[104] Our interdependence combines with our actual experiences of thirst and hunger to make this symbol still more powerful: Thirst and hunger are uncomfortable, and we view severe malnutrition and dehydration as extreme agony. This argument, then, stresses the similarities between nonmedical and medical acts of providing nutrition and hydration, rather than the similarities between MN&H and other medical treatments.

The assumptions underlying this argument may establish a presumption in favor of the provision of MN&H, but this presumption is rebuttable. For a few patients the burdens of MN&H outweigh their benefits, and MN&H may be withheld or withdrawn if they are not in the patients' best interests. The obligation to care for patients entails only that we must provide all treatments that are in accord with patients' preferences and interests (within the limits set by just allocation policies), not that we must provide treatments because of what they symbolize.

Some physicians start and continue intravenous lines at a rate that will result in dehydration over time.[105] Such an approach may represent a compromise for physicians who want to engage in symbolically significant actions and yet also act in accord with the patient's wishes and interests. However, this approach too is dangerous, because it appears to involve self-deception. The physician fails to acknowledge that the patient will become dehydrated and malnourished.

Self-deception also appears when agents disassociate themselves from their acts or from the consequences of their acts because of their sense of distance. For example, some professionals and commentators apparently favor withdrawing MN&H rather than the respirator because death is immediate when the latter is withdrawn. They note that, in contrast to "letting patients die" of later dehydration, discontinuing the respirator "creates an *immediate consequence of death* for which we must take responsibility."[106] However, it is not possible to avoid responsibility for discontinuing the IV on grounds that dehydration develops slowly, as a delayed consequence of actions. The act resulting in death is intentional, or—continuing our earlier discussion of the principle of double effect—death is at least a foreseen and avoidable consequence. There is often finality and near certainty about causing death when either form of withholding or withdrawal is adopted. Moral responsibility therefore cannot be evaded.

Concern for symbolic actions also appears in a third major argument, which is a version of the wedge or slippery slope argument.[107] The claim is that policies of not providing MN&H will lead to adverse consequences, because society will not be able to limit decisions about MN&H to legitimate cases, especially under pressures for cost containment in health care. The argument is that these decisions, although based on compassion, sow the seeds of potential abuse. Fears about the removal of an important clinical, psychological, and social barrier focus on a slide from acting in the patient's interests to acting in the society's interests, from considering the patient's quality of life to considering the patient's value for society, from decisions about dying patients to decisions about nondying patients, from letting die to killing, and from cessation of artificial feeding to cessation of natural feeding. The case for death with dignity emerged as a compassionate response to the threat of overtreatment, but now patients face the threat of undertreatment because of pressures to contain the escalating costs of health care.[108] The "right to die" thus might be transformed into the "obligation to die," perhaps against the patient's wishes and interests.

The fears underlying this third argument are legitimate and troubling because of uncertainties about whether lines can be drawn and maintained in order to prevent abuses. Perhaps eighty percent of the approximately two million people who die each year in the United States die in nursing homes or hospitals under the care of strangers, often at considerable cost to their families and to the society.[109] These patients and others, such as long-term care patients, are vulnerable, and it is essential that they be protected. But there is scant evidence that the protection of these patients requires that MN&H be provided in all circumstances. Daniel Callahan has defended the third argument with a stern warning—too stern in our view, despite its obvious merit.[110] He argues that it is possible to avoid "social disaster"—the movement from a right to die to an obligation to die and the subversion of the obligation to care for the poor who are hungry—only if there is widespread and "deep-seated revulsion at the stopping of feeding even under legitimate circumstances." His thesis is that it is a "dangerous business to tamper with, or adulterate, so enduring and central a moral emotion" as "repugnance against starving people to death." He does concede that we can morally differentiate acts of withholding or withdrawing MN&H, accepting some as right and rejecting others as wrong. However, he contends that we cannot avoid disaster unless all those acts routinely evoke revulsion and repugnance.

This approach could be described as sentiment or symbol utilitarianism, using an analogy to rule utilitarianism. There is a concern, and a serious one, about the potential loss of broad commitments and self-conceptions that form the cement of our social universe. But it is not clear that emotions underlying the symbol of providing nutrition and hydration are either necessary or sufficient to avert social disaster.

The interpretation of MN&H defended in this section is not as innovative or as deviant as some critics may suppose. In the early 1950s, Gerald Kelly, S. J., clarified the concepts and criteria of ordinary and extraordinary means of treatment, including intravenous nutrition, through appeal to the following case:

A patient almost ninety years of age, suffering from cardiorenal disease, had been in a coma for two weeks, during which time he received an intravenous solution of glucose and some digitalis preparation. The coma was apparently terminal. A member of the family asked that the medication and intravenous feeding be discontinued. With the approval of a priest, the doctor and Sisters acceded to the request, but they did so with some disquietude and they continued to be disturbed for some time after the patient's death.[111]

Disquietude and disturbance are appropriate emotions in struggling with the normal presumption in favor of treatments, but repugnance and revulsion are misplaced emotions.

The assessment of MN&H depends on the same criteria used to distinguish obligatory from optional treatments—criteria that focus on the patient's condition, interests, and preferences. The presumption in favor of MN&H can be successfully rebutted in the following sorts of situations. (1) The procedures are futile in that they would be highly unlikely to improve nutritional and fluid levels. (2) The procedures improve nutritional and fluid levels, but the patient will not benefit (e.g., the condition may be anencephaly or a permanent vegetative state). (3) The procedures improve nutritional and fluid levels and the patient benefits, but the burdens of MN&H outweigh the benefits (e.g., for a severely demented patient, essential physical restraints may cause fear and discomfort, especially as the patient struggles to break free of the restraints).[112]

Proxy decision makers: standards and procedures

We have thus far accepted the point of the distinction between *ordinary* and *extraordinary* forms of treatment but have replaced this language with *obligatory* and *optional*. Absent a patient's directive, the standard of what is obligatory or optional is the patient's best interests. This standard depends on the balance of benefits and burdens for the patient. Proxy decision makers must apply this standard for incompetent patients, whereas competent patients can determine their own best interests. In this section, we consider different proxy decision makers, and we elaborate the standard of the patient's best interests by comparing it to an alternative standard known as substituted judgment. Our intention is to analyze and assess standards and procedures that have either emerged in or could be developed for law and policy.

First consider these two questions about standards and procedures. (1) Is there a standard of a right or just outcome that is independent of the procedure for evaluating the outcome? (2) Can a procedure guarantee a right or just outcome? In response, John Rawls has analyzed three possible relations between procedures and outcomes:

	Independent Standard of Right Outcome	Procedure to Guarantee Right Outcome
Perfect procedural justice	Yes	Yes
Imperfect procedural justice	Yes	No
Pure procedural justice	No	Yes

In "perfect procedural justice," there is an independent standard of a right outcome, and it is possible to devise a procedure to guarantee that outcome. It is difficult to find examples of such a procedure, and Rawls settles on the distribution of a birthday cake at a children's party. The standard of a right outcome is equal shares, and it is possible to guarantee a right outcome by telling the child designated to cut the cake that he must take the last piece, after all the other children have chosen theirs. In "imperfect procedural justice," there is an independent standard of a right outcome, but the procedure is imperfect in some respect and thus cannot ensure the right outcome. For example, in criminal trials there is an independent standard of a right verdict (conviction of the guilty and only the guilty), but it is impossible to design a procedure that will guarantee the right verdict in every case. This relation between procedure and outcome is more common than either of the other two relations. In "pure procedural justice," any outcome of the procedure is right if the procedure has been followed, because there is no standard of rightness independent of the procedure itself. Rightness or justice inheres in the procedure, and any result is acceptable as long as the procedure has been followed. Gambling is an example because it does not matter who wins or loses if the game is fair.[113]

If our argument earlier in this chapter is correct, we can hope in life-and-death situations for imperfect procedural justice. There are, we have argued, some independent standards of decision making, but there is no procedure to guarantee that decisions or outcomes will match those standards. Competent patients who are sick or dying have a right to make their decisions, but no procedure based on rights of autonomy can guarantee right decisions. In the case of incompetent patients who cannot make their own decisions about life-sustaining treatment, the principles of nonmaleficence and beneficence require that we establish procedures to protect their interests. Because no procedure will guarantee that their interests will always be adequately protected, this state of affairs at best represents imperfect procedural justice.

Judgments about proxy decision makers for incompetent patients should generally be made first in terms of the principles of nonmaleficence and beneficence. (Respect for autonomy may also be applicable in cases of previously competent patients.) Specific criteria protecting the patient's interests should be employed, and if it can be determined that a family or another decision maker cannot be counted on to seek the patient's best interests, a replacement should be sought. Thus, it is important to determine standards for proxy decision making, as well as to establish procedures assigning decision-making authority to some parties.

Standards for proxy decision making

If a patient is not competent to choose or refuse treatment, a hospital, a physician, or a family member often goes before a court to seek resolution of the issues before a decision is implemented. Celebrated cases have emerged around several formerly competent patients, including Karen Ann Quinlan, Earle Spring, Brother Fox, Claire Conroy, and Paul Brophy, as well as patients such as Joseph Saikewicz and John Storar who have never been competent. Courts have split over the use of two proxy decision-making standards: best interests and substituted judgment. Paradoxically, the doctrine of parens patriae ("the state as parent"), which represents the underlying authority for the state's power to act in an incompetent's behalf, is the basis for both legal standards, as they are applied by courts in medical decision making for incompetents. The doctrine of *parens patriae* has traditionally rested on the principles of nonmaleficence and beneficence: the state's duty to protect persons under legal disability from harm they cannot themselves avoid.

BEST INTERESTS. Long before autonomy and privacy were applied to incompetents or minors, the responsibility of parents toward their children was legally defined as the responsibility to act in the best interests of those children. It was assumed in law that parents generally do act in their children's best interests and that the state should not interfere except in extreme circumstances in which the state and the parents disagree about some decision with potentially serious consequences for the child—for example, when Jehovah's Witness parents refuse lifesaving blood transfusions for their minor children. (See Case 12). When the court rather than the family decides, the court has thus already made a judgment about the unreasonableness of the family's proposed course of action.

The best interests test is sometimes interpreted as highly malleable and subject to incorporating intangible factors of questionable value to the child. For example, in some cases parents have sought court permission for a kidney transplant from an incompetent minor child to a competent sibling. Parental judgments about the best interests of the donor have on occasion taken into account projected psychological trauma from the death of a sibling and the psychological benefits of the unselfish act of donation.[114] Nonetheless, the most common application of the best interests standard concentrates on tangible factors—physical and financial risks, harms, and benefits—and makes use of such truisms as "Health is better than illness" and "Life is preferable to death."

SUBSTITUTED JUDGMENT. The second legal standard, substituted judgment, appears to be radically different from the best interests standard. Substituted judgment begins with the premise that decisions about treatment or nontreatment properly belong to the incompetent patient by virtue of rights of autonomy and privacy. (See Chapter 3 for a discussion of autonomy and Chapter 7 for privacy.) It would be unfair to deprive the incompetent patient of decision-making rights merely because he or she is incompetent. Nonetheless, another decision maker must be substituted because the patient is currently unable to decide. In legal terms, the patient has the right to decide but is incompetent to exercise it. Thus, the premise of the standard is a fiction: An incompetent person cannot literally be said to have the right to make medical decisions if the right can only be exercised by competent persons. This fictional quality makes substituted judgment controversial.

The substituted judgment standard requires the proxy decision maker to "don the mental mantle of the incompetent," as the Saikewicz court put it—that is, to make the decision the incompetent would have made if competent. In Saikewicz, the court had to consider evidence that most people with Saikewicz's illness choose treatment, but the court invoked the doctrine of substituted judgment to decide that Saikewicz, a never-competent patient, would not have chosen treatment had he been competent. The court defined its task as determining "how the right of an incompetent person to decline treatment might best be exercised so as to give the fullest possible expression to the character and circumstances of that individual." Asserting that what the majority of reasonable people would choose could differ from what this particular incompetent person would choose, the court proposed the following test:

[T]he decision in many cases such as this should be that which would be made by the incompetent person, if that person were competent, but taking into account the present and future incompetency of the individual as one of the factors which would necessarily enter into the decision-making process of the competent person.[115]

Both the *Quinlan* and the *Saikewicz* courts applied the substituted judgment standard—first determining the subjective wants and needs of the individual and then determining how a reasonable person with those wants and needs would decide. However, these two cases involve different applications of this standard. In *Quinlan*, the patient's father could draw on her life as a competent person to determine her expressed wants and needs. The count found that "if Karen herself were miraculously lucid for an interval . . . and perceptive of her irreversible condition she could effectively decide upon discontinuance of the life-support apparatus, even if it meant the prospect of natural death."[116] In *Saikewicz*, the lack of evidence about the incompetent's likely choice forced the court to look to what is known about other people in his particular circumstances to help determine what a reasonable person in his circumstances, with his needs and desires insofar as they are ascertainable, would decide.

John Robertson argues that it is desirable to treat incompetent persons as autonomous, despite the apparent absurdity of treating the incompetent in a way that "diverges" from his or her actual situation: "It is precisely such a divergence that respect for persons requires and which generally confers benefits on the incompetent. Eliminating this divergence would mean that we treat the incompetent in all respects as a nonthinking, nonchoosing, irrational being—in short, as a nonperson."[117] The courts in *Quinlan* and *Saikewicz* generally agree with this moral pronouncement, and they also ascribe to the incompetent the right of privacy. Ascription of this right makes a choice of either treatment or nontreatment potentially acceptable and frees the proxy decision maker to consider carefully all the individual and subjective features of each case, even if the incompetent patient has not expressed a relevant preference. The decision maker is not bound by the standard of best interests.

We believe that the standard of substituted judgment can and should be rejected for never-competent patients because of its fictional quality. It is conceptually and normatively dubious to treat never-autonomous patients as if they were autonomous. The gap between nonautonomy and autonomy is vast, and different degrees of autonomy constitute a relevant difference between patients. The principles of universalizability (see Chapter 1) and formal justice (see Chapter 6) require that we treat similar cases in a similar way; but the never-competent patient has had no autonomy and therefore should be treated as relevantly different from those who can now make or who have made autonomous choices. Exponents of substituted judgment have failed to established the relevance of the characteristic of autonomy for never-autonomous patients, and one court has held that trying to determine what a never-competent patient would have decided if competent is like asking, "If it snowed all summer, would it then be winter?"[118] The problems are also serious for previously competent patients, such as Karen Ann Quinlan, but they are more practical than conceptual and normative.

If a person has previously (and competently) expressed preferences with sufficient clarity, that person's autonomous preferences can and should be extended to situations of incompetence. Thus, the rule of substituted judgment is an appropriate guideline for previously competent patients whose relevant prior preferences can be discerned. However, this rule is inadequate for never-competent patients or for previously competent patients whose prior actions provide no reliable indication of their preferences. In the latter cases, nonmaleficence and beneficence require that we make treatment or nontreatment decisions according to patients' best interests, as judged by our best estimate of what reasonable persons would prefer, rather than by appeal to a phantom autonomy. Neither the principle of respect for autonomy nor the principle of justice is infringed by the standard of best interests in such cases.

OBJECTIVE AND SUBJECTIVE STANDARDS. In the *Conroy* case, we find an instructive approach to formerly competent patients. The New Jersey supreme court clarifies and combines the standards of best interests and substituted judgment and identifies three rather than two tests of decision making for incompetent patients.[119] Claire Conroy, an eighty-four-year-old resident of a nursing home, suffered from serious and irreversible physical and mental impairments, including arteriosclerotic heart disease, hypertension, and diabetes. She was awake but was severely demented and could not speak. Her condition had worsened so that she could not swallow enough food and water to sustain herself, and she received her nutrition and hydration through a nasogastric tube. She could move a little, but she could not control her excretory functions. Certain stimuli resulted in an occasional response. For example, she would sometimes smile when her hair was combed or when she received a comforting rub, and she would occasionally moan when moved or fed or when her bandages were changes. Conroy's nephew and only surviving blood relative was her guardian. He sought court permission to remove his incompetent aunt's nasogastric tube, which would result in her dehydration and death in about a week.

His petition was opposed by a guardian *ad litem* (a court-appointed guardian to represent the interests of an incompetent person). The trial court decided to permit removal of the feeding tube on the grounds that although her dying might be painful, her life had become impossibly and permanently burdensome. Conroy's guardian *ad litem* appealed. Although Conroy died during the appeal, the appellate court reversed the trial court's judgment on the grounds that removal of the feeding tube entailed killing her (and thus would be active euthanasia).

On further appeal, the court held that any medical treatment, including artificial nutrition and hydration, may be withheld or withdrawn from an incompetent patient under some circumstances. The court invoked the incompetent patient's right to accept or refuse medical treatment, a right that must be exercised by a substitute decision maker. Noting the rights of the competent patient, the court observed that

more difficult questions arise in the context of patients who, like Claire Conroy, are incompetent to make particular treatment decisions for themselves. Such patients are unable to exercise directly their own right to accept or refuse medical treatment. In attempting to exercise the right on their behalf, substitute decision-makers must seek to respect simultaneously both aspects of the patient's right to self-determination—the right to live, and the right, in some cases, to die of natural causes without medical intervention.

This court's language appears at first to accept only the standard of substituted judgment. It asserts that "the goal of decision-making . . . should be to determine and effectuate . . . the decision that the patient would have made if competent" and that "the right of an adult who, like Claire Conroy, was once competent, to determine the course of her medical treatment remains intact even when she is no longer able to assert that right or to appreciate its effectuation." However, in the full decision the court combines the substituted judgment and best interests standards. The court holds that life-sustaining treatment may be withheld or withdrawn from an incompetent patient when it is clear from a "subjective test"—substituted judgment—that this particular patient would have refused under the circumstances. If the subjective test is not met, a "best interests" test must be satisfied.

The court reasons that the subjective standard of substituted judgment may in principle be met by a written document (such as a living will); an oral directive to family member, friend, or health-care provider; durable power of attorney; the patient's convictions about medical treatment administered to others; religious beliefs and tenets of his or her religion; or the "patient's consistent pattern of conduct with respect to prior decisions about his own medical care." The court indicates that it had erred a decade earlier in *Quinlan* when it disregarded the evidence of "statements that Ms. Quinlan made to friends about ಚ൧e artificial prolongation of the lives of others who were terminally ill." Such evidence is "certainly relevant." But, the court notes, evidence has different degrees of probative value, "depending on the remoteness, consistency, and thoughtfulness of the prior statements or actions and the maturity of the person at the time of the statements or acts."

For example, advance directives by patients may involve a specification of standards, a designation of a decision maker, or some combination of the two. A so-called living will that specifies personal standards for decision making—such as, "I don't want to be kept alive by a respirator if I am permanently comatose"—can have high probative value, even though it may require interpretation in a particular situation. Such advance directives come close to making this use of substituted judgment an instance of the principle of respect for an incompetent patient's (previous) autonomy.

Ideally, a proxy conveys rather than substitutes a judgment. In many cases, however, there will be questions of reliability of evidence about the patient's earlier preferences, such as whether he or she was competent and clearly expressed preferences that would be relevant. In doubtful cases, as we have previously argued, it would be better to err on the side of preserving life. For this reason several statutes make it easier for a doubtfully competent person to abrogate an advance directive than to effectuate one. As the *Conroy* court notes, "in the absence of adequate proof of the patient's wishes, it is naive to pretend that the right to self-determination serves as the basis for substituted decision-making."

Nevertheless, the court holds that the absence of adequate proof for invoking substituted judgment does not entail that life-sustaining treatment must always be continued: "Life-sustaining treatment may also be withheld or withdrawn from a patient in Claire Conroy's situation if either of two types of 'best interest' test—a *limited-objective* or a *pure-objective* test—is satisfied." In this particular reliance on the patient's "best interests," the court does not substantially deviate from considerations of autonomy, at least in its "limited-objective test." The limited-objective test requires "some trustworthy evidence that the patient would have refused the treatment" along with the decision maker's conviction that "the burdens of the patient's continued life with the treatment outweigh the benefits of that life for him." If these conditions are satisfied, the treatment is deemed as only prolonging suffering. Any of the evidence mentioned under the subjective test could be sufficient in reaching judgments about the relevant burdens, although it would perhaps be "too vague, casual, or remote to constitute the clear proof of the patient's subjective intent that is necessary to satisfy the subjective test."

Even if there is no evidence about the patient's previous wishes, life-sustaining treatment may be justifiably withheld or withdrawn if decision makers satisfy the pure objective test of best interests: "The net burdens of the patient's life with the treatment should clearly and markedly outweigh the benefits that the patient derives from life" and "the recurring, unavoidable and severe pain of the patient's life with the treatment would be such that the effect of administering life-sustaining treatment would be inhumane." Although the New Jersey court limited its holding to previously competent patients in Claire Conroy's situation, its arguments extend to other classes of incompetent patients.[120]

The *Conroy* decision—which we have used as a case study—offers a sophisticated and helpful analysis of the relevance of substituted judgment and best interests in making decisions for incompetent patients, but it does not solve all problems. There are problems, for example, about the evidence that is satisfactory for substituted judgment and about the limits of such judgments. In the absence of explicit instructions, a proxy decision maker might selectively choose from the patient's life history those values that accord with the proxy's own values and then use only the selected values in reaching decisions. The proxy's findings might also be based on values of the patient that are only distantly relevant to the immediate decision—such as the patient's expressed dislike of hospitals. For example, what can a decision maker legitimately infer from Conroy's prior conduct, especially her fear and avoidance of doctors and her earlier refusal to consent to amputation of a gangrenous leg? Another problem concerns whether the burdens considered under the best interests standard should be limited to physical pain and suffering, as the court's language at points suggests. If pain and suffering were the only relevant burdens, it would be difficult to justify withholding or withdrawing life-sustaining treatment for a permanently comatose patient such as Karen Ann Quinlan.

There is also the problem of ensuring that proxies respect the patient's prior autonomous wishes, when known. Consider a study of decisions by proxies for elderly patients in nursing homes who were enrolled as research subjects in a study of morbidity associated with long-term urinary catheters. Refusal was significantly associated with the proxy's belief that research should not be conducted in nursing homes at all, that the proxy himself or herself would not consent to participate, that the research would disturb the patient, and that the patient, if competent, would not consent. Nonetheless, thirty-one percent of the proxies who believed that the patient would not consent if competent still consented for the patient. Because this discrepancy emerged only through interviews after the research project, the researchers did not have to confront the ethical dilemma of what to do when proxies act against what they believe the patient would do.[121]

In conclusion, we have argued in this section that previously competent patients who have autonomously expressed their preference can be fairly treated under the standard of substituted judgment, although many practical problems remain in implementing the standard. For previously competent patients whose prior preferences cannot be reliably traced and for never-competent patients, it is appropriate to rely on the best interests standard, based on nonmaleficence and beneficence, rather than on the substituted judgment standard, which is based on autonomy. It has been argued that substituted judgment is a standard that seeks "to implement the patients' best interests *as that patient would have defined them,*" and therefore "the substituted judgment approach is merely one way in which the best interests standard is given content."[122] This synthesis is, we think, too convenient and confusing. The best interests standard is not an autonomy-rooted conception and can in principle conflict with an autonomous preference or decision. It is best to keep the two standards as conceptually and normatively distinct as possible.

The selection of proxy decision makers

For any of these standards, fundamental questions concern procedures for decision making and who, finally, should decide for the incompetent patient. All we can hope for in treatment and nontreatment decisions for incompetent patients is imperfect procedural justice, while trying to improve our procedures so that they more closely approximate perfect procedural justice. This approach requires that we evaluate procedures in part according to their reliable production of right outcomes, as judged by the independent standards discussed in the previous section.

PERSONAL SELECTION OF A PROXY WHILE COMPETENT. In an increasingly important procedure, a person while competent may select a proxy or surrogate who can make decisions about treatment for him or her in periods of incompetence. We mentioned this possibility earlier in distinguishing two types of advance directives: the specification of standards of decision making and the designation of specific decision makers. Much of the early public discussion and legislative action on this topic (principally including natural death acts) focused on the agent's specification of standards through so-called living wills or advance directives to physicians. However, it has proved difficult to specify standards that adequately anticipate the full range of situations that might emerge.

Consider the following case. Mrs. Z., a fifty-five-year-old teacher of foreign languages, developed aspiration pneumonia, which required admission to the intensive care unit. Her aspiration pneumonia was probably caused by her diminished gag reflex, the result of twenty years of multiple sclerosis. To prevent future occurrence, after the immediate problem was brought under control, the staff discussed oversewing the patient's epiglottis (part of the larynx), which would require a permanent tracheostomy and entail loss of laryngeal speech capability. Because of her multiple sclerosis, Mrs. Z. was confined to a bed in her home, and her only interaction with friends involved speech. She also tutored students at home. If she did not have the procedure, a future episode of aspiration pneumonia would probably be fatal. Mrs. Z. stated that she would rather die than be unable to speak, but she was not clearly competent at the time, in part because of what was believed to be a mild organic brain syndrome. Mrs. Z.'s prior living will was then submitted by her sister. The document indicated Mrs. Z.'s wish not to be kept alive artificially if she could not lead a "useful life." The sister—in effect serving as a proxy—interpreted Mrs. Z.'s use of the phrase *useful life* to include the ability to relate to others meaningfully by verbal communication. The staff felt comfortable in accepting this judgment and in refraining from performing procedures they had been considering.[123]

Some states now offer the possibility of designating a surrogate or proxy decision maker as well as specifying standards for medical decision making. In addition, some commentators believe that the legal mechanism of "durable power of attorney" can be used effectively for medical decision making, including refusal of life-sustaining treatment. It involves a document to assign another person authority to perform specified actions on behalf of the signer. The power is "durable" because it continues in effect if the signer of the document becomes incompetent.[124] The main advantage is that a person while competent can designate someone who knows his or her values well and who will seek to apply them in a concrete situation that the patient might not have anticipated with sufficient clarity to guide a physician or hospital staff through written directives. This procedure of designating decision makers is not free of problems, because the designated decision maker may be unavailable when needed, may be incompetent to decide, or may have a conflict of interest (e.g., because of a prospective inheritance or a promotion in a family-owned business). Nonetheless, durable power of attorney is a promising way for competent persons to exercise their autonomy and extend their values into medical decision making when they are unable to make decisions.

QUALIFICATIONS OF PROXY DECISION MAKERS. When an incompetent patient has not designated a decision maker or has not left a directive to a physician, who should make the decision and with whom should that decision maker consult? We propose the following list of qualifications for decision makers for incompetent patients (including newborns): (1) ability to make reasoned judgments (competence), (2) adequate knowledge and information, (3) emotional stability, and (4) a commitment to the incompetent patient's interests that is free of conflicts of interest and free of controlling influence by others who may not seek the patient's best interests.[125]

The first three conditions on this list are familiar because they are necessary for a competent person making a decision about treatment. Our discussion of informed consent in Chapter 3 provides the relevant background: The ability to make reasoned judgments, the key ingredient in competence, may be independent of possession of adequate information and emotional stability, both of which may be decisively affected by the actions of physicians and others, who may be able to correct the deficiencies. More controversial on the list is item 4—a commitment to the incompetent patient's interests that is free of influences that might compromise the commitment. We are here endorsing a criterion of partiality (acting in the incompetent patient's best interests) rather than impartiality, which suggests neutrality in the consideration of the interests of various parties.[126]

FAMILY MEMBERS AS PRESUMPTIVE PROXIES. Four major classes of decision makers have been proposed and used in cases of withholding and terminating treatment of incompetent patients: families, physicians and other health-care professionals, institutional committees, and courts. We propose a structure of decision-making authority that places the family as the presumptive authority when the patient cannot make the decision and has not previously designated a decision maker. The family's role should be presumptively primary because of expectable identification with the patient's interests and intimate knowledge of his or her wishes. However, the authority of the family should not be final or ultimate.[127]

The general reasons for assigning priority to the family or next of kin in proxy decision making also suggests priority for some family members over others. An example we find acceptable is the ordering in the 1984 Virginia Natural Death Act. According to this act, if the patient is incompetent and has not specified standards through an advance directive, a decision to withhold or withdraw life-prolonging treatment must involve consultation and agreement between the attending physician and "any of the following individuals in the following order of priority if no individual in a prior class is reasonably available, willing and competent to act": judicially appointed guardian (if necessary in the circumstances); patient-designated decision maker; spouse; adult child or a majority of the adult children reasonably available; parents of the patient; nearest living relative of the patient.[128]

For a previously competent patient, this serial arrangement of family members—spouse, adult children, parents, and close relatives—rests on their presumed ability to use his or her preferences to make the decision or to interpret the standard of best interests as well as their presumed willingness to do so. For a newborn, the parents should generally be the primary decision makers, because they have made a series of decisions and engaged in a series of actions that have resulted in the birth of the infant. They may be presumed to choose and act in the infant's best interests, and they should be permitted to make the decision unless it is necessary to disqualify them as decision makers because of child abuse, abandonment, neglect, or the like.

This suggested ranking may be threatened by a decision maker's overriding personal interest. Serious conflicts of interest in the family may be more common than has generally been appreciated by either physicians or the courts. For example, a family member may simultaneously have an interest both in the patient's welfare and in the patient's death. A clear example is Case 17, the Earle Spring case. Spring's family was devoted to him but also was under a burdensome financial arrangement in paying for his care. As the debts mounted, a lien was placed on a family home. The court eventually appointed a guardian *ad litem* to investigate and protect Spring's interests. This case and many like it raise profound issues about valid decision making under conflict of interest.

Where a familial conflict of interest threatens the patient's previous wishes or interests and cannot be corrected, it will often be necessary to disqualify the family as proxy decision maker. The other conditions for disqualification simply reverse the conditions of qualification presented above: If a proxy's incompetence, inadequate information, or emotional instability are not correctable and threaten the incompetent patient's interests, the proxy should be disqualified.

THE ROLE OF HEALTH-CARE PROFESSIONALS. Physicians and other health-care professionals can and should help the family become adequate decision makers by imparting sufficient information and by imparting a proper climate for discussion. However, these health-care professionals remain moral agents, with a responsibility to safeguard the patient's interests and preferences (where known) by monitoring the quality of surrogate decision making. They should not violate the principle of nonmaleficence toward incompetent patients, which they can often discharge by withdrawing from the case or transferring the patient, and they also have obligations of beneficence to ensure that proxy decision makers do not violate obligations of beneficence and nonmaleficence. Mere withdrawal is not always morally adequate, because there may be a high probability of consequences seriously detrimental to the incompetent patient's interests.

In examining the role of physicians and other health-care professionals, empirical evidence about their willingness to override familial decisions and their reasons for doing so are relevant. Much of the available evidence is derived from parental decisions about neonates and may not be accurate beyond this class of patients. Some of this evidence indicates that physicians occasionally displace parents as decision makers in order to protect the parents rather than the infants. This practice is typically based on nonmaleficence and beneficence toward the family. One physician writes, "At the end it is usually the doctor who has to decide the issue. It is . . . cruel to ask the parents whether they want their child to live or die." [129] Such paternalistic actions toward the parents of seriously ill newborns usually involve nondisclosure or manipulation of information rather than coercion. For example, physicians may not inform the parents that they have a decision to make or may not provide enough information for them to make the decisions on the grounds that it would overburden them, upset them, or make them feel guilty. These paternalistic actions may in some cases be justified, but alternatives such as counseling also may alleviate the problems. (For conditions of justified paternalism, see Chapter 5.)

Another largely empirical question is whether physicians are too ready to acquiesce in the proxy's decisions. In one survey of pediatric surgeons and pediatricians, the following question was asked:

Would you acquiesce in parents' decisions to refuse to consent for surgery in a newborn with intestinal atresia if the infant also had (a) Down syndrome alone, (b) Down syndrome plus congenital heart disease, (c) anencephaly, (d) cloacal exstrophy, (e) meningomyelocele, (f) multiple limb or craniofacial malformations, (g) 13-15 trisomy, or (h) no other anomalies, i.e., normal aside from atresia?[130]

In their responses, 76.8 percent of the pediatric surgeons and 49.5 percent of the pediatricians indicated that they would acquiesce in parental decisions to refuse permission for surgery to correct intestinal atresia even if the infant's only other problem was Down syndrome. Of course, the term *acquiesce* does not imply approval of the decision, and it also fails to suggest the complexity of physician involvement in shaping the parents' understanding of the problem and the ultimate decision. But the term does indicate an unwillingness to override the decision.

The U.S. Department of Health and Human Services appealed to this survey as evidence that some mechanism is needed to protect handicapped infants against discrimination, although critics have charged that the survey is not statistically valid, is outdated, and may not reflect actual practice.[131] We cannot here moderate this empirical dispute. But we can offer the following normative generalization: If pediatric surgeons and pediatricians are willing to acquiesce in parents' decisions to let an infant with Down syndrome die rather than correct a life-threatening intestinal blockage, some procedure or mechanism is needed to protect the infant's interests. We have seen no sound argument that the interests of an infant with Down syndrome are better served by nontreatment than by surgery in such a case.

INSTITUTIONAL ETHICS COMMITTEES. If parents sometimes refuse treatment against the interests of their infants, and if physicians readily acquiesce, then some mechanism or procedure is needed to break the closed, private circle of refusal and acquiescence. One possible mechanism is the hospital ethics committee. It may not be sufficient to rely on an ethics committee only if a conflict emerges between parents and physicians, because of evidence about physician acquiescence to parental wishes. Thus, until we better understand the extent to which parents and physicians act or fail to act in accord with infants' best interests, it seems morally appropriate to mandate internal committee review whenever parents decide that life-sustaining therapy should be foregone.[132]

Although institutional committees were involved earlier in allocating time on kidney machines (see Chapter 6) and are now required for research involving human subjects (see Chapter 7), they are more controversial in decisions about treatment or nontreatment for incompetent patients. According to a survey in 1981, ethics committees existed in only one percent of all hospitals, in less than five percent of the hospitals with more than two hundred beds, and in no hospitals with fewer than two hundred beds.[133] There is evidence that they are more numerous now, partially as a result of the controversy over decisions about handicapped children.[134] However, they differ widely in their composition and function. Many recommend policies and serve educational functions in the hospital, but controversy centers on whether, apart from evidence of abuse of incompetent patients, committees are needed to make or facilitate decisions in particular cases.

Many argue that informal de facto committees already exist because decisions about treatment and nontreatment are not private whenever numerous caregivers are involved in the case. Several cases have reached the courts because some member of the health-care team, often a nurse, believed that the decision not to provide treatment violated the obligation of nonmaleficence.[135] From this perspective, committees may be unnecessary in actual decision making, they could diffuse responsibility, and they would impose another layer of bureaucratic delay insofar as they cannot be convened in a timely way. Unless they include independent parties, they could become pawns of powerful groups. These are, we believe, good reasons for caution. More research on the role and functioning of these committees is needed. For example, committees might serve as a forum for discussion without having power of veto, or they might engage in retrospective rather than prospective review of cases or in prospective review without veto power.

THE JUDICIAL SYSTEM. Beyond committees, the courts have also been proposed as final decision makers in these cases. Expressly departing from the *Quinlan* decision in New Jersey, the supreme judicial court of Massachusetts held in *Saikewicz* (Case 16) that questions of life and death require the "process of detached but passionate investigation and decision that forms the ideal on which the judicial branch of government was created." Achieving this ideal is the courts' responsibility and is "not to be entrusted to any other group." The Massachusetts court held that probate courts should make these decisions after considering all viewpoints and alternatives, including those of an ethics committee.[136]

In cases such as *Saikewicz* in which there is no involved family, or when the family is not interested, another decision maker—physicians, a committee, or the courts—is essential. There is nothing inherently objectionable about an appeal to probate courts as decision makers in such cases, but there is also no solid evidence to suppose that physicians and hospital ethics committees would be less satisfactory than the courts for many cases. There were early fears that the Massachusetts court had mandated regular judicial involvement and that such involvement would be slow, costly, and adversarial, as well as unnecessary. Later developments have indicated that the decision was intended to involve the courts only "from time to time" in decisions that are "fraught with difficulties" and where a court could serve as a safeguard.[137]

The courts, we suggest, should be invoked as a last resort, when there are good reasons to seek to disqualify the family in order to protect an incompetent patient's interests or to adjudicate conflicts over those interests. The courts may also need to intervene in nontreatment decisions for salvageable incompetent patients in mental institutions, nursing homes, and the like. If no family members are available or willing to be involved, and if the patient is confined to a state mental institution or is in a nursing home, it may be appropriate to establish various safeguards beyond the health-care team and the institutional ethics committee. For example, the New Jersey supreme court in *Conroy* recommended the involvement of the state ombudsman, already an established administrative office for the surveillance of nursing homes.[138]

Conclusion

In this chapter we have focused primarily on protecting the interests of incompetent persons, just as in Chapter 3 we focused primarily on respecting the autonomy of competent persons. We have reached several conclusions of substantive and procedural importance in this chapter. We have argued that the principle of double effect needs to be reconceived as a principle of nonmaleficence; that the distinction between killing and letting die is worth retaining in professional, social, and legal rules; and that the distinction between withholding and withdrawing life-sustaining treatments is morally irrelevant and potentially dangerous. We also proposed replacing the language of ordinary and extraordinary treatment with that of optional, obligatory, and wrong forms of treatment, and we argued that no form of life-prolonging medical treatment—including artificial nutrition or hydration—is always obligatory. The criteria for distinguishing obligatory, optional, and wrong treatments derive from the patient's wishes (a consideration of autonomy) and the patient's best interests (considerations of beneficence and nonmaleficence). These criteria include whether the treatment would provide a reasonable chance of benefit and whether the benefits would outweigh the burdens to the patient. Because decisions for incompetent patients must usually be made by proxy decision makers, we also proposed a structure of decision-making authority, assigning presumptive authority to the family in the absence of a previously competent patient's designation of a decision maker.

Implicit throughout Chapter 4 is the suggestion that morality is concerned with the harmfulness of harms *per se* and not simply with responsibility for causing harm. If it is conceded that we can and should, as a moral matter, protect against (some types and level of) harm and not merely avoid causing the harm, it is a short step to the conclusion that there is a positive obligation to provide benefits such as health care. The step may be shorter still because of the conceptual uncertainty that surrounds the distinctions between the obligation to avoid harm, the obligation to benefit, and the obligation to treat others justly. The last two topics are engaged in Chapters 5 and 6.

Notes

1. W. H. S. Jones, *Hippocrates*, Vol. I (Cambridge, Mass.: Harvard University Press, 1923), p. 165. See also Ludwig Edelstein, *Ancient Medicine* (Baltimore: Johns Hopkins University Press, 1967); and Albert R. Jonsen, "Do No Harm: Axiom of Medical Ethics," in *Philosophical and Medical Ethics: Its Nature and Significance*, ed. Stuart F. Spicker and H. Tristram Engelhardt, Jr. (Dordrecht: D. Reidel, 1977), pp. 27–41.
2. H. L. A. Hart, *The Concept of Law* (Oxford: Clarendon Press, 1961), p. 190.
3. W. D. Ross, *The Right and the Good* (Oxford: Clarendon Press, 1930), pp. 21–26; and John Rawls, *A Theory of Justice* (Cambridge, Mass.: Harvard University Press, 1971), p. 114.
4. William Frankena, *Ethics*, 2d ed. (Englewood Cliffs, N.J.: Prentice-Hall, 1973), p. 47.
5. Alan Meisel and Loren H. Roth, "Must a Man Be His Cousin's Keeper?" *Hastings Center Report* 8 (October 1978): 5–6.
6. Jonsen, "Do No Harm," pp. 27–41.
7. Ross, *The Right and the Good*, pp. 21–22.
8. See Joel Feinberg, *Harm to Others*, Vol. I of *The Moral Limits of the Criminal Law* (New York: Oxford University Press, 1984), pp. 32–36. Compare R. M. Hare, "Wrongness and Harm," in his *Essays on the Moral Concepts* (Berkeley: University of California Press, 1972).
9. See Bernard Gert, *The Moral Rules* (New York: Harper and Row, 1973), p. 125.
10. For a careful criticism of the priority of avoiding harm, see Nancy Davis, "The Priority of Avoiding Harm," in *Killing and Letting Die*, ed. Bonnie Steinbock (Englewood Cliffs, N.J.: Prentice-Hall, 1980), pp. 172–214.
11. See Eric D'Arcy, *Human Acts* (Oxford: Clarendon Press, 1963), p. 121.
12. William L. Prosser, *Handbook of the Law of Torts*, 4th ed. (St. Paul, Minn.: West Publishing, 1971), pp. 145–46. For a broader view of "moral negligence," see Ronald D. Milo, *Immorality* (Princeton, N.J.: Princeton University Press, 1984). Milo uses the term *moral negligence* to refer to "any kind of morally wrong act due to a particular kind of shortcoming on the part of the agent—namely, a culpable failure to take the precautions necessary to assure oneself, before acting, that what one proposes to do is not in violation of one's moral principles. Conduct due to such a shortcoming may take various forms, including not only conduct that involves an unreasonable risk of harm but also conduct that is undoubtedly harmful, as well as conduct that involves breaking a promise or deceiving someone" (p. 84).

13. See "Necessity and Sufficiency of Expert Evidence and Extent of Physician's Duty to Inform Patient of Risks of Proposed Treatment," *American Law Reports* 3d, 52 (1977): 1084; "Physician's Duty to Inform of Risks," *American Law Reports* 3d, 88 (1986): 1010–25; and Martin Curd and Larry May, *Professional Responsibility for Harmful Actions* (Dubuque: Kendall/Hunt, 1984).

14. Quoted in Angela Roddy Holder, *Medical Malpractice Law* (New York: John Wiley, 1975), p. 42.

15. The principle of double effect has some precedents that predate the writings of St. Thomas Aquinas (e.g., see Augustine and Abelard). However, the history primarily flows from Aquinas through theological writers in traditions such as that of the Jesuits. See Anthony Kenny, "The History of Intention in Ethics," *Anatomy of the Soul* (Oxford: Basil Blackwell, 1973), appendix; Stanley Windass, "Double Think and Double Effect," *Blackfriars* 44 (1963): 257–66; and Joseph T. Mangan, S. J., "An Historical Analysis of the Principle of Double Effect," *Theological Studies* 10 (1949): 41–61.

16. See David Granfield, *The Abortion Decision* (Garden City, N.Y.: Doubleday, 1969).

17. For literature on double effect, see Richard A. McCormick, S. J., *Ambiguity in Moral Choice* (Milwaukee: Marquette University, 1973); Paul Ramsey and Richard A. McCormick, S. J., eds., *Doing Evil to Achieve Good: Moral Choice in Conflict Situations* (Chicago: Loyola University Press, 1978); and Joseph M. Boyle, Jr., "Toward Understanding the Principle of Double Effect," *Ethics* 90 (July 1980): 527–38. For criticisms and attempts to redirect issues about the principle into another set of issues, see Jonathan Bennett, "Whatever the Consequences," *Analysis* 26 (1966): 83–102; Philippa Foot, "The Problem of Abortion and the Doctrine of Double Effect," *Oxford Review* 5 (1967): 5–15; Jonathan Glover, *Causing Death and Saving Lives* (London: Penguin Books, 1977); Susan Nicholson, *Abortion and the Roman Catholic Church* (Knoxville, Tenn.: Religious Ethics, 1978); R. A. Duff, "Intention, Responsibility, and Double Effect," *Philosophical Quarterly* 32 (1982): 1–16; R. G. Frey, *Rights, Killing, and Suffering* (Oxford: Basil Blackwell, 1983), chap. 13; Norvin Richards, "Double Effect and Moral Character," *Mind* 93 (1984): 381–97; and Nancy Davis, "The Doctrine of Double Effect: Problems of Interpretation," *Pacific Philosophical Quarterly* 65 (1984): 107–23.

18. For an emphasis on proportionality, see McCormick, *Ambiguity in Moral Choice*. For an emphasis on intention, see Charles Fried, *Right and Wrong* (Cambridge, Mass.: Harvard University Press, 1978); and Thomas Nagel, "The Limits of Objectivity," in *The Tanner Lectures on Human Values, 1980*, Vol. I, ed. S. McMurrin (Cambridge: Cambridge University Press, 1980), pp. 76–139. Various measures to reform the principle have been presented by Germain Grisez, Michael Walzer, and others. See Germain Grisez, "Towards a Consistent Natural Law Ethics of Killing," *American Journal of Jurisprudence* 15 (1970): 64–97; and Michael Walzer, *Just and Unjust Wars* (New York: Basic Books, 1977).

19. Here we think primarily of the philosophical analyses offered by G. E. M. Anscombe, John Finnis, and Joseph Boyle. See G. E. M. Anscombe, "War and Murder," in *Nuclear Weapons: A Catholic Response*, ed. Walter Stein (New York: Sheed and Ward, 1961), pp. 45–62; idem, "Modern Moral Philosophy," *Philosophy* (1958): 1–19; John Finnis, "The Rights and Wrongs of Abortions: A Reply to Judith Thomson," *Philosophy and Public Affairs* 2 (1973): 117–45; and Joseph Boyle, "Toward Understanding the Principle of Double Effect."

20. *Ethical and Religious Directives for Catholic Health Facilities* (St. Louis: Catholic Hospital Association, 1975).

21. Sacred Congregation for the Doctrine of the Faith, *Declaration on Euthanasia* (Vatican City, May 5, 1980), as reprinted in President's Commission for the Study of Ethical Problems in Medicine and Biomedical and Behavioral Research, *Deciding to Forego Life-Sustaining Treatment* (Washington, D.C.: U.S. Government Printing Office, 1983), pp. 300–307.

22. The most developed analysis of this description is Michael E. Bratman, *Intention, Plans, and Practical Reason* (Cambridge, Mass.: Harvard University Press, 1987). Bratman discusses problems of double effect in chap. 10. See also George A. Miller, Eugene Galanter, and Karl Pribram, *Plans and the Structure of Behavior* (New York: Holt, Rinehart, and Winston, 1960); and Alvin I. Goldman, *A Theory of Human Action* (Englewood Cliffs, N.J.: Prentice-Hall, 1970).

23. Goldman, *A Theory of Human Action*, pp. 49–85.

24. Hector-Neri Castañeda, "Intensionality and Identity in Human Action and Philosophical Method," *Nous* 13 (1979): 235–60, esp. 255.

25. Our analysis on this point borrows from Ruth R. Faden and Tom L. Beauchamp, *A History and Theory of Informed Consent* (New York: Oxford University Press, 1986), chap. 7.

26. We also follow John Searle in thinking that we cannot reliably distinguish in many situations among acts, effects, consequences, and events. John R. Searle, "The Intentionally of Intention and Action," *Cognitive Science* 4 (1980): 65.

27. Precisely this interpretation of double effect is defended by Leonard Gedden in "On the Intrinsic Wrongness of Killing Innocent People," *Analysis* 33 (1973): 94–95.

28. See the careful argument to this conclusion in Helga Kuhse, *The Sanctity-of-Life Doctrine in Medicine: A Critique* (Oxford: Clarendon Press, 1987), pp. 93–103. This book stimulated several of the arguments in this section.

29. Richards, "Double Effect and Moral Character"; and Kuhse, *The Sanctity-of-Life Doctrine in Medicine*, pp. 158–63.

30. American Medical Association Council on Ethical and Judicial Affairs, *Current Opinions* (Chicago: American Medical Association, 1986), 2.18.

31. See W. St. C. Symmers, Sr., "Not Allowed to Die," *British Medical Journal* 1 (1968): 442.

32. This 1973 statement, which was distributed by the AMA in reproduced typescript, is reprinted in James Rachels, *The End of Life: Euthanasia and Morality* (Oxford: Oxford University Press, 1986), pp. 88, 192–93.

33. James Rachels, "Active and Passive Euthanasia," *New England Journal of Medicine* 292 (1975): 78–80. For valuable articles on the distinction between killing and letting die, see Steinbock, *Killing and Letting Die;* and John Ladd, ed., *Ethical Issues Relating to Life and Death* (New York: Oxford University Press, 1979).

34. Richard L. Trammell, "Saving Life and Taking Life," *Journal of Philosophy* 72 (1975): 131–37.

35. Gilbert Meilaender, "The Distinction between Killing and Allowing to Die," *Theological Studies* 37 (1976): 467–70.

36. This distinction and our arguments are indebted to John Rawls, "Two Concepts of Rules," *Philosophical Review* 64 (1955): 3–32.

37. See G. J. Hughes, S. J., "Killing and Letting Die," *The Month* 236 (1975): 42–45; and David Louisell, "Euthanasia and Biothanasia: On Dying and Killing," *Linacre Quarterly* 40 (1973): 234–58.

38. For fuller discussions, see Sissela Bok, "The Leading Edge of the Wedge," *Hastings Center Report* 1 (December 1971): 8–10; Paul Ramsey, "The Wedge: Not So Simple," *Hastings Center Report* 1 (December 1971): 11–12; Trudy Govier, "What's Wrong with Slippery Slope Arguments?" *Canadian Journal of Philosophy* 12 (June 1982): 303–16; Frederick Schauer, "Slippery Slopes," *Harvard Law Review* 99 (1985): 361–83; and Bernard Williams, "Which Slopes are Slippery?" in *Moral Dilemmas in Modern Medicine*, ed. Michael Lockwood (Oxford: Oxford University Press, 1985), pp. 126–37. Williams further distinguishes two types of slippery slope argument: the *horrible result* argument objects to what is at the bottom of the slope; the *arbitrary result* argument objects to the fact that it is a slope and that there is no nonarbitrary way to get off. Even critics of the application of the slippery slope argument in debates about euthanasia may recognize that it has what James Rachels calls a "grain of truth," in that the reasons that support voluntary euthanasia may also support some forms of nonvoluntary euthanasia. However, he insists that they do not push toward acceptance of involuntary euthanasia. Rachels, *The End of Life*, chap. 10.

39. See Paul Ramsey, *Ethics at the Edges of Life* (New Haven: Yale University Press, 1978), pp. 306–7.

40. James Rachels, "Medical Ethics and the Rule against Killing: Comments on Professor Hare's Paper," in *Philosophical Medical Ethics*, ed. Spicker and Engelhardt, p. 65.

41. Rachels, "Active and Passive Euthanasia."

42. Leo Alexander, "Medical Science under Dictatorship," *New England Journal of Medicine* 241 (1949): 39–47.

43. Robert Jay Lifton, *The Nazi Doctors: Medical Killing and the Psychology of Genocide* (New York: Basic Books, 1986).

44. See Rachels, *The End of Life*. For the controversy about the appropriateness of the Nazi analogy, see the special supplement on "Biomedical Ethics and the Shadow of Nazism," *Hastings Center Report* 6 (1976), esp. the article by Lucy Dawidowicz.

45. For an important debate about these issues, see Yale Kamisar, "Some Non-religious Views against Proposed 'Mercy-Killing' Legislation," *Minnesota Law Review* 42 (1958); and Glanville Williams, " 'Mercy-Killing' Legislation—A Rejoinder," *Minnesota Law Review* 43 (1958). For the movement to legalize active, voluntary euthanasia in the Netherlands, see "Final Report of the Netherlands State Commission on Euthanasia: An English Summary," *Bioethics* 1 (1987): 156–62; and J. K. M. Gevers, "Legal Developments Concerning Active Euthanasia on Request in the Netherlands," *Bioethics* 1 (1987): 163–74.

46. "It's Over, Debbie," *Journal of the American Medical Association* 259 (1988): 272.

47. We owe most of this argument to James Rachels.

48. Marcia Angell, "The Quality of Mercy," *New England Journal of Medicine* 306 (1982): 98–99.

49. Eric J. Cassell, "The Nature of Suffering and the Goods of Medicine," *New England Journal of Medicine* 306 (1982): 639–45.

50. Charles Fried, "Rights and Health Care—Beyond Equity and Efficiency," *New England Journal of Medicine* 293 (1975): 245.

51. For a discussion of this case, see Paige Mitchell, *Act of Love: The Killing of George Zygmaniak* (New York: Knopf, 1976).

52. See Ramsey, *Ethics at the Edges of Life*, p. 217; and Robert Veatch, *Death, Dying, and the Biological Revolution* (New Haven: Yale University Press, 1976), p. 97.
53. See Antony Flew, "The Principle of Euthanasia," in *Euthanasia and the Right to Death: The Case of Voluntary Euthanasia*, ed. A. B. Downing (London: Peter Owen, 1969), pp. 30–48; and H. Tristram Engelhardt, Jr., *The Foundations of Bioethics* (New York: Oxford University Press, 1986), esp. chap. 7.
54. On the different conceptual problems in distinguishing between killing and letting die, see Kuhse, *The Sanctity-of-Life Doctrine*, pp. 41ff, 103ff, and 135ff.
55. Kenneth C. Micetich, Patricia H. Steinecker, and David C. Thomasma, "Are Intravenous Fluids Morally Required for a Dying Patient?" *Archives of Internal Medicine* 143 (May 1983): 975–78.
56. This case was presented to one of the authors during a consultation.
57. *In the matter of Spring*, 405 N.E. 2d 115 (1980), at 488–89.
58. See President's Commission, *Deciding to Forego Life-Sustaining Treatment*, pp. 73–77.
59. Robert Stinson and Peggy Stinson, *The Long Dying of Baby Andrew* (Boston: Little, Brown, 1983), p. 355.
60. President's Commission, *Deciding to Forego Life-Sustaining Treatment*, p. 235.
61. S. E. Bedell and T. L. Delbanco, "Choices about Cardiopulmonary Resuscitation in the Hospital," *New England Journal of Medicine* 309 (1983): 569–76.
62. S. E. Bedell and T. L. Delbanco, "Choices about Cardiopulmonary Resuscitation in the Hospital: When Do Physicians Talk with Patients?" *New England Journal of Medicine* 310 (1984): 1089–93. See also Marcia Angell, "Respecting the Autonomy of Competent Patients," *New England Journal of Medicine* 310 (1984): 1115–16.
63. See Ramsey, *Ethics at the Edges of Life*, p. 153; and Veatch, *Death, Dying and the Biological Revolution*, chap. 3.
64. See Paul Ramsey, *The Patient as Person* (New Haven: Yale University Press, 1970), p. 120.
65. See Diane Lynn Redleaf, Suzanne Baillie Schmitt, and William Charles Thompson, "The California Natural Death Act: An Empirical Study of Physicians' Practices," *Stanford Law Review* 31 (May 1979): 913–45.
66. Gerald Kelly, S. J., "The Duty to Preserve Life," *Theological Studies* 12 (December 1951): 550.
67. For a comprehensive statement of the issues in determining death, see President's Commission, *Defining Death* (Washington, D.C.: Government Printing Office, 1981).
68. See Sharon H. Imbus and Bruce E. Zawacki, "Autonomy for Burn Patients When Survival Is Unprecedented," *New England Journal of Medicine* 297 (1977): 390.
69. *Superintendent of Belchertown State School* v. *Saikewicz*, Mass. 370 N.E. 2d 417 (1977), at 428.
70. Ibid.
71. Ramsey, *Ethics at the Edges of Life*, p. 155.
72. We draw here from Richard McCormick, "The Quality of Life, the Sanctity of Life," *Hastings Center Report* 8 (February 1978): 32. See also Richard McCormick, "To Save or Let Die: The Dilemma of Modern Medicine," *Journal of the American Medical Association* 229 (1974): 172–76.
73. President's Commission, *Deciding to Forego Life-Sustaining Treatment*, chap. 5. See also the several articles on "The Persistent Problem of PVS [Persistent Vegetative State]," *Hastings Center Report* 18 (February–March, 1988): 26–47.

74. Ramsey, *Ethics at the Edges of Life*, p. 172.
75. President's Commission, *Deciding to Forego Life-Sustaining Treatment.*
76. See Norman L. Cantor, *Legal Frontiers of Death and Dying* (Bloomington: Indiana University Press, 1987), pp. 87–91. Cantor's book supports this conclusion and also provides a synthesis of legal materials relevant to the moral topics we are addressing in this chapter.
77. Fred M. Frohock, *Special Care: Medical Decisions at the Beginning of Life* (Chicago: University of Chicago Press, 1986). See also Jeanne Harley Guillemin and Lynda Lytle Holmstrom, *Mixed Blessings: Intensive Care for Newborns* (New York: Oxford University Press, 1986); and Jeffrey Lyon, *Playing God in the Nursery* (New York: W. W. Norton, 1986). For the fullest recent accounts of the ethical debates about decisions regarding seriously ill newborns, see Robert Weir, *Selective Nontreatment of Handicapped Newborns: Moral Dilemmas in Neonatal Medicine* (New York: Oxford University Press, 1984); Helga Kuhse and Peter Singer, *Should This Baby Live? The Problem of Handicapped Infants* (Oxford: Oxford University Press, 1985); Thomas H. Murray and Arthur L. Caplan, eds., *Which Babies Shall Live? Humanistic Dimensions of the Care of Imperiled Newborns* (Clifton, N.J.: Humana Press, 1985); Earl E. Shelp, *Born to Die? Deciding the Fate of Critically Ill Newborns* (New York: Free Press, 1986); and Richard C. McMillan, H. Tristram Englehardt, Jr., and Stuart F. Spicker, eds., *Euthanasia and the Newborn: Conflicts Regarding Saving Lives* (Dordrecht: D. Reidel, 1987).
78. Albert R. Jonsen and Michael J. Garland, "A Moral Policy for Life/Death Decisions in the Intensive Care Nursery," in *Ethics of Newborn Intensive Care*, ed. Albert R. Jonsen and Michael J. Garland (Berkeley: University of California, Institute of Governmental Studies, 1976), p. 148.
79. H. Tristram Engelhardt, Jr., "Ethical Issues in Aiding the Death of Young Children," in *Beneficent Euthanasia*, ed. Marvin Kohl (Buffalo, N.Y.: Prometheus Books, 1975), p. 187. Emphasis added.
80. See R. B. Zachary, "Ethical Social Aspects of Treatment of Spina Bifida," *Lancet* 2 (1968): 274–76; John M. Freeman, "To Treat or Not to Treat: Ethical Dilemmas of Treating the Infant with a Myelomeningocele," *Clinical Neurosurgery* 20 (1973): 134–46; John Lorber, "Selective Treatment of Myelomeningocele: To Treat or Not to Treat?" *Pediatrics* 53 (1974): 307–8; several articles in Chester Swinyard, ed., *Decision Making and the Defective Newborn* (Springfield, Ill.: Charles C. Thomas, 1978); and the discussions, with bibliographies, in Weir, *Selective Nontreatment of Handicapped Newborns*, and Kuhse and Singer, *Should the Baby Live?* esp. chap. 3 for the evolution of the debate.
81. Robert M. Veatch, "The Technical Criteria Fallacy," *Hastings Center Report* 7 (August 1977): 15–16.
82. See James M. Gustafson, "Mongolism, Parental Desires, and the Right to Life," *Perspectives in Biology and Medicine* 16 (Summer 1973): 529–30. A widely discussed British case involved an infant with Down syndrome but no life-threatening conditions. In 1980, a pediatrician, Dr. Leonard Arthur, was charged with murder (later modified to attempted murder) after he prescribed a strong painkilling medication and "nursing care only" for a newborn infant (John Pearson) with Down syndrome because the mother had rejected the newborn, who appeared to have no medical problems other than Down syndrome. Arthur was acquitted. For a discussion of the moral issues involved in the case, see Raanan Gillon, "An Introduction to Philosophical Medical Ethics: The Arthur Case," *British Medical Journal* 290

(1985): 1117–19; idem, "Conclusion: The Arthur Case Revisited," *British Medical Journal* 292 (1986): 543–45; and also Kuhse and Singer, *Should the Baby Live?* chap. 1.

83. President's Commission, *Deciding to Forego Life-Sustaining Treatment,* p. 218.

84. Raymond S. Duff and A. G. M. Campbell, "Moral and Ethical Dilemmas in the Special-Care Nursery," *New England Journal of Medicine* 289 (1973): 890–94.

85. "Child Abuse Prevention and Treatment and Adoption Reform Act Amendments of 1984," Public Law 98–457, 42 U.S.C. 5101 and following (1984); "Child Abuse and Neglect Prevention and Treatment Program: Final Rule," *Federal Register* 50 (April 15, 1985): 14878–901. For a discussion of the different stages in the evolution of the government's action, see Nancy M. P. King, "Federal and State Regulation of Neonatal Decision-Making," and Mary Ann Gardell and H. Tristram Engelhardt, Jr., "The Baby Doe Controversy: An Outline of Some Points in Its Development," in McMillan, Engelhardt, and Spicker, *Euthanasia and the Newborn,* pp. 293–99; and Cantor, *Legal Frontiers of Death and Dying,* chap. 6.

86. See Kuhse and Singer, *Should the Baby Live?* p. 46.

87. John Lantos, "Baby Doe Five Years Later: Implications for Child Health," *New England Journal of Medicine* 317 (1987): 444–47.

88. See, for example, David Sperlinger, ed., *Animals in Research* (London: John Wiley, 1981); Dale Jameson and Tom Regan, "On the Ethics of the Use of Animals in Science," in *And Justice for All,* ed. T. Regan and D. VanDeVeer (Totowa, N.J.: Rowman and Littlefield, 1982), pp. 169–96; a special issue on animal research of *Journal of Medicine and Philosophy* 13 (1988); Carl Cohen, "The Case for the Use of Animals in Biomedical Research," *New England Journal of Medicine* 315 (1986): 865–70; and R. G. Frey, "Animal Parts, Human Wholes," in *Biomedical Ethics Reviews—1987,* ed. J. M. Humber and R. F. Almeder (Clifton, N.J.: Humana Press, 1987), pp. 89–107.

89. This case has been adapted with permission from a case presented by Dr. Martin P. Albert of Charlottesville, Va.

90. *In the matter of Quinlan,* 70 N.J. 10 (1976).

91. In re *Conroy,* 486 A.2d 1209 (N.J. 1985).

92. *Brophy* v. *New England Sinai Hospital, Inc.,* 398 Mass. 417, 498 N.E. 2d 626 (1986).

93. See Joel Frader, "Forgoing Life-Sustaining Food and Water: Newborns," in *By No Extraordinary Means,* ed. Joanne Lynn (Bloomington: Indiana University Press, 1986), chap. 17.

94. See Joanne Lynn and James F. Childress, "Must Patients Always Be Given Food and Water?" *Hastings Center Report* 13 (October 1983): 17–21. See also the essays in Lynn, ed., *By No Extraordinary Means.*

95. President's Commission, *Deciding to Forego Life-Sustaining Treatment,* pp. 1, 90, 190, 288.

96. American Medical Association Council on Ethical and Judicial Affairs, *Current Opinions* (Chicago: American Medical Association, 1984), pp. 9–10.

97. See AMA, *Current Opinions* (1986), 2.180.

98. See D. W. Meyers, "Legal Aspects of Withdrawing Nourishment from an Incurably Ill Patient," *Archives of Internal Medicine* 145 (January 1985): 125–28.

99. G. E. M. Anscombe, "Ethical Problems in the Management of Some Severely Handicapped Children: Commentary 2," *Journal of Medical Ethics* 7 (1981): 122.

100. Sandra Bardinella, as quoted by John Paris, S. J., "Kaiser, Conroy, and the Withdrawal of IV Feeding: Killing or Letting Die," unpublished paper, p. 1.

101. *Federal Register* 48, No. 129, July 5, 1983.

102. See the summary of living will legislation in *The Physician and the Hopelessly Ill Patient* (New York: Society for the Right to Die, 1985).

103. Joyce V. Zerwekh, "The Dehydration Question," *Nursing '83* (January 1983): 47–51, reprinted in Lynn, ed., *By No Extraordinary Means,* chap. 2.

104. Daniel Callahan, "On Feeding the Dying," *Hastings Center Report* 13 (October 1983): 22. See also Ronald A. Carson, "The Symbolic Significance of Giving to Eat and Drink," in Lynn, ed., *By No Extraordinary Means,* chap. 8.

105. Micetich, Steinecker, and Thomasma, "Are Intravenous Fluids Morally Required for a Dying Patient?"

106. Ibid. For a strong criticism of withholding or withdrawing MN&H on the grounds that it involves the intention to kill, see Gilbert Meilaender, "On Removing Food and Water: Against the Stream," *Hastings Center Report* 14 (December 1984): 11–13.

107. See Mark Siegler and Alan J. Weisbard, "Against the Emerging Stream: Should Fluids and Nutritional Support Be Discontinued?" *Archives of Internal Medicine* 145 (January 1985): 129–32; and Patrick Derr, "Why Food and Fluids Can Never Be Denied," *Hastings Center Report* 16 (February 1986): 28–30.

108. For example, a substantial portion of the health-care dollar is spent during the last year and especially during the last few weeks of life. According to one study, Medicare expenditures in 1978 were six times higher for elderly recipients who died that year than for recipients who did not. However, of those who required major expenditures of Medicare funds, at least half survived. See Congress of the United States, Office of Technology Assessment, *Life-Sustaining Technology and the Elderly* (Washington, D.C.: U.S. Government Printing Office, 1987), chap. 2.

109. President's Commission, *Deciding to Forego Life-Sustaining Treatment,* pp. 17–18.

110. Callahan, "On Feeding the Dying."

111. Kelly, "The Duty to Preserve Life."

112. See Lynn and Childress, "Must Patients Always Be Given Food and Water?"

113. Rawls, *A Theory of Justice,* pp. 85–86.

114. *Strunk* v. *Strunk,* Ky 445 S.W. 2d 145 (1969).

115. *Superintendent of Belchertown State School* v. *Saikewicz,* Mass. 370 N.E. 2d 417 (1977). See the later case of In re *Mary Hier,* 18 Mass. App. Ct. 200 (1984); and for the full range of developments in the Massachusetts courts, see Sean M. Dunphy and John H. Cross, "Medical Decisionmaking for Incompetent Persons: The Massachusetts Substituted Judgment Model," *Western New England Law Review* 9 (1987): 153–67.

116. *In the matter of Karen Quinlan,* 70 N.J. 10, 355 A. 2d 647 (1976), at 663.

117. John Robertson, "Organ Donations By Incompetents and the Substituted Judgment Doctrine," *Columbia Law Review* 76 (1976): 65.

118. George Annas, "Help from the Dead: The Cases of Brother Fox and John Storar," *Hastings Center Report* 11 (June 1981): 19–20. See also Thomas G. Gutheil

and Paul S. Appelbaum, "Substituted Judgment: Best Interests in Disguise," *Hastings Center Report* 13 (1983): 8–11.

119. In re *Conroy,* 98 N.J. 321, 486 A. 2d 1209 (1985). All quotations immediately below are taken from this source.

120. In a series of decisions in June 1987, the New Jersey supreme court extended its analysis to three other types of cases: a thirty-seven-year-old, competent, terminally ill patient suffering from amyotrophic lateral sclerosis who wanted to have her respirator disconnected (In re *Farrell,* N.J. [1987]); a thirty-one-year-old woman who had been in a persistent vegetative state for several years in a nursing home and whose family wanted to withdraw her feeding tube (a jejunostomy tube) so that she could die (In re *Jobes,* N.J. [1987]); and a sixty-five-year-old nursing-home resident in a persistent vegetative state who had assigned durable power of attorney to a friend who wanted to remove her nasogastric tube (In re *Peters,* N.J. [1987]). The court authorized the withdrawal of life-sustaining treatment in each case.

121. John Warren et al., "Informed Consent by Proxy: An Issue in Research with Elderly Patients," *New England Journal of Medicine* 315 (1986): 1124–28. See also George Annas and Leonard Glantz, "Rules for Research in Nursing Homes," *New England Journal of Medicine* 315 (1986).

122. Paul S. Appelbaum, Charles W. Lidz, and Alan Meisel, *Informed Consent: Legal Theory and Clinical Practice* (New York: Oxford University Press, 1987).

123. S. J. Eisendrath and A. R. Jonsen, "The Living Will," *Journal of the American Medical Association* 249 (1983): 2084–88.

124. See President's Commission, *Deciding to Forego Life-Sustaining Treatment,* pp. 145–47.

125. See the somewhat different set of qualifications proposed by Weir, *Selective Nontreatment of Handicapped Newborns,* chap. 9.

126. Weir uses the criterion of impartiality. Ibid., p. 256.

127. For a careful assessment of the basis in common law and legislation for the family's right to refuse life-sustaining treatments for incompetent patients, see Judith Areen, "The Legal Status of Consent Obtained from Families of Adult Patients to Withhold or Withdraw Treatment," *Journal of the American Medical Association* 258 (1987): 229–35.

128. Virginia Natural Death Act, Va. Code 54-325, 8:1–13 (1983).

129. P. P. Rickham, "The Ethics of Surgery on Newborn Infants," *Clinical Pediatrics* 8 (1969): 251–53, as quoted in Anthony Shaw, "Dilemmas of 'Informed Consent' in Children," *New England Journal of Medicine* 289 (1973): 886. See also President's Commission, *Deciding to Forego Life-Sustaining Treatment,* pp. 210–11.

130. A. Shaw, J. G. Randolph, and B. Manard, "Ethical Issues in Pediatric Surgery: A National Survey of Pediatricians and Pediatric Surgeons," *Pediatrics* 60 (1977): 588–99. See also David Todres, "Pediatricians' Attitudes Affecting Decision-Making in Defective Infants,"*Pediatrics* 60 (1977): 197.

131. *Federal Register* 49 (January 12, 1984): 1645.

132. President's Commission, *Deciding to Forego Life-Sustaining Treatment,* p. 227. Contrast Raymond S. Duff and A. G. M. Campbell, "Moral Communities and Tragic Choice," in McMillan, Engelhardt, and Spicker, eds., *Euthanasia and the Newborn,* pp. 273–80.

133. President's Commission, *Deciding to Forego Life-Sustaining Treatment,* p. 446.

134. See Cantor, *Legal Frontiers of Death and Dying,* pp. 111–12.

135. Examples include a case of the Siamese twins in Danville, Illinois, and a case of two California physicians charged with murder after they disconnected a feeding tube from a patient who then died.

136. *Superintendent of Belchertown State School* v. *Saikewicz*, Mass. 370 N.E. 2d 417 (1977).

137. See the comments by Justice Liacos, the author of the opinion in *Saikewicz*, in his "Dilemmas of Dying," *Law, Medicine & Health Care* 7 (Fall 1979); reprinted in *Legal and Ethical Aspects of Treating Critically and Terminally Ill Patients*, ed. A. Edward Doudera and J. Douglas Peters (Ann Arbor, Mich.: Health Administration Press, 1982), pp. 149–58. In In re *Spring*, 405 N.E. 2d 115 (Mass. 1980) (Case 17 in the appendix), the supreme judicial court of Massachusetts identified several factors that determine when nontreatment decisions require judicial review—for example, whether the patient is in a state institution, whether a family member is available and is acting in good faith, what the patient's prognosis is, and whether there is a professional consensus about the case.

138. See In re *Conroy*, 486 A. 2d 1209 (N.J. 1985).

5

The Principle of Beneficence

Morality requires not only that we treat persons autonomously and refrain from harming them but also that we contribute to their welfare. These beneficial actions fall under the principle of beneficence. There are no sharp breaks on the continuum from the noninfliction of harm to the provision of benefit, but the principle of beneficence potentially demands more than the principle of nonmaleficence because it requires positive steps to help others.

In Chapter 4, we analyzed nonmaleficence in terms of the noninfliction of harm on others. The word *nonmaleficence* is sometimes used more broadly to include the prevention of harm and the removal of harmful conditions. However, because prevention and removal require positive acts to assist others, we include them under *beneficence* along with the provision of benefit. *Nonmaleficence* is restricted again in this chapter to the noninfliction of harm.

The concept and obligation of beneficence

Two principles of beneficence

In ordinary English the term *beneficence* can suggest acts of mercy, kindness, and charity. However, the concept of beneficent action should not be limited to mercy, kindness, or charity because it includes any form of action to benefit another. In its most general form, the principle of beneficence asserts an obligation to help others further their important and legitimate interests. The obli-

194

gation to confer benefits and actively to prevent and remove harms is important in biomedical contexts, but equally important is the obligation to weigh and balance the possible goods against the possible harms of an action. It is thus appropriate to distinguish two principles under the general principle of beneficence. The first principle requires the *provision* of benefits (including the prevention and removal of harm as well as the promotion of welfare), and the second requires a *balancing* of benefits and harms. The first may be called the principle of positive beneficence; the second is already familiar as a version of the principle of utility.

Because the moral life does not permit us simply to produce benefits without creating risks or to prevent or remove harms without creating risks, this second balancing principle is an essential addition to the principle of positive beneficence. For example, in our discussion in Chapter 4 of withholding or withdrawing life-sustaining treatment from incompetent patients, we noted the importance of considering a treatment's probable chance of success and then balancing its probable benefits against its probable costs or risks to the patient. And, as we saw in Chapter 2, both utilitarians and deontologists need a principle for balancing benefits and harms, balancing benefits against alternative benefits, and balancing harms against alternative harms.

This principle of utility might also be called the principle of proportionality. It is not identical in the structure of our moral theory to the classical utilitarian principle of utility, which is an absolute or preeminent principle. It thus should not be construed as the sole principle of morality or as one that justifies or overrides all other principles. It is one principle among others.

This principle is often rejected because it appears to allow the interests of society as a whole to override individual interests and rights. In the context of medical research, for example, the principle seems to imply that dangerous research on human subjects could be undertaken, and even ought to be undertaken, when the prospect of substantial benefit to society or other individuals outweighs the danger of the research to the individual. Although it is true that an unconstrained principle of utility carries this danger, there is no such danger in the moral theory we defend in this chapter. Utilitarianism does not offer the only basis on which our methods and conclusions might be justified. These same methods and conclusions can be and have been defended, for example, on the basis of a deontological theory of hypothetical consent and a deontological theory of individual rights.[1]

The assumption of beneficence in health care

The belief that there is an obligation to provide benefits is an unchallenged assumption in biomedicine: Promoting the welfare of patients—not merely avoiding harm—is the goal of health care and also of therapeutic research. This welfare objective expresses medicine's goal and justification: Clinical therapies are aimed at the promotion of health or the prevention of disease and injury.

Firmly established in the histories of medicine, health care, and public health is the belief that a failure to benefit others—and not simply the failure to avoid harm—in many circumstances violates social or professional or moral obligations. For example, the American Nurses' Association pledges that "The nurse's primary commitment is to the health, welfare, and safety of the client."[2] Preventive medicine and active public health interventions provide examples of concerted social actions of beneficence. Once methods of preventing yellow fever and cowpox were discovered in early modern medicine, it was universally agreed that it would be morally irresponsible not to take positive steps to establish public health programs.

We will treat the basic roles and concepts that give substance to the principle of beneficence in health care as follows. The positive benefit that physicians and other health-care professionals are obligated to seek is the promotion of health, as defined in part by the patient's own values. Health care aims at the restoration of the patient's health if there is a reasonable hope of cure; but often it will involve modes of care that fall short of cure (e.g., kidney dialysis for end-stage renal disease). The harms to be prevented, removed, or minimized include pain, suffering, disability, and death from injury and disease. In short, health care has many different modes, including critical, curative, chronic, and preventive. In therapeutic research the benefits presented to subjects parallel those in health care, with an additional goal of benefits to others from the generation of scientific knowledge. In nontherapeutic research, subjects do not stand to gain medical benefits, because the research is designed to generate generalizable knowledge to benefit society.

Social assistance for extremely dependent patients provides a clear case of societal action based on the obligation of beneficence. Consider Case 30. A bill has been introduced in a state legislature that would establish community-based homes for the care and education of the mentally retarded, thousands of whom live in unpleasant, impoverished, and medically unsatisfactory facilities. The motivation and moral basis of this bill is beneficence. However, as is typically the case, beneficence confronts limited resources, and controversies arise concerning how beneficent society can afford to be. Allocation rules and health policy decisions restrain or at least place limits on beneficence. These are primarily problems of distributive justice, the topic considered in Chapter 6.

The principle of beneficence could be understood to entail severe sacrifice and extreme altruism in the moral life—for example, giving a kidney or even both kidneys for transplantation. This implication has led some moral philosophers to argue that it is virtuous and morally ideal to act beneficently but not a moral obligation to do so. They have treated beneficent actions as akin to acts of charity and acts of conscience that exceed obligation. Beneficent acts are laudable, but persons are not morally deficient in discharging obligations if they fail of beneficence, and therefore there is no prima facie obligation of positive beneficence.

There is merit in this view, inasmuch as we are not always morally required to benefit persons, even if we are in a position to do so. Like all moral principles, beneficence has a limited scope. For example, we are not morally required to perform all possible acts of charity. The line between an obligation and a moral ideal is not easy to establish, and beneficence has proven to be a troublesome moral principle to place firmly in one (or both) of these categories. In what respects and within what limits, then, is beneficence a requirement of morality?

Consider public support of nontherapeutic biomedical research. The obligation to benefit members of society, including future generations, is commonly cited as the primary justification for scientific research. For example, the justification for using children as research subjects when they will not benefit individually from the research is that they are often the only subjects who can be used to study childhood disorders and development in order to help other children. In the Willowbrook case (see Case 26), we find this justification advanced by those who conducted hepatitis research involving institutionalized and mentally retarded children. Willowbrook administrators argued that successful research would produce generalizable knowledge about hepatitis that could benefit all potential victims of the disease.

Presume now (setting aside the controversy over the Willowbrook case) that support of biomedical research is morally justified. It is one thing to maintain that actions or programs are morally justified and another to maintain that they are morally required on grounds of a prima facie obligation. Even if the support of research is justified on grounds of beneficence, this does not demonstrate that the principle of positive beneficence establishes obligations. Another question is whether obligations of beneficence are general obligations or role-specific obligations that (in biomedicine) accrue to anyone who accepts certain positions, such as in the care of patients. This question is difficult, but we will argue that there are both general obligations of beneficence and role-specific obligations.

Several moral philosophers have proposed that beneficence is obligatory. In considering their proposals, we will concentrate first on obligations of beneficence for individuals, recalling that there are many possible agents of beneficence, including the society and the government, health-care institutions, and health-care professionals.

Obligatory beneficence

A first proposal accords a vital role in morality to beneficence but does not establish beneficence as obligatory. William Frankena has argued that ''Even if one holds that beneficence is not a *requirement* of morality but something supererogatory and morally *good,* one is still regarding beneficence as an important part of morality—as desirable if not required."[3] This contention is of little assistance for our immediate purposes. No one denies that beneficent acts, such as the donation of a kidney to a stranger, are morally praiseworthy when they exceed what is morally required. If a man gives more money to a charity than he has pledged, he performs a morally praiseworthy and generous action (at least as far as this feature of the action is concerned). Little is added by noting that beneficence forms an important part of morality, if the issue is whether some different part of morality, makes beneficence obligatory.

Frankena's observation can, however, be reconstructed for our purposes. To say we ought to do something in general may mean that (1) we ought to do it because it is a moral obligation, (2) we ought to do it because of a weak moral obligation, or (3) we ought to do it because of a self-imposed requirement, such as a rule of charity.[4] This schema leaves open whether beneficence is a strict moral obligation, a weaker form of moral obligation, or supererogatory, or some combination of all three, each one applying in some cases while not in others.[5] We believe all three are proper characterizations of beneficence in some contexts, and we will defend this view throughout this chapter and again in Chapter 8 (see pp. 371–72), as well as in Chapter 2 (see pp. 57–59).

A second and more pertinent proposal, offered by Marcus Singer is consistent with but moves beyond Frankena's modest formulation.[6] Singer argues that beneficent actions spring from a moral requirement to perform acts that avoid undesirable consequences—a requirement not so strong as to make it obligatory to produce good consequences. Thus, loss must be avoided, but there is no obligation to produce positive benefit. This approach has been defended in a more sweeping form by Peter Singer as "the obligation to assist."[7] He, too, relies on a distinction between preventing evil and promoting good. Assuming that it is bad to suffer and die from lack of food, shelter, and medical care, Peter Singer contends that "if it is in our power to *prevent something bad from happening,* without thereby sacrificing anything of comparable moral importance, we ought, morally, to do it."[8] This principle requires us to prevent what is bad, not to promote what is good.

These arguments may at first appear to be instances of the nonmaleficence-grounded thesis that society may not be able to impose affirmative obligations to provide benefits but may legitimately impose negative obligations not to cause harm. For example, we would generally agree that a corporation creating health hazards because of poor pollution control has an obligation to cease its harmful activities, but this obligation does not extend to a general corporate obligation to promote social welfare. However, this distinction does not capture the strategy of either Marcus or Peter Singer. Both argue that requirements of positive action are grounded in principles of preventing or acting to avoid bad outcomes.

Peter Singer's position is that we must always act to prevent what is bad, unless something of "comparable moral importance" must be given up by performing the action. We must always act to prevent harm, unless either a stronger prima facie moral obligation conflicts with and overrides that obligation or we would make ourselves worse off than the persons to whom we are discharging that obligation. That is, Singer requires that we give until we reach a level at which, by giving more, we would cause as much suffering to ourselves as we would relieve through our gift. This argument is controversial because it implies that we are morally obligated to make large sacrifices and reduce our standard of living substantially in the effort to rescue destitute persons around the world. Each of us would have to reduce his or her position to approximately that of the world's most destitute person.

This construal of an obligation of beneficence is overly demanding. Normal moral conventions establish limits to our obligations to help others by preventing harms and evils. That limit is exceeded, for example, if one's life plans are disrupted and possible achievements must be sacrificed in order to spend one's life helping sick or starving people. Our common, entrenched moral standards tend to assume that the level of cost or risk Singer seeks to make obligatory is beyond obligation—in the domain of moral sacrifice that we describe in Chapter 8 as a nonobligatory but commendable moral ideal. Common morality acknowledges that there is a threshold point at which our obligation to rescue and assist has been transcended. An action above the threshold line may not be so sacrificial as to be heroic, but it is more like heroic sacrifice than obligatory giving.

Michael Slote has argued, against Singer, that beneficent prevention of evil or harm must not require the sacrifice of a "basic life plan." He formulates the "principle of positive obligation" in this way: "One has an obligation to prevent serious evil or harm when one can do so without seriously interfering with one's life plans or style and without doing any wrongs of commission."[9] There may be ambiguities and even serious moral problems in Slote's formulation, but it is hard to imagine that for the person of modest life-style moral rules demand much more beneficence than his principles suggest. (We need to allow for qualifications in the case of frivolous millionaires and the like.) Individuals might accept a moral ideal of the sort proposed by Peter Singer, and society might conceivably be more advantaged by attempting to make his ideal an obligatory part of morality. However, this latter point is not obvious, given what we know about our abilities to live up to such high ideals.

Singer has attempted to take account of the objection that his principle of beneficence sets "too high a standard." He agrees in the abstract that the principle may need toning down. To the question "What level of assistance should we advocate?" he offers a more explicit and realistic answer:

Any figure will be arbitrary, but there may be something to be said for a round percentage of one's income like, say, 10%—more than a token donation, yet not so high as to be beyond all but saints. . . . No figure should be advocated as a rigid minimum or maximum. . . . [But] by any reasonable ethical standards this is the minimum we ought to do, and we do wrong if we do less.[10]

It is difficult to assess percentage of income as an expression of one's obligation, especially in light of vast differences in income and wealth and also in light of conditions we identify below. But Singer's revised thesis rightly attempts to set additional limits on the scope of the obligation of beneficence— limits that reduce required risk and impact on the agent's life plans.

The significance of such limits becomes evident when we consider how the idea of a threshold of obligation can crumble when an ethics of individual obligation confronts large-scale social problems. As James Fishkin argues, even if we normally assume that we are obligated to save a human life at minor cost if we can, this principle of minimal altruism, as weak as it is, will lead us step by step to enormous burdens that would ordinarily be considered heroic, when we consider the number of obligation-determining situations and the number of recipients who could benefit.[11] For example, an individual could provide food for a starving person for a small amount of money, but if there are numerous starving people, each of whom could be rescued by a small additional contribution, the burden would quickly surpass our resources.

This conclusion is both practically and theoretically puzzling and disturbing. It is practically bothersome because it becomes extremely difficult to pin down and discharge obligations of beneficence. We bounce back and forth between viewing actions as charitable and as obligatory; and we may feel guilty for not doing more, at the same time doubting that we are obligated to do more. The conclusion is theoretically puzzling because every time we try to formulate the nature of the obligation of beneficence in an abstract manner, the problem of incremental obligations tends to decimate the analysis. For example, a one-dollar gift to a famine relief organization would not make a noticeable dent in our standard of living, but if we gave away everything in our savings accounts most of us would regard the sacrifice as immense. Yet it would still be the case that only one more dollar from our pockets would make no dent in our standard of living. Thus, our ethical theory needs specific conditions of beneficence so that apparently faultless assumptions about obligations of minimal giving do not engulf us in a morass of obligations that exceed defensible limits. Let us see, then, if these conditions can be formulated.

The obligation to rescue

The obligation of beneficence is not strong enough, in our view, to require that the passerby who is a very poor swimmer try to swim a hundred yards to rescue someone who is drowning in deep water. But if the passerby does nothing— for example, fails to run several yards to alert a lifeguard—the omission is morally culpable. We would argue that apart from special moral relationships such as contracts, X has a determinate obligation of beneficence toward Y if and only if each of the following conditions is satisfied and X is aware of the relevant facts: (1) Y is at risk of significant loss or damage; (2) X's action is needed (singly or in concert with others) to prevent this loss; (3) X's action (singly or in concert with others) has a high probability of preventing it; (4) X's action would not present significant risks, costs, or burdens to X; and (5) the benefit that Y can be expected to gain outweighs any harms, costs, or burdens that X is likely to incur.[12]

Although morality includes a general obligation of beneficence, we have some discretion about discharging it. The obligation is indeterminate in that it does not require in many cases that we specifically benefit a particular person. As we saw in our discussion of rights in Chapter 2, Mill and Kant judged beneficence an imperfect obligation rather than a perfect obligation, thus leaving us free to direct our beneficence as we see fit. Nevertheless, if our argument is correct, under the five conditions identified above, a person can have a determinate obligation of beneficence toward Y, even apart from special moral relationships such as promises or professional roles. Only if one accepts significant risks, costs, or burdens—such as the disruption of one's life plans—is the act beyond the call of obligation (a supererogatory action, which we analyze in Chapter 8).

The fourth condition above is critical because it enables us to engage the problems that surround Peter Singer's and Slote's formulations of the obligation of beneficence. Although it is difficult to specify "significant risks, costs, or burdens," the implication of the fourth condition is clear: Even if X's action would probably save Y's life and would meet all conditions except the fourth, the action would not be obligatory on grounds of beneficence. We shall now test these theses about the demands of beneficence with two cases. The first is on the borderline of an obligation of beneficence, whereas the second, we believe, is a clear case of the obligation.

In Case 25, which we introduced in Chapter 4, Robert McFall was diagnosed as having aplastic anemia, which is usually fatal, but his physician believed that a bone marrow transplant from a genetically compatible donor could increase his chances of surviving one year from twenty-five percent to between forty and sixty percent. David Shimp, McFall's cousin, was the only relative willing to undergo the first test, which established tissue compatibility. However, Shimp then refused to undergo the second test for genetic compatibility. Clearly the first two conditions were met for an obligation of beneficence, independent of special moral relationships. The third condition was not as clearly satisfied, because McFall's chance of surviving a year would have only increased from twenty-five to between forty and sixty percent. These are the kinds of contingencies that make it difficult to determine whether the principle of beneficence demands a particular course of action. Shimp himself was especially concerned about the fourth condition, although most medical commentators agreed that the risks were minimal. The necessary one hundred to one hundred and fifty punctures of the pelvic bone can be painlessly performed under anesthesia, and the major risk is a one-in-ten-thousand chance of death from anesthesia. Shimp, however, believed that the risks were greater ("What if I become a cripple?") and that they outweighed the probability and magnitude of benefit to McFall, even though there was no medical evidence to support his fears. This case, then, is a borderline case.

A clear example of an obligation of beneficence is found if we slightly modify the *Tarasoff* case (Case 1), with which we began Chapter 1. The therapist learned of his patient's intention to kill a woman but maintained confidentiality and did not attempt to warn her. Suppose we modify the actual circumstances in this case in order to create the following hypothetical situation. A psychiatrist has told his patient that he does not believe in keeping any information confidential. The patient agrees to treatment under these conditions and subsequently reveals his intention to kill a woman. The psychiatrist may now either remain aloof or make some move to protect the woman (by calling her or the police). What does morality demand of the psychiatrist in this case? Only a remarkably narrow view of moral obligation would hold that the psychiatrist is under no obligation to contact the woman. The psychiatrist is not at risk (and, moreover, will suffer virtually no inconvenience or interference with his life plan). If morality does not demand this much beneficence, it is hard to see how morality creates any obligations at all. Moreover, even if there is a competing obligation such as the protection of confidentiality (which is indeed an obligation, as we show in Chapter 7), beneficence may outweigh it. This is a clear indication that beneficence is obligatory and not merely supererogatory.

In conclusion, we may express some doubt that our five conditions adequately solve the problem of incremental positive obligations that we raised, following Fishkin, in the previous section—that is, the problem of whether small gifts or acts of beneficence that are each morally required under our fivefold criteria can be required when they add up collectively to a large amount of giving. No doubt there can be a more refined analysis than the one we have presented, but we are inclined to think that it will also be a revisionary analysis in the sense that it will inevitably draw a new boundary or threshold for our obligations—a line that is much more explicit than any line that exists in common morality. Singer's ten percent criterion is such a revisionary line, and we believe any line created to specify the scope of our general obligation of positive beneficence will represent a significant change in and sharpening of our moral perspective. Ordinary morality is not sufficiently refined in the domain of positive beneficence to supply an answer, perhaps because most of our obligations of beneficence are discharged by specific and role obligations rather than by gifts to the anonymous needy.

To argue for a revisionary analysis of this sort is a worthy project, but not one that we can undertake in this book. (In Chapter 6 we reach a similar conclusion about the commitments of the rule of fair opportunity.) What we can do, however, is examine the distinction between a general obligation of beneficence owed to all persons and specific obligations owed to some persons such as patients.

Grounds of general and specific obligations of beneficence

Both the general obligation of beneficence and specific obligations of beneficence have been justified in several different ways. We need to examine the foundations of both the general obligation and specific obligations as they arise in medical practice.

Utilitarians such as Mill recognize the obligation of beneficence because it follows directly from the principle of utility, and deontologists such as Kant and Ross also recognize an obligation of beneficence—Kant because it is required by the categorical imperative, and Ross because it is a part of common morality. In another interpretation of the foundation of beneficence, David Hume argues that the obligation to benefit others arises from social interactions: ''All our obligations to do good to society seem to imply something reciprocal. I receive the benefits of society, and therefore ought to promote its interests.'' [13]

This view, which might be called the reciprocity theory of obligations of beneficence, correctly maintains that we incur obligations to help others at least in part because we have received or will receive beneficial assistance from them. If a person does not incur such obligations, then presumably he or she has no obligation to act beneficently, as in the case of a hypothetical, isolated individual who is ''an island unto himself.'' But the idea that we can be free of all indebtedness to our parents, to researchers in medicine and public health, to educators, and to other benefactors is as unrealistic as the idea that we can always act autonomously without affecting others. One appropriate justification, then, for the claim that beneficence is an obligation resides in the implicit arrangement underlying the necessary give-and-take of social life.

If we examine the obligations of health-care professionals in terms of reciprocity and fair play, we can see both the possibilities and the limitations of this approach. Codes of medical ethics traditionally have viewed physicians as independent, self-sufficient philanthropists whose beneficence is analogous to an act of gift-giving. These codes have sometimes distinguished between physicians' obligations to their patients and obligations to their teachers and colleagues. According to the Hippocratic oath, the physician's obligations to patients represent philanthropy and service, whereas obligations to teachers represent debts incurred in becoming a physician. But in the contemporary world, the professional is often indebted to society (e.g., for education and privileges) and to patients, past and present (e.g., for research and "practice").

Because of this indebtedness, the medical profession's role of beneficence is misconstrued as mere philanthropy. It is rooted in what William May calls the "reciprocity of giving and receiving."[14] Following May, it may be more appropriate to call this a covenant than a contract, because the relationship does not have a specific quid pro quo. It creates an obligation both to patients and to society, although the terms of that obligation are rarely specified. The professional usually has some discretion about discharging the obligation, and it is possible to have an obligation to Y without having specific obligations to do A, B, and C. Obligations to parents are often of this nature. That there is an obligation cannot be reasonably denied; however, the scope and content of the obligation may be disputed, particularly the specific actions it requires.

Even if the general obligation of beneficence derives largely from reciprocity, specific obligations of beneficence often derive from special moral relationships with persons, frequently through institutional roles and contractual arrangements such as those that bring the patient and the physician into a relationship. These obligations are not general and stem particularly from implicit and explicit commitments—for instance, making promises and accepting roles and positions that require beneficent actions—as well as from reception of benefits. To focus on the most relevant categories, we often ought to act to benefit someone either because of roles—our "station and its duties"—or because our promises require such acts. Thus, the lifeguard on duty is obligated to try to rescue a drowning swimmer, even at considerable personal risk, just as a physician has a strong obligation to accept some health risks in meeting the needs of patients. We might also believe that the father (in Case 3) has a stronger obligation to donate a kidney to his dying daughter than Shimp (in Case 25) has to donate bone marrow to his dying cousin. The claims that we make on each other as parents, spouses, and friends similarly stem not only from interpersonal encounters but also from fixed rules, roles, and relations that constitute the matrix of obligations and duties.[15]

When a patient engages a physician, the latter assumes a role-specific obligation of beneficent treatment that he or she would not have to this patient if there were no mutual agreement. According to the American Medical Association, its "body of ethical statements" was developed "primarily for the benefit of the patient," and the first principle is that "a physician shall be dedicated to providing competent medical service with compassion and respect for human dignity."[16] Human needs, actual or perceived, usually form the basis of this beneficent relationship. However, these actual or felt needs are not enough in most circumstances to impose either a legal or a moral obligation of service on the health-care professional. The AMA code affirms that "A physician shall in the provision of appropriate patient care, except in emergencies, be free to choose whom to serve.'' From a legal standpoint, both the patient (or the patient's representative) and the health-care professional must accept the relationship; the former's need is not sufficient to establish a contract for service.

Here we need to distinguish different roles a physician or other health-care professional may occupy in different contexts, and we need to determine whether the obligations that follow from the roles are legal or moral. If a physician is in private practice, he or she may have no legal obligation to see patients even in emergencies if no other physician is available. Again, a physician has no legal obligation to stop at the scene of an automobile accident or to answer affirmatively when the manager of a restaurant or theater asks, ''Is there a doctor in the house?'' By contrast, a physician on duty in a hospital emergency room may not legally refuse to care for a patient.

From a moral standpoint, the principle of beneficence often creates an obligation where the law is silent. A request or a need for help, as in the case of an automobile accident, imposes a moral responsibility on a health-care professional to respond with his or her special knowledge and skills, as long as there is only negligible or minimal risk and no major interference in life-style (subject to qualifications about a reasonable and appropriate life-style). However, it is not the case that the obligation to assist is itself specific or role-derived rather than an instance of acting under the general obligation of beneficence. If Janet James, a local lawyer, had happened on the scene of the accident in the same way, then she, too, would have had an obligation to assist, in whatever way she could. Anyone who falls under our five-condition analysis of the general obligation of beneficence would have an obligation to provide assistance, as he or she is able.

The physician is, however, in a position to lend more assistance in this instance than the lawyer, and should do so. Does the physician, then, have some specific obligation of assistance unique to persons with the skills and training of a medical professional? Here the answer seems to be that there is a gray area between being an instance of the general obligation and being an instance of a role-specific obligation. The physician at the scene of an accident is obligated to do more than the lawyer in accordance with the need for the skills and commitments of the medical profession; but the physician is not morally required to assume the same level of commitment and risk involved in the role-specific obligations entailed in a contractual relationship with a patient, hospital, and the like. This analysis suggests that we need to be careful in our use of the language of role or professional obligations. It also implicitly suggests, as health professionals and parents have long believed, that specific role obligations often can take priority over general obligations in cases of conflict.

A physician is also not morally obligated to emulate the Good Samaritan but rather to be what Judith Thomson calls ''a minimally decent Samaritan.''[17] What Good Samaritan laws may do best is not to require, under threat of a sanction, assistance by physicians or other health-care professionals, but rather to protect them from civil or criminal liability when they act in good faith to render aid in emergencies. For example, if there is a threat of civil or criminal liability for rendering medical assistance in an emergency, the professional may view the legal risk of intervening as a valid excuse for not fulfilling a moral obligation to intervene.

The uncertanties surrounding the principle of beneficence have now led us to examine its possible meanings, sources, and scope. Often the actions it requires, especially for individual risk-taking, hinge on other obligations, such as fair play, promise keeping, and role commitments. Although the distinction between beneficence and nonmaleficence is not always clear, the importance of the distinction is evident. The obligation of nonmaleficence is more independent of roles and relations, allows less discretion, and, in general, requires a higher level of risk assumption than the obligation of beneficence, which requires positive actions. For example, our obligation not to harm others must be observed uniformly in all roles, but some obligations to benefit others depend strictly on roles.

Positive beneficence and the donation of cadaver organs

The current debate about policies to increase the supply of cadaver organs for transplantation can be used to illuminate many subtleties that surround the obligation of beneficence when applied both to public policy and to individual responsibility.

Heart, liver, and kidney transplants have increased because of several improvements, especially in immunosuppressive medications, but organs for transplantation are still scarce. It is estimated that in the United States twenty thousand people die each year under circumstances in which their organs could be salvaged for transplantation to benefit others. For the most part these are patients who are brain dead and who are on life-support systems that can maintain their organs in good condition for transplantation. The 1985 figures for kidney transplantation might appear to suggest that a large number of the eligible donors who have died acted beneficently, because approximately seventy-seven hundred kidney transplants were performed in the United States that year. However, this figure is misleading. Approximately seventeen hundred kidneys came from living donors, and each cadaver usually provides two kidneys. If we take wastage into account (e.g., surgical error or lack of compatible recipients) and kidneys shipped abroad (approximately two hundred to two hundred fifty in 1985), the total number of actual donations was approximately thirty five hundred fifty (out of twenty thousand possible donations).

The figures establishing need are in sharp contrast: Of the approximately one hundred thousand patients now on kidney dialysis, approximately twelve thousand are on the active waiting list for kidney transplantation, and approximately ten thousand to fifteen thousand more could benefit from and would want transplants under appropriate circumstances. It should be noted that society, especially through the End-Stage Renal Disease Program of Medicare, has provided virtually universal coverage of treatment for patients suffering from kidney failure. Because in-center dialysis costs approximately twenty-five thousand dollars per patient year, society saves money over time if patients receive kidney transplants, which have a one-time cost of twenty-five thousand dollars to thirty-five thousand dollars followed by costs for immunosuppressive medications and follow-up care.

We believe that both individuals and their family members have an obligation of beneficence to donate cadaver organs to benefit patients suffering from end-stage organ failure. The donation of cadaver organs meets the five conditions of the obligation of beneficence depicted above. Even though the donor may not give to an identified patient in need, the donation has a high probability of benefit because of the large number of patients awaiting transplantation. Many waiting for hearts and livers die before a donor can be found because there is no backup or alternative treatment comparable to dialysis for patients suffering from end-stage renal failure. However, society should not enforce this obligation of beneficence against the decedent's prior wishes or the family's wishes, in order to respect autonomy and avoid offense and outrage. For example, some religious groups strongly oppose desecration of the corpse, and their refusal to donate should be respected.

All states in the United States have a version of the Uniform Anatomical Gift Act, which authorizes individuals to determine what will be done with their bodies after their deaths and authorizes family members to make a determination in the absence of the decedent's express wishes. However, the mechanism for making donations has presented a problem. Few people sign donor cards, apparently not because they want to refuse the use of their bodily parts for transplantation after their deaths but in part because they fear what will happen to them in the hospital if they have signed a donor card. They perceive signed donor cards as increasing their risks, and they worry that physicians will declare them dead prematurely or even hasten their deaths in order to benefit other patients.[18] Their distrust makes signing a donor card appear to them to be unduly risky beneficence. However, polls also indicate that people are generally more willing to donate a family member's organs, presumably in part because they are in a position to protect the dying or dead relative's interests.

Another problem is that physicians and other health-care professionals have difficulty asking grieving family members whether they want to donate the decedent's organs. Professionals worry about increasing the family's trauma, even though it has been demonstrated that many family members view donation as an opportunity to salvage some meaning out of tragic circumstances. We believe that physicians and other health-care professionals have an obligation to ask family members about the decedent's wishes and about their own wishes if the decedent's wishes are not known. Even though this obligation might be based in part on respect for the decedent's and the family's autonomy, it is also based on beneficence toward the family, as well as on beneficence toward patients suffering from end-stage organ failure. As always, there may be circumstances in which this obligation is outweighed by other obligations.

If, as we believe, society has a collective obligation of beneficence toward all its citizens, including those suffering from end-stage organ failure, which policy can society adopt to express beneficence by increasing the supply of organs for transplantation without violating other principles of nonmaleficence, respect for autonomy, and justice? Society has generally concentrated on educational efforts as part of a program of encouraged, voluntary beneficence. But it is difficult for educational efforts to overcome distrust and the associated perception of risks of vulnerability and abuse. Without dismantling the Uniform Anatomical Gift Act, the new major direction that has emerged is *required request*. Under this approach, hospitals set up procedures to ensure that the family members of each dying or dead person whose organs (and tissues) might qualify for transplantation are asked about donation. Most states have now adopted laws that require hospitals to set up such policies, and the U.S. federal government has mandated that hospitals receiving federal funds through Medicare and Medicaid establish such policies.

Many believe that policies of required request will increase the number of donated organs and thus benefit patients suffering from end-stage organ failure, without violating other principles. Under these policies, hospitals, rather than particular health-care professionals, are legally obligated to make the request, and individuals and family members retain their autonomy. Individuals who wish to do so can still sign a donor card (and proposed revisions will make it easier to indicate a wish not to donate). If individuals want to donate but fear the risks of being on record as a donor, they may instruct the family about their wishes. Finally, if individuals have not indicated their wishes, the family can decide. Room is thus allowed for individual autonomy and, in its absence, familial decision making. In this scheme, a legally enforceable requirement of beneficence falls on institutions, whereas professionals and potential donors have an opportunity of voluntary beneficence. All parties have a moral obligation of positive beneficence to ask for or to make donations.

Other policies have also been proposed, but they appear to be less effective and efficient or to be morally tenuous. A policy of actual conscription in taking organs—a stronger enforced beneficence—would violate respect for autonomy. A policy of presumed consent, which has been adopted in many countries for various organs and in several states for corneas, could be ethically acceptable if people were adequately informed that a failure to dissent or to refuse participation would be construed as consent. But vigorous educational efforts would be required. Furthermore, in view of current attitudes, a policy of presumed consent is likely to be ineffective, because more potential donors would decline in advance because of their fears of abuse.

We conclude that the obligation of positive beneficence—for society, hospitals, health-care professionals, individuals, and families—can best be discharged, at least for the time being, by a policy of required request, which appears to be effective and efficient without threatening or violating other ethical principles.[19]

Paternalism: conflicts between beneficence and autonomy

Disputes about the primacy of beneficence

We have seen that the aim of the relationship between health-care professionals and patients can be understood in terms of beneficence and that the principle of beneficence can be invoked to express the primary obligation in medicine and health care. In an inchoate form, this outlook is an ancient one. Throughout the history of healing, the health professional's obligations and virtues, as expressed in codes and didactic writings on ethics, have been understood in terms of the professional commitments of beneficence. In the Hippocratic work *Epidemics* we find perhaps the most celebrated expression of beneficence as the core principle in medicine: "As to disease, make a habit of two things—*to help, or at least to do no harm.*"[20]

The primacy of beneficence—usually understood to include nonmaleficence—has had an immense impact on the history of medical ethics. Thomas Percival, perhaps the most influential writer in medical ethics in the modern period, moved from the premise that the patient's best medical interest is the proper goal of the physician's actions to descriptions of the physician's proper behavior, including those traits of character that maximize the patient's welfare. Percival's *Medical Ethics* supplies a short list of recommended virtues of the physician all of which are associated with benevolence and professional responsibility. Recognizing the dependence of patients, Percival counsels physicians to discard feelings of pride and dignity and to attend strictly to the patient's medical needs. In Percival's work, the profession's understanding of its obligations is invariably beneficence-based. For example, the physician is encouraged in difficult circumstances to manipulate the truth if it is in the best medical interests of the patient.

As long as beneficence retained unchallenged primacy in medical ethics, physicians were able to rely almost exclusively on their own judgment about their patients' needs for treatment, information, and consultation—where "needs" is primarily construed as "needs for medical care." However, medicine has increasingly been confronted—especially in the last thirty years—with a different kind of need, namely the patient's asserted need to make an independent judgment. Values in patients' judgments often differ from the medical values of care and healing. Various assumptions of the claimed primacy of the obligation of beneficence have thus been challenged in the name of a patient-centered medical ethics that emphasizes autonomy rights over professional obligations of beneficence when they conflict.

One result of these developments has been to introduce both confusion and constructive change in medicine, which continues as a profession to struggle with unprecedented challenges to its authority in the control and treatment of patients. The central problem in these discussions is whether the principle of respect for autonomy that gives primary decision-making authority to patients should have priority in medical practice over the principle of beneficence that gives authority to providers to implement sound principles of health care. For proponents of the primacy of autonomy, the physician's obligations to the patient of disclosure, confidentiality, privacy, and seeking consent are established primarily (perhaps exclusively) by the principle of respect for autonomy.

Proponents of the priority of beneficence, by contrast, ground the physician's obligations of disclosure, seeking consent, and the like on the principle of beneficence; the physician's primary obligation is to provide medical benefits. From this perspective, the management of information is generally understood in terms of the medical management of patients. That is, the physician's primary obligation is to handle information so as to maximize the patient's medical benefits.

A typical statement of the priority of respect for autonomy in the event of conflict with beneficence (toward the patient) is found in the following statement by the President's Commission for the Study of Ethical Problems in Medicine and Biomedical and Behavioral Research:

> The primary goal of health care in general is to maximize each patient's well-being. However, merely acting in a patient's best interests without recognizing the individual as the pivotal decisionmaker would fail to respect each person's interest in self-determination. . . . When the conflicts that arise between a competent patient's self-determination and his or her apparent well-being remain unresolved after adequate deliberation, a competent patient's self-determination is and usually should be given greater weight than other people's views on that individual's well-being. . . .
>   Respect for the self-determination of competent patients is of special importance. . . . The patient [should have] the final authority to decide.[21]

So influential is this autonomy model at the present time that it has become difficult to find clear commitments to the traditional beneficence model in contemporary biomedical ethics. The debate has often been confused by the failure of a number of discussants to distinguish clearly between a principle of beneficence that actually *competes* with a principle of respect for autonomy and a principle of beneficence that *includes* respect for patient autonomy. For example, two exponents of the preeminence of beneficence—Edmund Pellegrino and David Thomasma—argue as follows:

None of [the court cases favoring patient autonomy] can be seen as an objection to the beneficence model. It might be tempting to think that these cases give precedence to patient wishes or presumed wishes over physician paternalism, but that is not so. Instead, they emphasize patient wishes . . . as a means for protecting the patient's best interests. This is a critical point. While autonomy is not a clear winner in these cases, neither is paternalism. Rather, the best interests of the patients are intimately linked with their preferences. From these are derived our primary duties toward them.[22]

This formulation and defense of the beneficence model is little more than a dressed-up defense of one form of autonomy model. If the content of the physician's obligation to be beneficent is set exclusively by the patient's choices and preferences, the principle of autonomy has triumphed. Elsewhere, however, Pellegrino and Thomasma expand on their thesis:

Both autonomy and paternalism are superseded by the obligation to act beneficently; that is to say, the choice of whether one acts to foster autonomy or instead acts paternalistically should be based on what most benefits the patient. . . .

Any critical reflection on beneficence must include limitations on autonomy. There are too many clinical situations in which freedom—either the physician's or the patient's—must be curtailed. In the real world of clinical medicine, there are no absolute moral principles except the injunction to act in the patient's best interest.[23]

These writers go on to list a number of circumstances in which medical beneficence overrides respect for patient autonomy because patients have made irresponsible choices. For example, "autonomy would be wrongly exercised if [the patient] rejected penicillin treatment for pneumococcal or meningococcal meningitis."[24] The reason is that these infections are life-threatening and can produce serious central nervous system damage if the patient recovers. The patient has made an irresponsible choice that a caring physician would disallow. Here we do have a defense of a genuine beneficence model, although not one in which beneficence necessarily overrides respect for autonomy in a bona fide situation of conflict. Pellegrino and Thomasma construe their absolute principle "Act in the patient's best interest" so that in some circumstances the physician should act on what the patient prefers even if it conflicts with what is medically indicated.

We believe that this general problem of which principle should be overriding in medical practice is not amenable to solution by defending one principle against the other principle. According to the structure of the argument we have developed throughout this book, there is no premier and overriding authority in either the patient or the physician and no preeminent principle in biomedical ethics— not even the admonition to act in the patient's best interest. However, the implications of our position for authority in health care will be unsettled until we come to terms with the problem of paternalism.

The nature of paternalism

When the health-care professional has an assessment of benefits, harms, and their balance that differs from the patient's assessment, this circumstance may be complicated by an additional problem. Some patients—for example, those who are depressed or are addicted to potentially harmful drugs—are unlikely to reach adequately reasoned decisions. Other patients who are competent and deliberative may make poor choices about courses of action recommended by their physicians. When patients of either type choose harmful courses of action, some health-care professionals are inclined to respect autonomy by not interfering beyond attempts at persuasion, whereas others are inclined to act beneficently by protecting patients against the potentially harmful consequences of their choices. The problem of which principle to follow and whether and how to intervene in the decisions and affairs of such patients is the problem of medical paternalism.[25]

Analyses of paternalism in terms of the restriction of either autonomy or freedom are at least as old as Kant, who denounced paternalistic government ("imperium paternale," he called it) for benevolent limitations of the freedoms of its subjects. When Kant denounced paternalistic government as "the worst conceivable despotism," he meant a government that "cancels the freedom of subjects." He never considered the possibility that a *parens patriae* or parental model of intervention—one that likens the state to a protective parent in caring for an incompetent minor—might be considered paternalistic. Nor did John Stuart Mill's influential rejection of paternalism in *On Liberty* contemplate the possibility that paternalism might encompass intervention with those who have limited or no autonomy.[26]

Yet the model they did not contemplate subsequently became and remains the most widely accepted model of justified paternalism. The *Oxford English Dictionary* dates the term *paternalism* from the 1880s (after the writings of Kant and Mill), giving the root meaning as "the principle and practice of paternal administration; government as by a father; the claim or attempt to supply the needs or to regulate the life of a nation or community in the same way a father does those of his children." When the analogy with the father is used to illuminate the role of professionals or the state in health care, it presupposes two features of the paternal role: that the father acts beneficently (i.e., in accord with his conception of the interests of his children) and that he makes all or at least some of the decisions relating to his children's welfare rather than letting them make those decisions. In professional relationships the argument is that a professional has superior training, knowledge, and insight and is in an authoritative position to determine what is in the patient's best interests. In short, from this perspective, a professional is like a parent when dealing with dependent and often ignorant and fearful patients.

Medical paternalism poses significant moral questions because (on some formulations) it holds that beneficence can legitimately take precedence over respect for autonomy. The principle of nonmaleficence has likewise been viewed as outweighing respect for autonomy in discussions of medical paternalism. For example, physicians have traditionally taken the view that disclosing certain forms of information can cause harm to patients under their care and that medical ethics obligates them not to cause harm. In a classic article, L. J. Henderson argues that "the best physicians" use the following as their primary guide: "So far as possible, 'Do No Harm.' You can do harm by the process that is quaintly called telling the truth. You can do harm by lying. . . . But try to do as little harm as possible, not only in treatment with drugs, or with the knife, but also in treatment with words." Henderson and others in the medical community argue that for the patient's good, some information should be withheld or should be disclosed only to the family and that deference to the autonomy rights of patients is dangerous because it compromises clinical judgment and presents a hazard to the patient's health.[27]

The following case illustrates these problems. A woman had a fatal reaction during urography (visualization of the urinary tract after injection of an opaque medium). The radiologist had not informed her of the possible fatal reaction on grounds that his obligation was to do "what is best for our patients medically." He conceived the doctor's role as that of judging whether the presentation of information is more or less harmful to the patient. In this particular case, he determined that it was not in the best interest of the patient to be informed because the risk of death was slight, while the possibility of causing undue alarm was great.[28] This paternalistic attitude is clearly grounded in nonmaleficence and beneficence.

The case just considered is one of many types of truth-telling cases involving paternalism. Other cases arise when unwelcome news might lead to suicide, as when a cancer victim is told the truth about his or her condition. In Case 6, an inoperable, incurable carcinoma is discovered in a sixty-nine-year-old male. Because of a long relationship with this patient, the physician knew that the patient was fragile in several respects. The patient was neurotic, had a history of psychiatric disease, and had recently suffered a severe depressive reaction, during which he had behaved irrationally and attempted suicide. When he blurted out, "Am I OK?" and, "I don't have cancer, do I?" the physician answered, "You're as good as you were ten years ago," knowing that the response was a paternalistic lie but also believing it justified. The physician was obviously worried that a truthful disclosure would seriously disrupt the man's life plans and possibly cause mental instability or lead to suicide.

Cases of paternalism, then, involve overriding a person's wishes or intentional actions in order to benefit *or* to avoid or prevent harm to that person. Paternalistic actions generally involve force or coercion on the one hand or deception, lying, or nondisclosure of information on the other. According to some definitions, a paternalistic action, whatever its form, necessarily infringes autonomous choice. While one author of this text prefers this definition,[29] we will here follow the mainstream of the literature on paternalism and accept the broader definition suggested by the *Oxford English Dictionary*. We thus understand paternalism as the overriding of a person's wishes or intentional actions for beneficent reasons. If these wishes or intentional actions do not derive from a substantially autonomous choice, overriding them can still be paternalistic. For example, if a man wholly ignorant of his fragile, life-threatening condition and sick with a raging fever expresses his intention to leave the hospital, it would be paternalistic to detain him even if we judged that his expressed wish did not derive from a substantially autonomous choice.

Despite his opposition to paternalism, Mill considered temporary beneficent interventions in a person's intentional actions to be justified on some occasions. He argued that a person who is ignorant of a potential risk or is otherwise temporarily encumbered may justifiably be restrained in order to ensure that he or she is acting intentionally with adequate knowledge of the consequences of the action. Once warned, the person should be free to choose whatever course he or she desires. Because Mill did not regard this temporary intervention as a "real infringement" of liberty, he did not view it as paternalistic. However, under the definition of paternalism we have accepted, even such temporary intervention would be paternalistic because the restricted action is intentional, even though it has unintended effects of which the person is ignorant. Protection against the unintended effects of an intentional action is one of the primary reasons for defending paternalism.

Because "paternalistic interventions," in our usage, do not necessarily override autonomy, it is easier to justify some paternalistic interferences with a person's actions than it would be if these actions (by definition of paternalism) had to be autonomous. However, we will later argue that both autonomous and nonautonomous actions may be justifiably restricted on grounds of beneficence. We thus will argue for a broader form of paternalism than has generally been supported in literature on the subject.

One preliminary caution is that in some cases a justification for an action may appear to be paternalistic when in fact it is nonpaternalistic. An example is found in research involving prisoners. In 1976, the National Commission for the Protection of Human Subjects of Biomedical and Behavioral Research issued a report on research involving prisoners.[30] It argued that the closed nature of prison environments creates a strong potential for abuse of authority and therefore invites the exploitation and coercion of prisoners. However, a commission study indicated that most prisoners do not regard their consent to research as obtained under coercion or undue influence. The commission nonetheless argued that the inherent coercive possibilities in prisons justify regulations prohibiting many prisoners from engaging in research, even if they wish to do so.

This justification may appear to be paternalistic, but closer analysis of the commission report shows that it is not. The commission explicitly maintained that if an environment were not exploitative or coercive (and if a few other conditions were met), then prisoners should be free to choose to participate in research. The commission's justifying ground was the factual claim that most prisons could not be rendered sufficiently free of coercion and exploitation by drug companies and prison officials, not the moral claim that the prisoners should be protected from their wishes and choices. The argument is that we cannot predict whether prisoners will be exploited in settings that render them vulnerable, but research to which they might validly consent should nonetheless be prohibited because we cannot adequately monitor the consent process.

Competing moral theories of paternalism

In the literature on paternalism, two main positions have been defended by moral arguments: justified paternalism and antipaternalism.

THE JUSTIFICATION OF PATERNALISM BY CONSENT. Any supporter of the paternalistic principle will specify precisely which goods, needs, and interests warrant paternalistic protection. In recent formulations, it has been maintained that an individual or the state is justified in interfering with a person's action if that interference protects the person against his or her extremely and unreasonably risky actions—such as dangerous self-administered medical experiments. Thus, paternalism can be justified only if (1) the harms prevented from occurring or the benefits provided to the person outweigh the loss of independence and the sense of invasion caused by the interference, (2) the person's condition seriously limits his or her ability to choose autonomously, and (3) the interference is universally justified under relevantly similar circumstances.

Roughly this position is defended by a number of recent writers, some of whom regard paternalism as a form of "social insurance policy" that fully rational persons would take out in order to protect themselves.[31] Such persons would know, for example, that they might be tempted at times to make decisions that are far-reaching, potentially dangerous, and irreversible, while at other times they might suffer irresistible psychological or social pressures to do something they believe too risky to be worth performing, such as placing their honor in question by a challenge to fight. In still other cases, persons might not sufficiently understand or appreciate dangers, such as medical facts about the effects of smoking. Thus, some conclude, we ought to consent to a limited authorization for others to control our actions by paternalistic policies and interventions.

Case 10 presents an example of one kind of action that fits this form of justified paternalism. An involuntarily committed mental patient wishes to leave the hospital, although his family is opposed to his release. The patient argues that his mental condition does not justify confinement, but after one release he plucked out his right eye, and after another release he severed his right hand. The patient functions fairly normally in the state hospital, where he sells news materials to fellow patients and handles limited financial affairs. The source of his "problems" is apparently his religious beliefs. He regards himself as a true prophet of God and believes that "it is far better for one man to believe and accept an appropriate message from God to sacrifice an eye or a hand according to the sacred scriptures rather than for the present course of the world to cause even greater loss of human life." Acting on this belief, he engages in self-mutilation. According to the paternalist, this person generally functions normally, by usual behavioral or observational criteria, yet needs and deserves help. His capacities are too diminished and his dangerousness to himself is too severe to leave him without confinement and custodial care.

John Rawls and Gerald Dworkin espouse a form of justified paternalism in which the justification of the position rests on an argument that completely rational agents fully aware of their circumstances would "consent to paternalism" and would even "consent to a scheme of penalties that may give them a sufficient motive to avoid foolish actions." This position relies on a "but for" theory of consent, according to which those whose autonomy is reduced would consent but for their compromised condition.[32] Some form of consent is thus a necessary, though not sufficient, condition of justified paternalism. Rawls and Dworkin do not propose a subsequent or predictive consent theory, according to which a consent would be given if only a present impairment were removed. They argue from a Kantian conception of the rational and autonomous agent, rather than from empirical predictions about what particular agents would do.

An appeal to some kind of consent for justification—be it rational consent, subsequent consent, or some other type of consent—is central to the strategy of the most prominent theories of justified paternalism. As Dworkin puts it, "the basic notion of consent is important and seems to me the only acceptable way to try to delimit an area of justified paternalism." Rosemary Carter agrees with this common sentiment, arguing that "consent plays the central role in justifying paternalism, and indeed . . . no other concepts are relevant."[33]

The justifying ground of paternalism in this type of theory is rational informed consent. Even though such an autonomy-based theory has some appealing features, we will not defend this form of paternalism. Our thesis is that beneficence alone is the justification of paternalism, just as it is of parental actions that override the preferences of children. We do not interfere in the lives of our children because we believe that they will subsequently consent or would rationally approve. We interfere because we think the intervention gives them a better life, whether they know it or not.

ANTIPATERNALISTIC INDIVIDUALISM. Some believe that paternalistic intervention cannot be justified because it violates individual rights and unduly restricts free choice. The serious adverse consequences of giving such power to the state, or to any class of individuals, such as physicians, also motivate antipaternalists to reject the view that the completely rational person would accept paternalism under some circumstances. But the dominant reason why paternalism is unacceptable is that rightful authority resides in the individual whose life is controlled, not in the controller. The argument for this conclusion is found in the analysis of the principle of respect for autonomy in Chapter 3.

Antipaternalists argue that paternalistic principles are too broad and hence would justify or institutionalize too much intervention if made the basis of policy. Using an extreme example, Robert Harris has argued that paternalism would in principle "justify the imposition of a Spartan-like regimen requiring rigorous physical exercise and abstention from smoking, drinking, and hazardous pastimes."[34] The more thoughtful restrictions on paternalism accepted by some paternalists would disallow these extreme interventions but, according to antipaternalists, would still leave unacceptable latitude of judgment in contexts where power is likely to be abused and also would leave unresolved problems concerning the scope of the principle. On the latter point, suppose that a man risks his life for the advancement of medicine by submitting to an unreasonably risky experiment, an act most would think not in his best interests. Are we to commend him, ignore him, or coercively restrain him? Paternalism suggests that it would be permissible and perhaps even obligatory to restrain such a person. Yet if so, antipaternalists argue, the state is permitted in principle to coerce its morally heroic citizens, not to mention its martyrs, if they act—as such people sometimes do—in a manner "harmful" to themselves.

Physicians and nurses would be authorized by the principle of beneficence to treat patients in parallel paternalistic ways. Antipaternalists worry about the power paternalism gives health-care professionals in the full range of their interactions with patients. The medical example with the most extensive antipaternalistic literature is the involuntary hospitalization of persons who have neither been harmed by others nor actually harmed themselves but who are thought to be at risk of such harm. These cases involve a double paternalism, a paternalistic justification for both therapy and commitment.

A widely discussed case is that of Catherine Lake, Case 9. Lake suffers from arteriosclerosis, which has caused temporary confusion and mild loss of memory, interspersed with periods of mental alertness and rationality. All parties agree that Lake has never harmed anyone or presented any threat of danger, yet she was committed to a mental institution because she often seemed confused and defenseless. At her trial, while apparently rational, she testified that she knew the risk of living outside the hospital and preferred to take that risk rather than be in the hospital environment. The court of appeals denied her petition, arguing that she is "mentally ill," "is of danger to herself . . . and is not competent to care for herself." The legal justification cited by the court was a statute that "provides for involuntary hospitalization of a person who is 'mentally ill and, because of that illness is likely to injure himself.' . . ."[35] Antipaternalists argue that since Lake is not causing harm to others and understands the dangers under which she is placing herself, she should be free to proceed as she wishes.

Strong and weak paternalism

Supporters of limited paternalism and opponents of paternalism often disagree in particular cases about a person's competence both for decision making and for stating preferences. (See the discussion of competence in Chapter 3.) Supporters of paternalism tend to cite examples of persons of diminished capacity—for example, persons in severe depression. By contrast, opponents cite examples of persons who are capable of autonomous choice, at least in some contexts—for example, those involuntarily committed merely for eccentric behavior, those in prison who are not permitted to volunteer for research on drugs, and those who rationally elect to refuse treatment in life-threatening circumstances. A critical factor in the dispute between paternalists and antipaternalists thus turns on the quality or degree of personal autonomy.

Joel Feinberg's distinction between strong and weak paternalism illuminates this disagreement.[36] In weak paternalism, one "has the right to prevent self-regarding conduct only when it is *substantially nonvoluntary* or when temporary intervention is necessary to establish whether it is voluntary or not." To say that conduct is substantially nonvoluntary is to say, in our language, that the person's action is substantially nonautonomous, even if it is autonomous in some respects. The class of nonvoluntary or nonautonomous actions includes cases of consent that are not adequately informed. By the standards of weak paternalism, it is morally appropriate to intervene when a person's judgment is impaired by an illness, a person suffers from serious depression, and the like—even though such persons have some degree of capacity for judgment and action. Weak paternalism thus requires some degree of compromised ability.

Strong paternalism, by contrast, holds that it is sometimes proper to intervene in order to benefit a person even if that person's risky choices are informed and voluntary. Strong paternalism overrides autonomy: It restricts the information available to a person or overrides the person's informed and voluntary choices. These choices might not be fully autonomous or voluntary, but in order for the interventions to qualify as strong paternalism the choices must be substantially autonomous or voluntary. Unlike weak paternalism, strong paternalism is not built on a conception of compromised ability, dysfunctional incompetence, or encumbrances in deciding, willing, or acting.

Virtually everyone acknowledges that some acts of weak paternalism are justified acts of beneficence, such as preventing a man under the influence of LSD from killing himself. Weak paternalism thus may not be a form of paternalism that is controversial; it may not be an intervention to which even antipaternalists would object, because it does not involve an intervention in a substantially autonomous action, which is the primary form of intervention of concern to the antipaternalist. If the only justification of paternalistic intervention always rests on preventing harm to substantially nonautonomous persons, then paternalism of this sort will not violate the antipaternalist's principle of respect for autonomy or liberty. Rather, the antipaternalist will view these interventions as justified by the principle of beneficence, which in this context does not conflict with the principle of respect for autonomy. In weak paternalism there is no substantial autonomy to be restricted, and since antipaternalists are only interested in protecting substantial autonomy, there appears to be no moral conflict between weak paternalism and antipaternalism. It is not even clear that weak paternalism as a moral position can be distinguished from antipaternalism, inasmuch as they eventuate in the same moral recommendations for the same general moral reasons.

An alternative formulation of justified paternalism

Strong paternalism, then, seems to be the only controversial form of paternalism. To the present writers, strong paternalism is a dangerous moral position to espouse without careful qualification, because of its potential for abuse, but some individual acts of strong paternalism are justified.[37] For example, consider the following case. A physician obtains the results of a myelogram (a graph of the spinal region) following examination of a patient. The results are inconclusive enough to require that the test be repeated, but there is a suggestion of a serious pathology. When the patient asks about the test results, the physician determines on grounds of beneficence to withhold this relevant information, knowing that upon disclosure the patient would be distressed and anxious. Based on her experience with other patients and her ten-year knowledge of this patient, the physician is confident that the information would in no way affect the patient's decision to consent to another myelogram. Her sole motivation in withholding the information is to spare the patient the emotional distress of having to think through a painful decision prematurely. The physician does, however, intend to be fully truthful with the patient about the results of the second test, no matter how negative the findings; and the truthful disclosure will be made well in advance of the time when the patient will need to make a decision about surgery. This physician's act of temporary nondisclosure seems to us morally justified, even though beneficence is (temporarily) given priority over respect for autonomy. Had the patient requested "the whole truth" and been denied it, the paternalism would be more questionable because the physician would be lying and not merely without information. Nevertheless, we think this second action might also be an instance of morally justified paternalism.

A still more commonplace example of justified strong paternalism is found in the following case reported by Mary Silva:

> After receiving his preoperative medicine, Mr. D., a 23 year old male athlete scheduled for a hernia repair, states that he does not want the side rails up. Mr. D. is of clear mind and understands why the rule is required; however, Mr. D. does not feel that the rule should apply to him because he is not the least bit drowsy from the preoperative medication and he has no intention of falling out of bed. After considerable discussion between the nurse and patient, the nurse responsible for Mr. D.'s care puts the side rails up. Her justification is as follows: Mr. D. is not drowsy because he has just received the preoperative medication and its effects have not occurred. Furthermore, if he follows the typical pattern of patients receiving this medication in this dosage, he will become drowsy very quickly. A drowsy patient is a risk for a fall. Since there is no family at the hospital to remain with the patient, and since the nurses on the unit are exceptionally busy, no one can constantly stay with Mr. D. to monitor his level of alertness. Under these circumstances, the patient must be protected from the potential harm of a fall, despite the fact that he does not want this protection. . . . The nurse restricted this autonomous patient's liberty based on . . . . protection of the patient from potential harm . . . and *not* as a hedge against liability or to protect herself from criticism.[38]

Minor paternalistic actions against the preferences of patients and careful monitoring of potentially upsetting information are common in hospitals, and where there is no reasonable alternative they are justified examples of strong paternalism. The weight of beneficence in these cases is substantial, whereas infringement of the principle of respect for autonomy is minimal. These and other paternalistic actions are appropriate in health care only if

(1) a patient is at risk of injury or illness,
(2) the risks of the paternalistic action (e.g., intervention or nondisclosure) to the patient are not substantial,
(3) the action's projected benefits to the patient outweigh its risks,
(4) there is no feasible and acceptable alternative to the paternalistic action,
(5) infringement of the principle of respect for autonomy is minimal, and
(6) the action involves the least infringement necessary in the circumstances.

The crucial fifth condition can be satisfied only if vital autonomy interests are not at stake. For example, if a Jehovah's Witness refuses a blood transfusion because of a deeply held conviction, a vital autonomy interest is at stake. To intervene coercively by providing the transfusion would be a substantial infringement of autonomy and thus would be unjustifiable.

The fifth condition may be too restrictive in the eyes of some strong paternalists. A plausible kind of case favoring strong paternalistic intervention that infringes autonomy more than minimally (and thus exceeds our six conditions) is the following. A psychiatrist is treating a patient like the patient in Case 10 who plucked out his eye and cut off his hand for religious reasons. Presume that this patient is not insane and acts conscientiously on his unique religious views. Suppose further that this patient asks the psychiatrist a question about his condition, a question that has a definite answer but which, if answered, would lead the patient to engage in self-maiming behavior in order to fulfill what he believes to be the requirements of his religion. Many, including the present authors, are inclined to say that the doctor acts paternalistically but justifiably by concealing information from the patient, even if the patient is rational and relevantly informed. Because a good case can be made that the infringement of the principle of respect for autonomy is more than minimal in this case, our fifth condition may need modification. However, defenders of that condition might also challenge whether the patient's autonomy is intact in this case.

There are, of course, many examples of justified weak paternalism. Everyone familiar with the practice of medicine knows that some patients who are mentally alert nonetheless suffer from nonvoluntary conditions, such as depression and drug addiction, that affect their behavior. These persons are generally capable of making judgments that affect their lives, but their limitations can have profound effects on their decisions. Cases involving adult patients on dialysis and suffering from uremia (retention in the blood of toxic urinary constituents) or suicidal patients suffering from serious depression likewise invite paternalistic treatment. It would be callous, uncaring, and wrong to allow such persons to die through their own decisions when certain conditions substantially reduce the autonomy of their actions.

It can be argued that on some occasions the physician actually protects a patient's autonomy by overriding his or her immediate wishes. For example, as discussed earlier, in Case 6, a sixty-nine-year-old man unaware that he has prostate cancer asks his physician for the results of recent tests. The physician tells him that he is as healthy as he was ten years ago. The physician is attempting to protect this very fragile patient, who has a psychiatric history, from the potential loss of the capacity to choose autonomously. Few would say that the doctor made an utterly indefensible choice, yet his action is a paternalistic lie. Moreover, it is a particularly interesting lie because it straddles the boundary between strong paternalism and weak paternalism. Although the patient acts (as the case is described) autonomously in requesting the information, the physician believes he would not be able to act autonomously if he were given the information. This case illustrates how complex the interactions sometimes become in the attempt to balance considerations of respect for autonomy, beneficence, and nonmaleficence in the treatment of patients.

We conclude that weak paternalism is a defensible moral position but that it applies only to the range of cases in which persons are clearly endangered and are not adequately autonomous. Weak paternalism thus may be compatible with an antipaternalism that includes a principle of beneficence. Strong paternalism is more difficult to justify but can sometimes be justified. The possibilities for abuse inherent in a defense of strong paternalism seem to outweigh its possible benefits, unless the lines can be more carefully drawn than they have been in the past. This conclusion follows from the general line of moral argument in previous chapters. We have argued for a pluralism of moral principles, equally weighted in advance of information about particular circumstances. It therefore cannot be assumed that even an autonomous choice can never be validly overridden on grounds of beneficence to the chooser; and it is possible to imagine cases in which the weight of respect for autonomy is minimal, while the weight of beneficence is maximal, and the other conditions for overriding a prima facie obligation are also met.

Problems of suicide intervention

Intervention in an intentional act of suicide poses some of the sharpest controversies about paternalism. We will now explore suicide intervention in order to assess and develop the conclusions we have reached about the justification of paternalism. The primary problems are whether the suicide's circumstances render the act less than substantially autonomous, and under which conditions, if any, the principle of beneficence justifies intervention.

There are approximately twenty-eight thousand certified suicides in the United States each year, but many other suicides probably get classified as accidental deaths simply because too little is known about the decedents' intentions. There is also a reluctance in uncertain cases to label deaths as suicides in order to protect the survivors from the stigma of suicide, the sense of failure to provide adequate care for the decedent, and the possible loss of life insurance benefits.

There are also difficult conceptual questions about suicide.[39] When Barney Clark, age sixty-two, became the first human to receive an artificial heart on December 2, 1982, he was also given a key that he could use to turn off the compressor if he wanted to die. As Dr. Willem Kolff noted, if the patient "suffers and feels it isn't worth it any more, he has a key that he can apply. . . . I think it is entirely legitimate that this man whose life has been extended should have the right to cut it off if he doesn't want it, if life ceases to be enjoyable."[40] There would have been vigorous debate about the characterization of Clark's action if he had used the key to turn off his artificial heart. If Clark had refused to accept the artificial heart in the first place, few would have characterized his act as one of suicide, because of his overall condition and the experimental nature of the artificial heart; but if he had shot himself while on the artificial heart, it would have been difficult to avoid characterizing the act as one of suicide. If he had used the key to turn off his artificial heart, controversy would have erupted about whether to characterize his act as forgoing life-sustaining treatment, as withdrawing from an experiment, or as suicide. We often shield acts of which we approve (or at least acts that are not disapproved) from the stigmatizing label of "suicide." It would take us too far afield to pursue these conceptual points farther, and in assessing suicide intervention we will concentrate on cases that would generally be viewed as acts of suicide or attempted suicide, noting that questions of paternalism still arise for related acts such as refusal of life-sustaining treatment.

A clear example of attempted suicide appears in Case 11. Recently two neurologists independently confirmed that John K.'s facial twitching, which has been evident for three months, is an early sign of Huntington's chorea, a neurological disorder that becomes progressively worse, leads to irreversible dementia, and is uniformly fatal in approximately ten years. This thirty-two-year-old lawyer's mother suffered a horrible death from the same (autosomal dominant) disease, and John K. has often said that he would prefer to die than to suffer the way his mother suffered. Over several years he has been anxious, has drunk heavily, and has sought psychiatric help for intermittent depression. After the confirmed diagnosis, John K. told his psychiatrist about his situation and asked for help in committing suicide. After the psychiatrist refused to help him commit suicide, he attempted to take his life by ingesting all of his antidepressant medication, leaving a note of explanation to his wife and child.

Several interventions were possible in this case. First, the psychiatrist refused to assist John K.'s suicide but did not seek to have him involuntarily committed because the patient assured him that he did not plan to attempt suicide anytime soon. The psychiatrist probably also thought that he could provide appropriate psychotherapy over time. Second, John K.'s wife found him unconscious and rushed him to the emergency room. Third, the emergency room staff decided to treat him despite the note indicating attempted suicide. Which of these possible or actual interventions could be justified? And were they obligatory on the basis of paternalistic beneficence?

One widely held account of our obligations is based on a modification of the principle of respect for autonomy defended by Mill: Intervention is justified to ascertain or to establish the quality of autonomy in the person; and any further intervention is unjustified. Glanville Williams has expressed this argument as follows:

If one suddenly comes upon another person attempting suicide, the natural and humane thing to do is to try to stop him, for the purpose of ascertaining the cause of his distress and attempting to remedy it, or else of attempting moral dissuasion if it seems that the act of suicide shows lack of consideration for others, or else again from the purpose of trying to persuade him to accept psychiatric help if this seems to be called for. . . . But nothing longer than a temporary restraint could be defended. I would gravely doubt whether a suicide attempt should be a factor leading to a diagnosis of psychosis or to compulsory admissions to a hospital. Psychiatrists are too ready to assume that an attempt to commit suicide is the act of mentally sick persons.[41]

This kind of antipaternalistic rule has been criticized on two grounds. First, failure to intervene indicates a lack of concern about others and a diminished sense of moral responsibility in a community. From this perspective, a policy of nonintervention may symbolically communicate to potential suicides a lack of communal care and diminishes our sense of communal responsibility. Second, many persons who commit suicide are either mentally ill, clinically depressed, or destabilized by a crisis and are therefore not acting autonomously. From a clinical perspective, many suicidal persons are under intense strains or under the influence of drugs or alcohol, are beset with ambivalence, or simply wish to reduce or interrupt anxiety. These common clinical circumstances have led many mental-health professionals to conclude that suicides are almost always the result of maladaptive attitudes, pressures, or illnesses needing therapeutic attention and social support. Their conviction is that "reasons" for suicide are rationalizations that derive from pathological conditions preventing autonomous choice.[42] These professionals believe that medicine and behavioral therapy have a responsibility to prevent the patient's self-destruction and to cure the problem.

Early studies indicate that people who have been diagnosed with AIDS commit suicide at a rate many times greater—one study suggests sixty-six times greater—than the general population.[43] In the case of patients who have AIDS and want to commit suicide rather than face the process of suffering and dying from their disease, the medical condition that to the patient appears to justify suicide often causes central nervous system complications such as delirium or dementia that may render the patient unable to make a substantially autonomous choice. Thus, while recognizing the case for "rational suicide" on the part of patients with AIDS, one physician contends that "from the clinical point of view, careful evaluations of suicides, even in terminally ill patients, almost invariably reveal evidence that the suicide occurred as a manifestation of a psychiatric disorder rather than as a rational choice. . . . I would urge that the physicians continue to consider suicide, in AIDS patients as in others, as an untoward illness outcome to be diagnosed, treated, and prevented."[44] The prevention in view includes social support systems, along with opportunities for open discussion of emotional reactions to the illness and death.

Many people attempt suicide when they find their situations "unbearable"—

for example, when they have experienced a personal loss or believe that they have no alternatives or options. Arthur Koestler faced such circumstances. He was seventy-seven years old, in very poor health, and suffering from both Parkinson's disease and leukemia. His literary agent indicated that Koestler found his situation "intolerable." Koestler committed suicide from barbiturate overdose, as did his fifty-six-year-old wife, for whom he was "her whole world." These kinds of cases do not necessarily indicate that the person is not acting autonomously, but many such cases do involve persons who have been patients seeking relief from a serious psychiatric or medical problem.

The grave circumstances under which many patients take their lives have had a deep impact on current law. Although the act of suicide has been decriminalized, a suicidal attempt, irrespective of motive, almost universally gives a legal basis for intervention by public officers and for involuntary hospitalization.[45] In most jurisdictions involuntary hospitalization is permitted to establish whether a person is mentally ill and a threat to his or her own person or to others. In law the burden of proof of mental illness, dangerousness to oneself, and dangerousness to others is not as heavy as the burden of proof involved in depriving persons of liberty in criminal convictions, where the standard of evidence is "beyond a reasonable doubt." However, the standard is not as modest as in civil law, which uses the standard of "preponderance of the evidence." For involuntary hospitalization the standard is generally that of clear and compelling evidence.[46] This, we believe, is an appropriate standard. In practice it is easier to satisfy the burden of proof for brief periods than for longer involuntary commitments.

Virtually everyone agrees—for reasons already established above—that nonautonomous suicidal actions may be justifiably prevented and that there are often good reasons to intervene temporarily to determine the competence and the actual wishes of persons attempting suicide. There remain deep problems, however, about how to assess the quality of autonomy in patients and about the proper role of mental-health professionals. Contrary to Williams's perspective, mental-health professionals often see a patient who expresses an interest in suicide—for example, a person with a painful life-threatening illness or grave physical handicap and with little or no will to live—as a person needing treatment. Indeed, many mental-health professionals view a patient's statement of a desire to commit suicide as a plea for help in resisting suicide. Thus, they would approach John K.'s statement (in Case 11) as a request for help not in committing suicide but in preventing suicide.[47] In any event, they often view their obligation of beneficence as preventing suicide, at least temporarily. Others, by contrast, view the patient as acting autonomously in electing suicide. Thus, they could hold that John K. is acting autonomously and even reasonably, particularly in view of his life prospects. These competing accounts will not always be reconcilable, as the following case suggests.

Ida Rollin, seventy-four years old, suffered from ovarian cancer, and her physicians indicated that she had only a few months to live, that chemotherapy would not arrest her cancer, and that her dying would be very painful. The chemotherapy produced baldness and perpetual nausea with vomiting. Rollin indicated to her daughter, Betty Rollin, that she wanted to commit suicide and asked her assistance in doing so as efficiently and as painlessly as possible. The daughter secured the pills and passed on a doctor's instructions about how they should be taken. When the daughter expressed reservations about these plans, her husband reminded her that they "weren't driving, she [Ida Rollin] was" and that they were only "navigators."[48] This metaphor-laden reference to rightful authority is a reminder that the burden of proof is on those who claim that the patient's judgment is not autonomous. And if she is autonomous, an even greater burden of proof rests on those who believe that her family or her physicians are under an obligation to intervene to prevent her action.

In considering such cases as Ida Rollin with terminal cancer or John K. with Huntington's chorea, it is important to distinguish *justifying* an act of suicide or attempted suicide from *excusing* it. If an act is morally justified, it is right, all things considered. But having a right to do X does not establish that it is right (or virtuous) to do X. Whether John K.'s act was, all things considered, right or virtuous would depend on his responsibilities to others, including his wife and child, the probable impact of his suicide on them, and the like. Sometimes in focusing too narrowly on rights, we lose sight of what is right, dignified, courageous, and honorable. Acts may be substantially autonomous but, at the same time, irresponsible or deficient in such virtues as courage. (See our discussion of virtues in Chapter 8.)

Even a morally unjustified act may be excused if the agent is not responsible for that act. For example, rather than retrospectively justifying an act of suicide, religious communities have often held that the agent was not responsible for the act of suicide. It is plausible to hold that some suicides are excusable because they are premised on false information (e.g., a misdiagnosis of a fatal disease such as AIDS), caused by uncontrollable desires, or prompted by overwhelming depression. A suicide may be seriously misguided, and even wrong, yet may not be morally blameworthy.[49] If known at the time of the act, such conditions of excusability would often justify vigorous intervention to prevent the suicide. Rarely, however, will it be appropriate to intervene beyond efforts at dissuasion in an autonomous act of suicide on the grounds that it is morally unjustified. Nevertheless, manipulative or coercive intervention would be justified in extreme cases in which the autonomous act of suicide would seriously threaten others—such as if the potential suicide alone had vital information that could prevent serious harm to others.

We conclude that paternalistic interventions in attempted suicides can be justified, at least temporarily, in order to express care, to act beneficently, and to determine whether the person is acting autonomously. Beneficence may even require interventions in suicide attempts, at least temporarily. In the case of John K., depending on the information available, the psychiatrist might have had an obligation to have John K. involuntarily hospitalized for a brief period; and the responsibility of John K.'s wife also depended on what she knew about his condition, his preferences, and so on. Because the emergency room staff presumably did not know John K., they had an obligation based on beneficence and respect for autonomy to treat him vigorously when he was brought to the hospital. If, as appears likely in this case, John K. over time could establish that his act of suicide was autonomous, then others' moral rights or obligations to intervene would diminish, although the legal right and obligation might persist for some parties. Rarely would (strong) paternalistic beneficence to the patient justify overriding an autonomous suicide.

We also conclude that there are conditions in health care (and elsewhere) under which it is appropriate to step aside and let a person commit suicide. Such nonintervention is appropriately characterized as allowed suicide rather than assisted suicide. *Assistance* usually implies aid in reaching a decision or in implementing a decision. In the case of Ida Rollin, her daughter went beyond nonintervention to secure pills and obtain a doctor's instructions about their use. Aiding and abetting suicide remains illegal throughout the United States, even though the act of suicide or attempted suicide has been decriminalized.[50] In one famous case, a woman was bedridden with advanced multiple sclerosis and asked her husband to put a cup of poison by her bed so that she could kill herself. When she took the poison and died, he was prosecuted and convicted of murder on the grounds that he had assisted a suicide.[51]

It has been argued that acts of assisted suicide may sometimes be justified and even required by the principle of beneficence, in conjunction with the principle of respect for autonomy.[52] However, when applied to social and legal rules, the principle of beneficence also justifies the legal and social prohibition of assisted suicide, primarily to prevent abuse and exploitation of victims. Our claim here draws on our earlier argument against rules to permit voluntary, active euthanasia in medicine. Assisted suicide and voluntary, active euthanasia differ only in their final agency—in the former the final agent is the one whose death is brought about; in the latter it is another party. Although beneficence, coupled with respect for autonomy, can justify some acts of assisted suicide— perhaps Betty Rollin's action on behalf of her mother—these principles, in conjunction with nonmaleficence and justice, nonetheless support a social and legal prohibition of assisted suicide. Even when there is no prosecution, as in the Rollin case, a social and legal prohibition provides a valuable warning and deterrent.

Balancing costs, risks, and benefits

Thus far we have concentrated primarily on the role of the principle of benefi-cence in clinical medicine. But many public and institutional policies turn no less on considerations of beneficence. Particularly prominent are various forms of cost- and risk-benefit analysis, which are now frequently employed to imple-ment the principle of utility. These forms of analysis are morally unobjection-able and may be morally required if they can help make reasoned assessments and judgments about trade-offs more perspicacious than they otherwise might be. That is, their value and justification are found in their capacity to imple-ment the demands of the principle of utility in our policies.

Questions commonly arise in biomedicine about the comparison and relative weights of costs—including risks—and benefits. Questions about the most suit-able medical treatment are routinely decided by reference to the probable ben-efits and harms, and questions about the justification of research involving hu-man subjects are resolved, in part, by determining whether the risks to subjects are outweighed by the probable overall benefits. For example, in submitting a research protocol involving human subjects to an institutional review board (IRB) for approval, an investigator is expected to array the risks to subjects and the benefits to both subjects and society, and then to explain why the probable benefits outweigh the risks. The IRB then offers its own assessment. If the research is approved, the investigator is expected to describe the risks and benefits to potential subjects so that they can make an informed decision about participation in the research.[53] This application of the principle of benef-icence to research can, with only slight reformulation, be extended to the treat-ment of patients and to the delivery of health services. Societal assessments of technologies, including medical technologies, provide another area of frequent application.

Various informal strategies have evolved to help make decisions about costs, risks, and benefits. These strategies include expert judgments based on the most reliable data that can be assembled and analogical reasoning based on prece-dents. The latter strategy attempts to establish new policies on the basis of policies that have already proved their worth in the past. These are important and widely used methods of analysis. When IRBs array risks and benefits, determine their respective weights, and reach decisions on this basis, they use informal techniques; they virtually never use techniques that manipulate num-bers in order to express the objective probability that an event will result in a benefit or a harm. However, our focus in this section is on techniques that employ formal, quantitative analysis of costs, risks, and benefits. These tech-niques are now widely used in health policy and raise more pointed moral issues than those raised by informal techniques.

The nature of costs, risks, and benefits

Costs are the resources required to bring about a benefit, as well as the negative effects of pursuing and realizing that benefit. These resources may be financial, or, if they involve time and energy, they may be statable in monetary terms. Both opportunity costs and risks play a prominent role in discussions of costs, particularly when they are translated into monetary terms. We will concentrate on costs expressed in monetary terms—the primary and generally the exclusive interpretation of costs in cost-benefit and cost-effectiveness analysis.

The term *risk*, by contrast, refers to a possible future harm, where *harm* is defined as a setback to interests such as those in life, health, and welfare. The probability of a harm's occurrence is only one way of expressing a risk and should be distinguished from the magnitude of the potential harm. When such expressions as *minimal risk* or *high risk* are used, they usually refer to both the chance of experiencing a harm—its probability—and the severity of the harm—its magnitude—if it occurs.

Expressions of risk are descriptive inasmuch as they are descriptions of the probability that events resulting in harm will occur. However, expressions of risk are also normative, inasmuch as a value is necessarily attached to the occurrence or prevention of the events. There is no risk unless there is a prior negative evaluation of conditions. Thus, risk is both a descriptive and an evaluative concept. At its core, a circumstance of risk is one in which there is both a possible occurrence of something that has been evaluated as harmful and an uncertainty about the occurrence that can be expressed in terms of probability of occurrence.[54]

There are many types of risk: physical, psychological, financial, legal, and so on. Case 19 illustrates the range of types of risk that correlate with human interests that may be set back. In this case, a baby girl suffers from Seckel or "bird-headed" dwarfism, a recessive genetic disease, as well as multiple other medical complications. The child is at risk of starvation if an operation is not performed, but she also is at risk of severe suffering and serious medical complications if the operation is performed. The family is at risk of psychological harm and perhaps of economic harm (because of the extremely low per capita funding for state institutions that house the retarded). Eventually, the parents decide against the surgery—a decision that in some states places them at legal risk.

The term *benefit* is sometimes used to refer to cost avoidance and risk reduction, but more commonly in biomedicine it refers to something of positive value such as life or health. Unlike *risk*, *benefit* is not a probabilistic term. Probability of benefit is the proper contrast to risk, and benefits are comparable to harms rather than to risks of harm. Thus, risk-benefit relations are best conceived in terms of a ratio between the probability and magnitude of an antici-pated benefit and the probability and magnitude of an anticipated harm.

Use of the terms *cost, risk,* and *benefit* always involves making an evalua-tion. Values are necessary to determine what will count as costs and benefits as well as how much particular costs and benefits will count—that is, how much weight they will have in our calculations.

Cost-effectiveness and cost-benefit analysis

Cost-effectiveness analysis (CEA) and benefit-cost or cost-benefit analysis (CBA) are two controversial tools of formal analysis. They have been increasingly used in decision making about societal policies regarding health and safety and about medical technologies for patient care, especially because of burgeoning demands for expensive medical care and the need to contain the costs of health care.[55] As analytic approaches, CEA, CBA, and related approaches have been praised as new tools for making or assisting in making decisions. They present trade-offs with as much rigor and objectivity as possible, using quantified terms. These techniques have also been praised as ways of reducing intuitive weighing of options and avoiding political decisions.

However, these tools have also been sharply criticized, especially as used in health care and in policy decisions about health, safety, and the environment. Critics claim that these methods are not sufficiently comprehensive to include all relevant values and options, that they are often subjective and biased, and that they are sometimes ad hoc rather than derived from a general and defen-sible theory. Critics also charge that decision-making authority is concentrated in the hands of narrow technical professionals who fail to understand moral, legal, and political constraints that legitimately limit use of these methods. We address and criticize these powerful objections below. However, the defense we offer of formal analysis should not be understood as a defense of all forms and all applications of these methods.

Both CEA and CBA aim to identify, measure, compare, and evaluate all relevant costs and consequences of policies, programs, and technologies in quantitative terms.[56] They can be distinguished by the terms in which they state the value of the consequences. In CBA both the benefits and the costs are measured in monetary terms, such as dollars, whereas in CEA the benefits are measured in nonmonetary terms, such as years of life, quality-adjusted life years, or cases of disease. CEA does not attempt to convert all benefits into a common measure for comparison with costs. Thus, CEA offers a bottom line such as ''cost per year of life saved,'' whereas CBA offers a bottom line of a benefit-cost ratio stated in monetary figures, which form the common measure-ment. Although CBA often begins by measuring different quantitative units—such as number of accidents, statistical deaths, dollars expended, and number of persons treated—it attempts in the end to convert and express these seemingly incommensurable units of measurement into a common one. This goal of an ultimate reduction gives the method its appeal, because judgments about trade-offs can be made on the basis of comparable quantities. As it is often metaphorically put, costs and benefits can be "weighed" and "balanced" and shown to be "in a favorable ratio."

Consider as an example an early study by Klarman of the benefits of eradicating syphilis in the United States.[57] Benefits in this case include reductions in the costs of medical care expenditures, economic deprivation from loss of employment, and pain and disability during and after the disease. In this study, the costs incurred in 1962 were measured at $117.5 million. The value of the disease's total eradication is equivalent to this annual sum projected in perpetuity. By employing discount rates, Klarman argued that the present capital value of this eradication is several billion dollars. Having arrived at these benefits (based on cost eradication), analysts could then figure the costs of treatment programs for purposes of comparison. Different but parallel studies could also be provided—such as cost-benefit calculations for a control program that reduced the incidence of the disease but did not attempt to eradicate it. Because of the rapid emergence of highly resistant strains of syphilis, the latter more complicated CBA would be the most useful (although Klarman unfortunately did not provide it).

Through its benefit-cost ratio, CBA can provide an evaluation of a program on its own terms and an evaluation of different programs with different aims. For example, through the common metric of money, it permits a comparison of programs that save lives with programs that reduce disability. By contrast, CEA functions best to compare and evaluate different programs with the same aim, such as saving life years. It does not permit an evaluation of the inherent worth of programs or a comparative evaluation of programs with different aims. The point of CEA is to display which among the possible alternatives either maximizes the desirable consequences, given a fixed set of resources such as money, or minimizes the costs, in order to achieve a desired consequence.

Thus, many CEAs involve comparing alternative courses of action that have similar health benefits in order to determine which is most cost-effective. A good example (see Case 35) is the Weinstein-Stason cost-effectiveness analysis of programs to control hypertension in the population. According to their CEA, the most cost-effective program is not (as many had thought) public screening to find hypertensives but rather "improving the adherence of known hypertensives."[58] Their data indicate that screening programs aimed at identifying people who are not aware that they have high blood pressure are not cost-efficient, because those not already under a physician's care either are unlikely to report to a physician for treatment when informed of their condition or, if they report, are unlikely to follow what the physician suggests.

Another good example in medical practice is the use of the guaiac test, an inexpensive test for detecting minute amounts of blood in the stool. Such blood may result from several problems, including hemorrhoids, benign intestinal polyps, or colonic cancer. The last problem is a major killer, but it may be curable if diagnosed very early. A guaiac test cannot identify the cause of the bleeding, but if there is a positive stool guaiac and no other obvious cause for the bleeding, physicians undertake other tests. The American Cancer Society in 1974 proposed that six sequential stool guaiac tests be used to screen for colorectal cancer. This proposal was based on the fact that any single stool guaiac detects only approximately ninety-two percent of the colorectal cancers. Two analysts prepared a careful CEA of the six stool guaiac tests. Assuming that the initial test costs four dollars and that each additional test costs one dollar, and noting that many fewer cases of cancer are detected with each successive test, they determined that the marginal cost per case of detected cancer increased dramatically: $1175 for one test; $5492 for two tests; $49,150 for three tests; $469,534 for four tests; $4.7 million for five tests; and $47 million for the full six-test screen.[59]

These findings do not dictate a conclusion, but the analysis is relevant for a society allocating resources, for insurance companies and hospitals setting policies, for physicians making recommendations to patients, and for patients considering diagnostic procedures. This is a CEA rather than a CBA because it does not attempt to convert the benefit of detection of colorectal cancer into a measure, such as dollars, that can then be compared with the costs. It also does not include effects such as reassurance that may be hard to measure.

There has, however, been some conceptual confusion about the nature of CEA. According to some analysts, CEA should not be confused with either a reduction of costs or an increase of effectiveness alone, because it often depends on an examination of both together. In some cases, when two programs are compared, the cost savings offered by one may be sufficient to view it as more cost-effective than the other. However, some analysts insist, a program may be more cost-effective than another even if it costs more—because it may greatly increase medical effectiveness—or even if it leads to a decrease in medical effectiveness—because it may greatly reduce the costs. For these reasons, Doubilet, Weinstein, and McNeil have argued that the term *cost-effective* should be used for cases in which "one strategy is more 'cost effective' than another if it is (a) less costly and at least as effective; (b) more effective and more costly, its additional benefit being worth its additional cost; or (c) less effective and less costly, the added benefit of the rival strategy not being worth its extra cost."[60]

Although plausible, this definition is not the only available one. A competitive definition is simpler and less sweeping: Cost-effectiveness should be restricted to cases in which one strategy is more cost-effective than another if it costs less and achieves the same goal. In this conception, CEA requires that a uniform goal has already been established by an independent assessment of the benefits of reaching that goal. We will not here choose between these two very different definitions. Our reason for comparing them is simply to note that the choice of a definition can make a major difference to one's understanding of methodology, goals, and results in using CEA.

Diagnostic or therapeutic procedures may be more or less cost-effective in comparison with others that have the same outcome. If both procedures produce an equal outcome—in, say, life years—but one is less expensive, then that procedure is more cost-effective. To say that it is cost-effective, apart from such a comparison, is to presuppose a value placed on the health outcome relative to the monetary cost. This evaluation takes a step in the direction of CBA, though perhaps without converting the benefit into a measure common to the costs, such as dollars. For instance, according to a study of leukocyte transfusion during chemotherapy for acute leukemia, prophylactic transfusion costs $2431 more than therapeutic transfusion and increase the patients' life expectancy by 0.0285 years.[61] But whether it is appropriate to say that prophylactic transfusion is more or less cost-effective than therapeutic transfusion depends on the value assigned to the additional benefit relative to the additional cost. Stated simply, is it worth $85,300 for an additional statistical year of life gained? Without answering this question one cannot determine whether prophylactic transfusion is cost-effective.

The principle of utility does not dictate a procedure simply because it has the lowest cost-effectiveness ratio (e.g., because it provides the greatest benefit for each dollar). To assign priority to the lowest cost-effectiveness ratio is to endorse a minimalist approach to medical diagnosis and therapy.[62] For example, such an approach would stop with the first stool guaiac test, because the cost-effectiveness ratio is the lowest for that first test and increases for subsequent tests. This approach to decision analysis is too narrow, because it omits from the calculation the value of the additional health benefits, including reassurance, provided by the additional tests.

Prevention of accident, disease, and illness has often been touted as the best way to contain the costs of health care. However, prevention is not always better than cure from the standpoint of CEA. For example, one study of hypertension indicated that the cost per year of life gained for hypertensives was approximately the same for prevention (screening and drug therapy) as for bypass surgery after their problem became serious.[63] Prevention may produce savings in particular treatments, but it may also add medical expenditures for other health problems.[64] Similarly, successful strategies to reduce risky lifestyles and behavioral patterns generally result in an increase rather than a decrease in social expenditures, including retirement funds.[65] Here an exclusive focus on costs may downplay the value of health itself, because preventive strategies, if effective, have the advantage of maintaining health over time, even if they have an increased net cost.

Risk assessment

Risk assessment is another important technique of analysis. We need to consider risk assessment before offering an overall evaluation of CBA, because one of the most controversial forms of CBA involves valuing lives. This form of CBA takes risk reduction as the main benefit and then proceeds to balance that benefit against the costs, asking how much it is worth to save a life.

Whereas risk analysis identifies risks, risk assessment estimates the probability of a negative event and may also evaluate the risk's acceptability and significance in itself and in relation to other objectives. Assessment of risk in relation to possible benefits is often labeled risk-benefit analysis (RBA), which may be formulated in terms of a ratio of benefits to risks. Finally, risk management is the set of responses to the analysis and assessment of risk, including decisions to reduce or control risks. For example, risk management in hospitals includes setting policies to reduce the risk of medical malpractice suits.

In this section we will focus on risk assessment, which is frequently used for technology assessment, environmental impact statements, medical care, and public policies protecting health and safety. Risk assessment may be charted in the following schema of magnitude and probability of harm:

		Magnitude of Harm	
		Major	*Minor*
Probability	*High*	1	2
of Harm	*Low*	3	4

For purposes of medical decision making and public policy, the acceptability of risks should be determined in view of the most objective estimates of probability and magnitude together with all of the relevant values, including the benefits that are sought.

As category 4 suggests, there is a question about whether some risks are so insignificant, in terms of either probability or magnitude of harm, as not to merit attention. Is there a category of *de minimus* risks which are acceptable because they can be treated as effectively zero?[66] For example, according to the Food and Drug Administration, a risk of less than one cancer per million persons exposed is *de minimus*.[67]

Risk assessment also may focus on the acceptability of risks relative to benefits that are sought. With the exception of *de minimus* risks, most risks will be considered acceptable or unacceptable according to their significance in relation to the benefits that can be derived from the actions that carry those risks—

for example, the benefits of radiation or a surgical procedure in health care or the benefits of nuclear power or toxic chemicals in the workplace.[68]

THE PROBLEM OF UNCERTAINTY. Risk should be distinguished from uncertainty, even though we speak of uncertain risks and sometimes use the two words interchangeably. Both assume a lack of predictability or knowledge of future events, but *risk* refers to the probability and magnitude of a setback to interests, whereas *uncertainty* refers to a lack of predictability or knowledge because of insufficient evidence. Risk analysis, assessment, and management are all fraught with uncertainty. For example, there may be large margins of error in quantifying risks, and it may be difficult to extrapolate information about the effects of a chemical on human beings, even though the chemical is demonstrably carcinogenic at high dose levels in rodents. A fundamental question, then, is which way to err in situations of uncertainty. Here values clearly play a role. Whether uncertainty will be resolved optimistically or pessimistically depends on the value judgments of those who perform the analysis.[69] Regulators, for example, typically assume the most conservative estimate by taking a worst-case scenario.[70]

There may be several elements of uncertainty, one of which may be the way technologies will combine and interact. Even though it may be possible to give reasonable estimates of the risks of a new technology by itself, society may be ignorant of how that technology may combine and interact with other technologies to produce unanticipatable effects.[71] For example, it may be uncertain which effects simultaneous exposure to several chemicals will have on individuals, because the interaction of the chemicals may produce synergistic rather than additive effects. Other uncertainties about technologies include how they will be used—for example, how physicians will manage them and whether patients will follow instructions. Proposals for safer sex in the AIDS crisis hinge not only on the quality of the condoms used but also on care by users. Thus, evidence based on laboratory studies on the effectiveness of condoms in preventing the transmission of HIV (human immunodeficiency virus) is insufficient as a predictive basis for the effectiveness of condoms in actual sexual intercourse.

Other uncertainties stem from the social and cultural context of technological advances. For example, Lynn White insists that technology assessment requires social analysis, because the impact of a technology is filtered through the society and its culture. His analysis directs our attention away from easily measured factors to what he calls ''imponderables.'' His case studies include alcohol, which was distilled from wine as a pharmaceutical in the twelfth century at Salerno, the site of Europe's most famous medical school. It was praised as a pharmaceutical with beneficial effects for chronic headaches, stomach trouble, cancer, arthritis, sterility, falling or graying hair, and bad breath. It was hailed as good for people with a "cold temperament." But then widespread drunkenness and disorder became problems, and we now confront alcohol-related diseases and automobile accidents. As White observes, "a study group eight centuries ago, equipped with entire foresight, would have failed at an assessment of alcohol as we today fail."[72]

To take another example, if we attempt to assess technologies for sex selection—or perhaps the use of several technologies for sex selection—we will have to consider how their impact may affect and be affected by social beliefs and institutions. Whether prospective parents, for instance, would prefer more male or female children or prefer to have a male or female first born may depend on cultural attitudes and on social policies such as whether males or females have more or equal opportunities and rewards. Some of the main risks of techniques for sex selection will be their social effects. For example, widespread sex selection could reinforce sexual stereotypes and sex discrimination, while setting back social policies of equal opportunity.

RISK PERCEPTION. An individual's perceptions of risks may differ from an expert's view. Variation may hinge not only on their goals and "risk budgets," but also on their qualitative assessment of risks, including whether the risks are voluntary, controllable, or dreaded.[73] Consider different perceptions and assessments of the risks of coronary artery bypass surgery. One to two patients die out of every one hundred undergoing the operation. An active sportsperson might view this risk of death from surgery as insignificant in view of the active life sought; another person might choose medical treatment because of a fear of dying on the operating table.[74] In addition, as we saw in Chapter 3, the patient's perception of risks and benefits may depend in part on how the physician presents them—for example, whether the presentation is in terms of probability of dying or probability of surviving.[75]

The problem of risk perception points to certain limitations in attempts to use only objective, quantitative statements of probability and magnitude in reaching conclusions about the acceptability of risk. The perceived or subjective quality of a harm may be more important than the relevant objectively quantified data. As Raanan Gillon observes, "The quantity of breast tissue to be lost in a mastectomy cannot provide an adequate measure of the harm to be anticipated from the loss of that breast or part of that breast."[76]

Individual and societal perceptions also play a large role in the assessment of new technologies. For example, a vigorous debate has accompanied the development of recombinant DNA technologies. Early fears about the escape of genetically modified organisms from laboratories have now abated, but debate continues over the genetic engineering of plants and animals, in part because of uncertainty about the risks. The most intense debate has centered on the prospect of human genetic engineering. The main considerations in the debate turn on the risks of 1 through 4 in the following representation suggested by LeRoy Walters:

	Human Genetic Engineering	
	Somatic Cell	Reproductive Cells (Germline)
Correction of Disease	1	2
Enhancement of Qualities	3	4

Despite persistent general fears, the public appears to accept the risks of 1, which involves human gene therapy aimed at somatic cells (i.e., nonreproductive cells) in order to correct serious diseases for which there is no other cure, such as adenosine deaminase (ADA) deficiency, which results in severe combined immune deficiency, and Lesch-Nyhan syndrome, which leads to mental retardation and self-mutilation in children.[77] This therapy is analogous to standard medical treatments. However, before it is attempted on human beings, it must pass the risk-benefit tests required for research involving human subjects. There is debate about the appropriateness of this requirement in the absence of other treatments for these patients, and some argue that physicians and patients or their families should be able to decide to pursue human gene therapy even in the absence of evidence of a high probability of benefit based on laboratory and animal studies.

Critics worry that it will be impossible to confine human genetic engineering to somatic cell therapy aimed at the correction of disease. They predict that once genetic engineering is accepted for human beings—and many have concerns about plants and animals as well—it will be used as soon as technically feasible for 2, 3, or 4, that is, to alter reproductive cells or to enhance such qualities as height, strength, and intelligence. The risk perception is that all controls will be lost when a threshold of minimal risk is crossed and that dangerous programs of eugenics will emerge.[78] Thus, for some critics the risks are sufficiently large that it would be better not to cross the threshold into human genetic engineering and to forgo the projected benefits of this biotechnology.

After a risk analysis and assessment, including determining a risk-benefit ratio, the results may be compared with the anticipated costs. Alternatively, when the benefit is the reduction of risks (i.e., prevention or removal of a risk of harm), then the CBA itself takes a different form, the most dramatic and debated version involving the assignment of an economic value to human life.

Valuing lives

One of the most controversial uses of CBA is to determine the value of human life. The benefit sought in this use of CBA is risk reduction, and the question is whether the benefit outweighs the costs of realizing it. Analysts try to determine the monetary value of human life in order to state the benefit (a reduction of risk) in terms that can then be balanced against the costs. Effort has been put into determining the value of life in order to develop consistency across practices and policies. As analysts note, the society may spend X to save a life (i.e., reduce the risk of death from such causes as cancer or mining accidents) in one setting but only Y to save a life in another setting. Of course, these different expenditures reflect an inconsistency of policy only if life has a certain value and death a certain disvalue across the two settings that can be quantitatively compared.[79]

METHODS FOR VALUING LIVES. Several methods have been developed to determine the value of human life.[80] According to the discounted future earnings (DFE) or human capital approach, the value of life can be determined by considering what people at risk of some disease or accident could be expected to earn if they survived. Future income is discounted, because money earned now could be invested and thus is worth more than future income. In the simplest terms, the value of a life is equivalent to the sum of money that would have to be invested at the present time in order to pay dividends equal to the sum the person would earn over the course of an expected lifetime. On these economic assumptions, those who have no income have no value, and those who drain society's resources have a negative value (e.g., thieves, the institutionalized mentally ill, and retirees all qualify).

This approach can help measure the economic costs of disease, accidents, and death, but it biases health policy in favor of such classes as young, adult white males and those who are already wealthy, because they can be expected to earn more. Thus, a public health policy to encourage motorcyclists to wear helmets might be selected over a cervical cancer program. This first approach also raises moral questions because it gauges, for policy purposes, the social value of human lives in terms of economic value—a problem we discuss as an issue of justice in Chapter 6.

A second, more defensible approach has been developed out of dissatisfaction with the DFE approach and is known as willingness to pay (WTP). This approach considers how much individuals would be willing to pay to reduce the risks of death (first by summing up the amounts reported by individuals, and then dividing by the anticipated number of deaths that could be prevented). This approach resembles and may be reducible to preference utilitarianism, as is the case with a number of forms of decision analysis that proceed by quantifying preferences on the basis of reported or observed behavior. Subjective preferences are called utilities in decision analysis, and in principle any preference can be quantified.

One version of WTP focuses on revealed preferences by analyzing preferences that are well established in society and can be revealed by empirical research. This research attempts to determine how much risk individuals now assume in order to obtain a certain benefit. Their preferences, as exhibited in their balancing of risks and benefits, become the basis for establishing the level of risk that should be permitted in that group when a new technology is introduced or a new hazard is discovered. For example, Thaler and Rosen studied the behavior of workers who make trade-offs between occupational risks and economic benefits. They determined that a job carrying approximately a two-hundred-dollar yearly increase over the workers' current salary was sufficient to induce workers to accept an increase of .001 in annual probability of death by accident. This and other figures derived from the study were then used to reach conclusions about acceptable risk, the value of a life, and what society should be willing to pay to avert a death.[81]

Although this version of WTP appears to reflect the preferences of individuals as revealed in their conduct, it is reliable only if the workers understand the risks and voluntarily assume them. That is, the conclusions are acceptable only if the conditions of informed consent are met, as established in Chapter 3. If the workers do not adequately understand and appreciate the risks—for instance, it may be more difficult for them to understand and to appreciate long-term risks to health than risks to safety—and if they have few choices—for instance, if they would find it almost impossible to relocate to find another job—then this version of WTP is unreliable. In any event, this approach takes what is desired or accepted by individuals as the measure of what is desirable or acceptable, a methodology that might be criticized as normatively flawed.

Another version of WTP focuses on expressed preferences by considering how people respond to hypothetical questions designed to determine how much they are willing to pay to reduce the risk of death. For example, Jan Acton used the following question, among others, to determine how people value life:

They are thinking about putting ambulances and other devices in communities around the country, but only if people are willing to pay enough for them. This program would be for you and 10,000 people living around you. In your area there are about 100 heart attacks per year. About 40 of these persons die. With the heart attack program, only 20 of these people would die. How much would you be willing to pay in taxes per year for the ambulance so that 20 lives could be saved in your community?[82]

Such questions are relevant in decisions about developing and funding expensive technologies. However, individuals' answers to hypothetical questions may not adequately indicate how much they would be willing to spend on an actual program in order to reduce their (and others') risk of death.

MORAL APPRAISAL OF VALUING LIVES. Several moral objections have been registered against these efforts to place a value on human life. Some of these problems, as discussed below, are versions of problems that plague CBA and

RBA generally. Deontologists tend to have more trouble with such approaches, especially those who follow Kant in arguing that persons have dignity but not a price.[83] Consequentialist theories that take a broad view of types of consequences beyond purely economic ones—for example, by considering the impact of acts and policies on practices and character—have also raised questions about putting an economic value on human life. However, these reservations need to be placed in perspective or they will seem trifling and unduly obstructive for social policy.

No ethical theory known to us requires individuals or society to do everything possible, regardless of the costs, to reduce risks to human life. From a religious or humanistic perspective, the slogan that human life has infinite value or sanctity does not imply that it is to be preserved irrespective of other values. An examination of individual risk budgets indicates that people are willing to risk life for various values, including salvation, recreation, friendship, fame, and fortune. Religious traditions recognize the possibility—and in some cases the obligation—of martyrdom in preserving faith. Many kinds of trade-offs are also involved in determining the value to be placed on human life. If economic analysis can help clarify the nature of some of the trade-offs and options, there is nothing intrinsically wrong with such analysis, and it may even be morally required.

We do not suggest that a monetary value should be put on human life. In many cases qualitative factors may be far more important than the purely economic factors at work in CBA. For example, how the death occurs, by what means, and with what symbolic features may legitimately lead society to allocate its resources differently in order to reduce various risks of death. Studies of subjective perceptions of risk, as we have seen, reflect many qualitative factors such as dread and unfamiliarity, which justifiably play a role in some determinations of acceptable risk.[84]

Society also may justifiably expend large amounts of time, energy, and money to rescue individuals from peril. Such unstinting acts of beneficence as rescuing trapped coal miners symbolize society's benevolence and reassert the value of the victims to society. These social goods and acts of rescue focus on identified lives in peril, whereas preventive measures to reduce the risk of death focus on statistical lives, on unnameable persons in positive future danger.[85] We may not know in the latter cases which persons will be saved from actual harm, including death, by preventive measures, but we know that some will be saved statistically by reducing their risk of death. Concentrating resources on identified individuals in peril may turn out to be less efficient than a preventive strategy designed to maximize the number of lives, or life years, or quality-adjusted life years saved, but the preference is not thereby irrational. Policies may be rational not because they achieve desired goals efficiently but because they express or symbolize significant values.

It has been argued that the symbolic value of rescuing identified individuals in part accounts for the 1972 U.S. congressional decision—following widespread publicity in the media about particular individuals who were dying of renal failure—to make funds available for almost all citizens who need renal dialysis or renal transplantation.[86] This decision also reflected the value of equality, because hospital committees had to decide which identified individuals would live and which would die. The end-stage renal disease program now costs approximately three billion dollars a year, and serious questions have been raised about its justifiability from the standpoint of CBA.[87] However, it is not unreasonable to violate efficiency criteria derived from CBA in order to protect and symbolize commitment to a precious social value.

Consequences of the use of CBA should also be considered. For example, putting a price on a nonmarket entity such as human life can reduce its perceived value, and society may choose to value human life more highly in public, collective decisions than some individuals would in their private decisions. It is not, then, legitimate to infer from individuals' conduct or from their answers to hypothetical questions how much human life should be valued in society's policies.[88] Data gathered by these techniques are relevant to the formation of public policies, but the data provide only one set of premises among others in a complex argument.

We are convinced that techniques of CBA present a rational and defensible approach to public policy that is grounded in the principle of beneficence. But we are no less convinced that these techniques cannot be turned into a narrow prescriptive formula to direct decision making without considering a wide variety of qualitative factors. It also may not be necessary to put a value on human life in order to evaluate possible risk-reduction policies and to compare their costs. Evaluation may reasonably focus on the life years or quality-adjusted life years saved without conversion into monetary measures.

The decision-making process: who decides?

Whether the focus is on decisions in medical practice or on public policies, there are important questions about who rightly decides. This issue is not identical with, but often overlaps with, questions of which and whose values should be considered in the calculus of CBA and RBA. These issues are not identical, because a decision maker may make decisions in terms of others' values. However, the best guarantee that a set of values will be represented is to incorporate its proponents into the decision-making process itself. Thus, in technology assessment and public policy, a major problem is how to ensure democratic representation.[89] The main tension is between those who emphasize decision making by experts engaged in objective analyses and those who put a premium on public participation. We believe that the expert has an important role to play, particularly in arraying the costs, risks, and benefits involved, but that there are legitimate reservations about allowing the expert to make the final decision.

Many proponents of CEA, CBA, and RBA who rely on expert judgment deny that they are nondemocratic or antidemocratic. The argument is that experts respect consumer sovereignty and derive values from expressed, revealed, or implied preferences of consumers; costs, risks, and benefits are then assessed in relation to those values. However, experts often find the public's perception to be less reliable in political processes, which can be unpredictable and erratic, careening wildly in response to "popular perceptions and whims of the moment." The defenders of CBA contend that their methods make it possible for the government to regulate risks "by finding, developing, and legitimating methods for making centralized decisions."[90] Although there is much to commend the corrective powers of CBA, it would be odd to respect individuals' values as expressed economically but not as expressed politically. Appropriate mechanisms for public participation in decisions that incorporate CEA, CBA, and RBA are at least as socially valuable as the methods themselves.

Many proponents of formal methods of analysis rightly distinguish between these methods and their use in decision making. Some also recognize that "for many societal decisions that affect life-threatening activities, the procedure by which the decision is made may be as important as the actual dollar numbers employed to value the lives involved."[91] Processes of public participation in such matters as technology assessment are essential to embody the rights of citizens and affected parties to treatment as equals. The principle of justice often supports specific procedures used for public participation—such as adversary hearings and testimonies at public forums. A fair and acceptable process of decision making is defensible because of the principles it embodies as well as the hope that it will produce a good decision or outcome. At the same time, it is important for society to address the implications of CEA, CBA, and RBA through its democratic processes.

In confronting the question whether formal techniques should be viewed as methods of decision making or as mere aids for decision makers, we believe no unqualified answer can be given. But it would be a serious error in many contexts to view these methods of analysis as more than aids, especially if moral principles lead us to different conclusions. Formal methods of analysis are fashioned for specific goals and should be evaluated strictly in light of their service to those goals. However, those goals are not our only goals.

Cost-effectiveness analysis—which we have seen to be among the most widely practiced methods—is often imperiled by the narrowness of its goals and focus, because it does not require a broad comparison in terms of costs and benefits. Often one assumes a fixed budgetary amount in order to apply this method— for instance, a fixed amount of money to treat a population of hypertensives. The method does not promote questions such as whether the amount budgeted is inadequate to solve the real problems, whether the allocated resources might be more profitably rebudgeted in alternative ways, whether cost-effectiveness may cause rather than alleviate injustices, or whether costs saved in the sphere under examination might not produce even greater costs elsewhere. For these reasons it is especially hazardous to permit CEA to operate without broader external constraints on its use. We shall now look more closely at one particular constraint on all of these analytical approaches—CBA and RBA, as well as CEA.

Constraints of distributive justice

Even though we discuss the principle of justice more fully in the next chapter, the above argument leads to a consideration of some special problems at this juncture. Utilitarianism and analytic techniques are commonly said to fail to take account of problems of justice because they focus on the net balance of benefits over costs, without considering the distribution of those benefits and costs. (Such criticisms do not work well against certain rule-utilitarian theories, but act utilitarianism does seem open to these objections.) For example, in Case 35, as discussed earlier, Weinstein and Stason argue that the most cost-effective approach for control of hypertension is to concentrate resources on known hypertensives, yet they recognize that this approach might be criticized on grounds of injustice. Many poor people and blacks (who have a higher rate of hypertension than whites) would not learn of their hypertension because they would not already be in the health-care system. Similarly, a study of the costs and benefits of treating mental retardation in small institutions emphasizing advanced individual training might show that the costs outweigh the benefits, while justice might demand that special benefits be extended to mentally retarded persons. In both examples, justice may require a different distribution of resources than CBA or CEA would support.

RBA is no less subject to constraints of justice. Consider four possible patterns of distribution of risks and benefits. (1) The risks and benefits may fall on the same party. For example, in most therapy, the patient bears the major risks and stands to gain the major benefits. (2) One party may bear the risks, while another party gains the benefits. For example, in nontherapeutic research, the subject bears the risks, while others in the future will gain the benefits. Or one generation may gain the benefits of technologies that will adversely affect future generations—for instance, if nuclear power produces nuclear waste stored in hazardous sites. (3) Both parties may bear the risks, while only one party stands to benefit. For example, a nuclear-powered artificial heart would primarily benefit the user, but its risks would also be imposed on other parties in contact with the user. (4) Both parties may gain the benefits, while only one party bears the risks. For example, persons in the vicinity of a nuclear power plant may bear significantly greater risks than other persons who also benefit from the plant.

We conclude that for RBA, as well as for CEA and CBA, it is not sufficient merely to consider the aggregation of benefits and costs or risks without simultaneously considering patterns of distribution. We do not argue, however, that principles of justice must always triumph over economic efficiency. Here our views stand in contrast to those of some theorists who assign principles of justice absolute priority over consequentialist principles. For us these principles are all prima facie binding, and a practical judgment is required, subject to the conditions of the framework of moral reasoning developed throughout this book.

As an example of the balancing required in order to apply principles of beneficence and distributive justice in programs of risk reduction, consider the use of genetic screening and monitoring in the workplace. Workers may be screened for a genetic predisposition toward diseases that may be more likely to occur as a result of exposures to chemicals in a plant. There is nothing inherently objectionable about genetic screening and monitoring to determine workers' susceptibility to diseases. These tests may be based on beneficence toward workers as well as on reduction of costs to the company and the society. But the company may be able to reduce risks in several different ways, some of which are morally preferable to others. The options may be (1) barring workers from certain jobs by not hiring them or by assigning them to other jobs, (2) devising protective equipment for the workers, or (3) altering the work environment.[92] In some cases the latter two may be deemed too costly for the benefits to be derived in the reduction of risks, but the first raises questions about how to balance fair access to jobs against the reduction of risks. If a worker's condition interferes with job performance or endangers others, there is no serious ethical problem in the first policy. But if health risks are limited to the worker, the ethical problems are more serious. Here it is morally reasonable (although, we acknowledge, not always feasible) to require the company to consider reducing the risk for all workers (perhaps by options 2 and 3) rather than denying employment to those whose risks may be increased by their genetic predisposition.

Related questions of beneficence and justice have also arisen in the debate about reproductive risk in the workplace. There is a complex set of obligations of nonmaleficence and beneficence in the workplace, including the society's and the employers' obligations to workers and to workers' offspring, as well as the workers' obligations to their offspring.[93] Workers may believe that the health hazards to a fetus or future offspring are outweighed by benefits they can provide for their offspring through their income, such as housing, food, and health care. Faced with the options identified above for reducing risk exposure in the workplace, some employers have excluded women of childbearing age from certain jobs or, in some cases, have made "voluntary" sterilization a condition of employment. Questions have naturally been raised about the fairness of policies of prohibition of employment, elective sterilization, and selective exclusion of women if occupational exposure has a toxic effect on the reproductive cells of both sexes.

Similar questions emerge about hiring practices toward people with the sickle-cell trait, which affects approximately seven to thirteen percent of the black population but rarely appears in the rest of the population. Those with the sickle-cell trait do not have sickle-cell disease, but they are sometimes barred from some occupations because of the possibility that they are at greater risk from exposure to substances that might compromise the oxygen-carrying capacity of blood. Nevertheless, before anyone is denied work because of an association with a so-called high-risk group, scientific evidence should demonstrate that the person is hypersusceptible to hazards and that there is no reasonable way to protect against the hazards.[94]

It is sometimes held that monetary compensation, whether prospective or retrospective, satisfies the principles of justice when benefits and risks are unequally distributed. One argument is that fair compensation for employment—or even additional compensation for risky jobs—makes the imposition of risks on workers fair. This argument requires the premise that these workers have voluntarily assumed the risks of their jobs. However, before this argument can be taken seriously, it must be shown that the conditions for autonomous choice are met, including both adequate understanding and substantial voluntariness. There is less understanding of health hazards than safety hazards, in part because health problems such as cancer often develop over time and may result from several factors. It may also be difficult to disclose what is known in a way that facilitates an informed choice, and the worker's voluntariness may be compromised by the lack of available alternatives. Thus, in the employment situation voluntary acceptance of a job and hazard pay may be unjust substitutes for what should be done, namely correcting dangerous working conditions.[95]

A second argument is that retrospective monetary compensation—for example, through tort claims—is a valid substitute for prevention of exposure to hazards. The proposal is that an adequate system of compensation for injury satisfies the conditions of fairness. We would argue, however, that even if a CBA would favor the compensation scheme, fairness requires both employers and society to undertake to reduce the hazards to the lowest level that is feasible or practicable, because compensation cannot restore victims to the health they enjoyed prior to their exposure.[96] This is another example of how the principle of justice constrains CBA, although we again acknowledge the prima facie character of this constraint when justice conflicts with utility.

More subtle but equally important questions of justice arise in discounting some people's interests by the methods used to assign positive or negative values to consequences. Proponents of analytic techniques usually agree with Jeremy Bentham that each person is to count as one and only one in the calculus, but the technique of discounted future earnings considers social value measured in economic terms, and the technique of willingness to pay tends to reflect a person's economic status. Such approaches are problematic if used to determine how resources should be allocated among programs that will have a differential impact on groups. For example, when society is considering whether to adopt a program by using criteria of extended life years or quality-adjusted life years, there is a danger that the elderly will be unfairly treated because the life years gained will be fewer and their quality will often be lower. In a sharp critique of CBA and CEA in health-care allocation, Jerry Avorn notes that "as usually applied, these methods embody a set of hidden value assumptions that virtually guarantee an anti-geriatric bias to their purportedly objective data."[97] (We will consider the possible relevance of age in the distribution of health care when we examine the principle of justice in Chapter 6.)

Our point in this section has been that analytic methods must be carefully scrutinized to avoid settling questions of justice on the basis of value assumptions that are unfair to such groups as workers, women, minorities, or different age cohorts. Even when the methods are free of such biases, assessing the weight of beneficence as expressed in these analytic techniques against the claims of justice is essential.

Other problems

These techniques also may attach exaggerated importance to quantifiable values while ignoring values that are not easily quantifiable, such as relief of pain and suffering or the symbolic significance of actions and policies. For instance, a hospice program caring for dying patients may be defensible because of its intangible benefits, including dying with dignity and without pain and suffering, but a formal CEA/CBA based solely on economic considerations may dismiss these considerations.[98]

A related concern is the impact of analytic techniques, especially CBA, on personal and social values, perspectives, and attitudes. Stuart Hampshire maintains that many believe "large-scale computations in modern politics and social planning bring with them a coarseness and grossness of moral feeling, a blunting of sensibility, and a suppression of individual discrimination and gentleness, which is a price that they will not pay for the benefits of clear calculation."[99] Some critics worry that these analytic tools may even come to dominate their users. They fear that economic language, already evident in the discussion of "the health care industry," "providers," and "consumers," as well as CEA and CBA, will corrupt or even replace the traditional language of the doctor-patient relationship, including humanity and decency, especially under pressures of cost containment.[100] It is important, then, to pay attention to the social (as well as economic) costs of such approaches, including their possible negative effects on important attitudes, outlooks, and social practices. At the same time, we believe these possible negative effects can be avoided if the analytic techniques are limited in the ways we have proposed.

We conclude that these analytic techniques are not ethically neutral and may suffer from defective uses of an unconstrained principle of utility.[101] Beyond the moral problems we have noted, there are also obvious practical difficulties in predicting consequences and in assigning probabilities to both harms and benefits. In addition, there are problems in computing discount rates, psychological and social effects, and indirect effects of certain personal and social interventions. These problems, while important, are not fatal to analytic techniques; they do, however, suggest caution in the use of those techniques. These techniques are nevertheless acceptable and often useful, as long as their limitations and limits are recognized, especially the limits set by other principles such as respect for autonomy and justice.

Conclusion

We have fought several battles in this chapter. In the middle sections we defended a version of paternalism that permits some strong paternalistic interventions—despite our acknowledgment that strong paternalism is a moral quicksand with constant dangers of engulfing us. Parallel to the position about mercy killing that we defended in Chapter 4, we might say that strong paternalism can be justified in particular cases, but a policy or rule permitting strong paternalism in professional practice is not worth the risk of abuse the policy or rule invites. We also argued that the distinction between antipaternalism and weak paternalism is less significant than has generally been thought and may be a distinction that makes no moral difference. These conclusions are significant inasmuch as the consensus view in the literature on biomedical ethics seems to be either that paternalism is unjustified or that weak paternalism alone is justified.

We have also maintained that paternalistic interventions are seldom justified, because the right to act autonomously almost always outweighs obligations of beneficence toward the autonomous agent. Justified paternalistic interventions involve a balancing of the demands of both beneficence and respect for autonomy, and the balance seldom allows beneficence to override respect for autonomy. But when the balance does fall on the side of beneficence, the justification of paternalism does not rest on the consent of the person—either actual or hypothetical consent. It rests on the importance of the benefits conferred or the harms avoided, and it must also satisfy the other conditions for justified infringements of prima facie principles.

It is vital in the moral life to protect areas of autonomous action from intrusion. The alternative—to recognize no zones protected by autonomy rights—is morally perilous. Within the protected areas infringements of autonomy are virtually always wrong. These areas are, however, only heavily protected zones. They are not impenetrable shields if they conflict with other areas that are also protected. No protected area has an ironclad moral security.

Second, in the final section we argued that formal techniques of analysis— CEA, CBA, and RBA—can be morally unobjectionable and can even be morally demanded by the version of the principle of utility developed in the first section. Many critics correctly argue that these forms of analysis can be morally objectionable in the way they are applied, especially if they conceal underlying moral premises that bias the results achieved by use of the methods. Our claim has been that these criticisms present serious but surmountable problems.

Many of the attacks on these analytic techniques have been directed at the utilitarian perspective they encourage. However, any adequate moral theory, deontological or otherwise, must have a large place for consequentialist and utilitarian considerations, that is, for prediction and assessment of the consequences of actions and determination of effective and efficient means to maximize desired outcomes. Insofar as a moral theory recognizes a principle of beneficence, it must recognize, we have argued, a balancing principle to deal with the relation of means, ends, and consequences and particularly to balance costs, risks, and benefits. This recognition of the importance of consequences does not entail a commitment to utilitarianism as an ethical theory. We have emphasized the importance of other moral principles, particularly respect for autonomy and justice, which are prima facie binding in the same way the principle of utility is. Both respect for autonomy and justice set limits on the use of the analytic techniques we have examined. As we argued in Chapter 2, all four principles can in theory be derived from the utilitarians' principle of utility as well as from deontological sources, but in our framework no principle is more than a prima facie principle.

Third, we have argued against moral philosophers who contend that the only general moral obligations are negative and who maintain that morality is confined to our obligations not to disrespect persons, not to deprive them of goods to which they are entitled, and not to inflict harm on them. From their perspective, respect for autonomy and nonmaleficence are genuine moral principles, but beneficence is a fabrication. Some recent writers in bioethics have even argued that respect for autonomy is the only foundational moral principle in bioethics.

We have countered these claims by arguing that there are positive obligations to provide goods and services. We believe that no defensible ethical theory would, in all circumstances of conflict, place respect for autonomy absolutely above beneficent promotion of human welfare. We have also raised conceptual and normative questions about whether it is advisable to draw a sharp distinction in ethical theory between nonmaleficence and beneficence. Because omissions to act can inflict harms on others and because failures to assist can be as morally blameworthy as inflicting harms, it is doubtful that a morality erected on negative obligations alone could be satisfactory. However, there are complexities in this controversy that we have not considered, and we cannot claim to have resolved the larger problem of the status of positive and negative obligations.

We do hope, however, to have shown that there are some positive obligations in biomedical ethics. In Chapter 6 we will build on this foundation by arguing that there are general social obligations of distributive justice strong enough to support a right to health care.

Notes

1. See Douglas MacLean, "Risk and Consent: Philosophical Issues for Centralized Decisions," in *Values at Risk,* ed. D. MacLean (Totowa, N.J.: Rowman and Allanheld, 1986), pp. 17–30. MacLean argues that the justification of formal methods of risk analysis should rest on consent rather than social efficiency or individual rights.
2. American Nurses' Association, *Code for Nurses with Interpretive Statements* (Kansas City, Mo.: American Nurses' Association, 1985), sec. 3.1, p. 6.
3. William Frankena, *Ethics,* 2d ed. (Englewood Cliffs, N.J.: Prentice-Hall, 1973), p. 47. Frankena includes moral ideals under the umbrella of "the ingredients of morality" (pp. 67f).
4. See Joel Feinberg, "The Nature and Value of Rights," *Journal of Value Inquiry* 4 (1970): 243–57, esp. 244ff.
5. Frankena does say later (*Ethics,* p. 47) that principles of beneficence specify "prima facie duties," but it remains unclear whether this means that they are moral requirements (as Ross's theory of prima facie duties entails that they are), because Frankena allows for an extremely lengthy list of possible prima facie duties (pp. 48, 56). See also Frankena's subsequent essay, "Moral Philosophy and World Hunger," in *World Hunger and Moral Obligation,* ed. W. Aiken and H. LaFollette (Englewood Cliffs, N.J.: Prentice-Hall, 1977), pp. 66–84, esp. pp. 70, 73.
6. Marcus G. Singer, *Generalization in Ethics* (New York: Alfred A. Knopf, 1961), pp. 180–89.
7. Peter Singer, *Practical Ethics* (Cambridge: Cambridge University Press, 1979), pp. 168ff.
8. Peter Singer, "Famine, Affluence, and Morality," *Philosophy and Public Affairs* 1 (1972). This article is updated in "Reconsidering the Famine Relief Argument," in *Food Policy: The Responsibility of the United States in the Life and Death Choices,* ed. Peter Brown and Henry Shue (New York: Free Press, 1977); and in *Practical Ethics.*
9. Michael A. Slote, "The Morality of Wealth," in *World Hunger and Moral Obligation,* ed. Aiken and LaFollette, pp. 125–27.
10. Singer, *Practical Ethics,* p. 181.

11. James Fishkin, *The Limits of Obligation* (New Haven: Yale University Press, 1982), pp. 4–9 for a summary of the full argument.

12. Our formulation of these conditions is indebted to Eric D'Arcy, *Human Acts: An Essay in their Moral Evaluation* (Oxford: Clarendon Press, 1963), pp. 56–57. We have added the fourth condition. Richard Brandt and Rick McCarty have offered provocative criticisms of our statement of the obligation to rescue, and we have not done justice to their criticisms. For recent major defenses of the obligation to rescue, see Alan Gewirth, *Reason and Morality* (Chicago: University of Chicago Press, 1978), pp. 217–30; Ernest J. Weinrib, "The Case for a Duty to Rescue," *Yale Law Journal* 90 (December 1980): 247–93; and Joel Feinberg, *Harm to Others* (New York: Oxford University Press, 1984), chap. 4. The last two focus on the justification of a legal obligation to rescue.

13. David Hume, "On Suicide," as reprinted in Samuel Gorovitz et al., *Moral Problems in Medicine* (Englewood Cliffs, N.J.: Prentice-Hall, 1976), p. 386.

14. William F. May, "Code and Covenant or Philanthropy and Contract?" in *Ethics in Medicine*, ed. Stanley Joel Reiser, Arthur J. Dyck, and William J. Curran (Cambridge, Mass.: MIT Press, 1977), pp. 65–76, has greatly influenced this paragraph. See also William F. May, *The Physician's Covenant: Images of the Healer in Medical Ethics* (Philadelphia: Westminster Press, 1983).

15. John Reeder even claims that "the beneficence which is proper to the therapeutic role is a duty of justice." "Beneficence, Supererogation, and Role Duty," in *Beneficence and Health Care*, ed. Earl E. Shelp (Dordrecht: D. Reidel, 1982), p. 101.

16. American Medical Association, "Principles of Medical Ethics," in *Current Opinions of the Council on Ethical and Judicial Affairs* (Chicago: American Medical Association, 1986).

17. Judith Jarvis Thomson, "A Defense of Abortion," *Philosophy and Public Affairs* 1 (1971): 47–66. Slote acknowledges an indebtedness to this essay for part of his analysis of the obligation of beneficence.

18. See Gallup Survey, "The U.S. Public's Attitudes toward Organ Transplants/Organ Donation" (Princeton, N.J.: Gallup Organization, January 1985).

19. For a fuller discussion of issues in organ procurement and donation, see James F. Childress, "Some Moral Connections between Organ Procurement and Organ Distribution," *Journal of Contemporary Health Law and Policy* 3 (1987): 85–110; Hastings Center, *Ethical, Legal and Policy Issues Pertaining to Sold Organ Procurement* (Hastings-on-Hudson, N.Y.: Hastings Center, 1985); and Task Force on Organ Transplantation, *Organ Transplantation: Issue and Recommendations*, April 1986, U.S. Department of Health and Human Services. A market in organs has been proposed, but federal law prohibits it, as do several state laws. The major arguments against a market in organs focus on potential exploitation and abuse and, even if those problems could be avoided, on the larger harm that the society and individuals within it would experience over time through viewing the body and its parts as commercial property. In addition, a market might not increase supply, for it might drive out donations based on beneficence to needy patients.

20. *Epidemics*, 1:11, from W. H. S. Jones, ed., *Hippocrates* (Cambridge, Mass.: Harvard University Press, 1923), Vol. I, p. 165.

21. President's Commission for the Study of Ethical Problems in Medicine and Biomedical and Behavioral Research, *Deciding to Forego Life-Sustaining Treatment* (Washington, D.C.: U.S. Government Printing Office, 1983), pp. 26–27, 44.

22. Edmund Pellegrino and David Thomasma, *For the Patient's Good: The Restoration of Beneficence in Health Care* (New York: Oxford University Press, 1988), p. 29.

23. Ibid., pp. 32, 25, 46.

24. Ibid., p. 47.

25. The term *paternalism* is not wholly felicitous, especially because it is sex-linked. Although it might seem desirable to use another term, such as *parentalism*, the term *paternalism* is established by usage and philosophical discussion, and it reflects the role of the father in the family in the nineteenth century. For recent literature on paternalism, see James F. Childress, *Who Should Decide? Paternalism in Health Care* (New York: Oxford University Press, 1982); Rolf Sartorius, ed., *Paternalism* (Minneapolis: University of Minnesota Press, 1983); John Kleinig, *Paternalism* (Totowa, N.J.: Rowman and Allanheld, 1984); Donald Van DeVeer, *Paternalistic Interventions: The Moral Bounds on Benevolence* (Princeton: Princeton University Press, 1986). Kleinig's book contains an outstanding bibliography.

26. Immanuel Kant, *On the Old Saw: That May Be Right in Theory but It Won't Work in Practice*, trans. E. B. Ashton (Philadelphia: University of Pennsylvania Press, 1974), pp. 290–91; John Stuart Mill, *On Liberty*, available in several editions.

27. L. J. Henderson, "Physician and Patient as a Social System," *New England Journal of Medicine* 212 (1935): 819–23. See the similar arguments in Charles C. Lund, "The Doctor, the Patient, and the Truth," *Annals of Internal Medicine* 24 (1946): 959; and Steven R. Kaplan et al., "Neglected Aspects of Informed Consent," *New England Journal of Medicine* 303 (1980): 1127.

28. Robert W. Allen, "Informed Consent: A Medical Decision," *Radiology* 119 (April 1976): 233–34.

29. See Tom L. Beauchamp and Laurence B. McCullough, *Medical Ethics: The Moral Responsibilities of Physicians* (Englewood Cliffs, N.J.: Prentice-Hall, 1984), p. 84.

30. National Commission for the Protection of Human Subjects of Biomedical and Behavioral Research, *Report and Recommendations: Research on Prisoners* (Washington, D.C.: DHEW Publication No. OS 76-131, 1976). See also DHEW, Office of the Secretary, "Additional Protections Pertaining to Biomedical and Behavioral Research Involving Prisoners as Subjects," *Federal Register* 43, Part IV: HEW 53652–56, November 16, 1978; and DHHS, Food and Drug Administration, "Protection of Human Subjects; Prisoners Used as Subjects in Research," *Federal Register* 45:36386–91, May 30, 1980.

31. See especially Gerald Dworkin, "Paternalism," *The Monist* (January 1972): 64–84; and John Rawls, *A Theory of Justice*, (Cambridge, Mass.: Harvard University Press, 1971), pp. 248–49. See also Charles Culver and Bernard Gert, *Philosophy in Medicine* (New York: Oxford University Press, 1982), chaps. 7–9; Jeffrie Murphy, "Incompetence and Paternalism," *Archiv für Rechts-und-Sozialphilosophie* 60 (1974): 466, 485; and Childress, *Who Should Decide?*

32. See Rawls, *A Theory of Justice;* and Dworkin, "Paternalism."

33. Dworkin, "Paternalism"; and Rosemary Carter, "Justifying Paternalism," *Canadian Journal of Philosophy* 7 (1977): 133–45, esp. 135. For criticisms, see Childress, *Who Should Decide?*

34. Robert Harris, "Private Consensual Adult Behavior: The Requirement of Harm to Others in the Enforcement of Morality," *UCLA Law Review* 14 (1967): 585n. Similar complaints, situated in the context of political philosophy, are found in Isaiah Berlin, *Four Essays on Liberty* (Oxford: Oxford University Press, 1969), pp. lxi–lxii, 132–33, 137–38, 149–51, 157.

35. Jay Katz, Joseph Goldstein, and Alan M. Dershowitz, eds., *Psychoanalysis, Psychiatry, and the Law* (New York: Free Press, 1967), pp. 552–54, 710–13; and Robert A. Burt, *Taking Care of Strangers* (New York: Free Press, 1979), chap. 2.

36. Joel Feinberg, "Legal Paternalism," *Canadian Journal of Philosophy* 1 (1971): 105–24, esp. 113, 116. See also Joel Feinberg, *Social Philosophy* (Englewood Cliffs, N.J.: Prentice-Hall, 1973), p. 33; and Joel Feinberg, *Harm to Self*, Vol. III of *The Moral Limits of Criminal Law* (New York: Oxford University Press, 1986).

37. This thesis is argued in Tom L. Beauchamp, "Paternalism and Biobehavioral Control," *The Monist* 60 (January 1977): 62–80; and in Childress, *Who Should Decide?*

38. Mary C. Silva, *Ethical Decisionmaking in Nursing Administration* (Norwalk, Conn.: Appleton and Lange, 1989), chap. 3.

39. We do not here address the major conceptual problems surrounding suicide. See, for example, Tom L. Beauchamp, "Suicide," in *Matters of Life and Death*, ed. Tom Regan (New York: Random House, 1980), pp. 67–108, esp. part I.

40. See James Rachels, "Barney Clark's Key," *Hastings Center Report* 13 (April 1983): 17–19.

41. Glanville Williams, "Euthanasia," *Medico-Legal Journal* 41 (1973): 27.

42. A useful discussion of "Criteria for Rational Suicide" is found in Margaret Pabst Battin, *Ethical Issues in Suicide* (Englewood Cliffs, N.J.: Prentice-Hall, 1982), pp. 132–53. A reply to our view about rational, autonomous suicide is found in Stanley Hauerwas, "Rational Suicide and Reasons for Living," in *Rights and Responsibilities in Modern Medicine: The Second Volume in a Series on Ethics, Humanism, and Medicine*, ed. Marc D. Basson (New York: Alan R. Liss, 1981), pp. 185–99.

43. See Peter M. Marzuk et al., "Increased Risk of Suicide in Persons with AIDS," *Journal of the American Medical Association* 25 (1988): 1333–37.

44. See Richard M. Glass, "AIDS and Suicide," *Journal of the American Medical Association* 259 (1988): 1369–70.

45. See President's Commission, *Deciding to Forego Life-Sustaining Treatment*, 37.

46. See *Addington* v. *Texas*, 441 U.S. 418 (1979).

47. Psychiatrist Jerome A. Motto writes: "I make the assumption that if a person has no ambivalence about suicide he will not be in my office, nor write to me about it, nor call me on the telephone. I interpret, rightly or wrongly, a person's calling my attention to his suicidal impulse as a request to intercede that I cannot ignore." Jerome A. Motto, "The Right to Suicide," in *Suicide: The Philosophical Issues*, ed. M. P. Battin and D. J. Mayo (New York: St. Martin's Press, 1980), p. 217.

48. Betty Rollin, *Last Wish* (New York: Linden/Simon and Schuster, 1985).

49. See Richard B. Brandt, "The Morality and Rationality of Suicide," in *A Handbook for the Study of Suicide*, ed. Seymour Perlin (New York: Oxford University Press, 1975), p. 124.

50. See L. P. Francis, "Assisting Suicide," in *Suicide: The Philosophical Issues*, ed. Battin and Mayo.

51. *People* v. *Roberts*, 211 Mich. 187, 178 N.W. 690 (1920).

52. Brandt, "The Morality and Rationality of Suicide."

53. The functions and moral obligations of such committees are analyzed in a report on the subject of the National Commission for the Protection of Human Subjects, *Report and Recommendations: Institutional Review Boards*, including a separate appendix (Washington, D.C.: DHEW Publication Nos. OS 78-0008 and OS 78-0009, 1978). This study includes considerations of cost-benefit analysis.

54. See the modestly different analysis in William D. Rowe, *An Anatomy of Risk* (New York: John Wiley, 1977), pp. 18–24.

55. A comprehensive source for economists' accounts of cost-benefit analysis is E. J. Mishan, *Cost-Benefit Analysis,* expanded ed. (New York: Praeger, 1976). For a critique, see Steven E. Rhoads, *The Economist's View of the World: Government, Markets, and Public Policy* (Cambridge: Cambridge University Press, 1985).

56. U.S. Congress, Office of Technology Assessment, *The Implications of Cost-Effectiveness Analysis of Medical Technology: Background Paper #1: Methodological Issues and Literature Review* (Washington, D.C.: U.S. Government Printing Office, 1980), p. 4. We have drawn on this document in this paragraph. See also Kenneth E. Warner and Bryan R. Luce, *Cost-Benefit and Cost-Effectiveness Analysis in Health Care* (Ann Arbor, Mich.: Health Administration Press, 1982).

57. H. E. Klarman, "Syphilis Control Problems," in *Measuring Benefits of Government Investments,* ed. R. Dorfman (Washington, D.C.: Brookings Institution, 1965).

58. See Milton Weinstein and William B. Stason, "Allocating Resources: The Case of Hypertension," *Hastings Center Report* 7 (October 1977): 24–29. See also their other works, including *Hypertension* (Cambridge, Mass.: Harvard University Press, 1976); "Foundations of Cost-Effectiveness Analysis for Health and Medical Practices," *New England Journal of Medicine* 296 (1977): 716–21; and "Cost-Effectiveness of Interventions to Prevent or Treat Coronary Heart Disease," *American Review of Public Health* 6 (1985): 41–63.

59. Duncan Neuhauser and Ann M. Lewicki, "What Do We Gain From the Sixth Stool Guaiac?" *New England Journal of Medicine* 293 (1975): 226–28. See also "American Cancer Society Report on the Cancer-related Checkup," *CA—A Cancer Journal for Clinicians* 30 (1980): 193–240, which recommends six stool guaiac tests. For a discussion of some of the issues, see Norman Daniels, "Cost-Effectiveness and Patient Welfare," in *Rights and Responsibilities in Modern Medicine,* ed. Basson, pp. 159–70.

60. Peter Doubilet, Milton C. Weinstein, and Barbara J. McNeil, "Use and Misuse of the Term 'Cost Effective' in Medicine," *New England Journal of Medicine* 314 (1986): 253–56, which has influenced this paragraph and the next two paragraphs.

61. M. S. Rosenshein, V. T. Farewell, T. H. Price, et al., "The Cost Effectiveness of Therapeutic and Prophylactic Leukocyte Transfusion," *New England Journal of Medicine* 392 (1980): 1058–62.

62. Doubilet, Weinstein, and McNeil, "Use and Misuse of the Term 'Cost Effective,' " p. 255.

63. Milton G. Weinstein, "Economic Impact and Cost-Effectiveness of Medical Technology," paper presented at the 1981 Frank M. Norfleet Forum for the Advancement of Health, University of Tennessee Center for the Health Sciences, Memphis; summarized in Louise Russell, *Is Prevention Better Than Cure?* (Washington, D.C.: Brookings Institution, 1986), p. 111.

64. Russell, *Is Prevention Better Than Cure?*

65. See Howard Leichter, "Public Policy and the British Experience," *Hastings Center Report* 11 (October 1981): 32–39.

66. The term *de minimus* has been drawn from the common law tradition, where it appears in the maxim, *De minimus non curat lex* ("The law does not concern itself with trifles"). For an early use in risk analysis, see C. Comer, "Risk: A Pragmatic *De Minimus* Approach," *Science* 203 (1979). See also Chris G. Whipple, "Dealing with Uncertainty about Risk in Risk Management," in National Academy of En-

gineering, *Hazards: Technology and Fairness* (Washington, D.C.: National Academy Press, 1986), pp. 45–59.

67. Nicholas Rescher, *Risk* (Washington, D.C.: University Press of America, 1983), p. 37.

68. See Richard Wilson and E. A. C. Crouch, "Risk Assessment and Comparisons: An Introduction," *Science* 236 (1987): 267–70.

69. Harold P. Green, "The Risk-Benefit Calculus in Safety Determinations," *George Washington Law Review* 43 (1975): 799.

70. Lester B. Lave, "Health and Safety Risk Analyses: Information for Better Decisions," *Science* 236 (1987): 292–93.

71. Ian Hacking, "Culpable Ignorance of Interference Effects," in *Values at Risk,* ed. MacLean, chap. 7.

72. Lynn White, Jr., "Technology Assessment from the Stance of a Medieval Historian," *Medieval Religion and Technology: Collected Essays* (Berkeley: University of California Press, 1978), pp. 261–76. For a cultural theory of risk perception, see Mary Douglas and Aaron Wildavsky, *Risk and Culture* (Berkeley: University of California Press, 1982).

73. Paul Slovic, "Perception of Risk," *Science* 236 (1987): 280–85.

74. Lave, "Health and Safety Risk Analyses," p. 291.

75. See the discussion in Chapter 3 of this problem, pp. 102–3.

76. Raanan Gillon, "Risk," *Journal of Medical Ethics* 8 (1982): 171–72.

77. For an ethical analysis, see LeRoy Walters, "The Ethics of Human Gene Therapy," *Nature* 320 (1986): 225–27; and several articles, particularly those by W. French Anderson and John C. Fletcher, in the *Journal of Medicine and Philosophy* 10 (1985). For public attitudes, see U.S. Congress, Office of Technology Assessment, *New Developments in Biotechnology—Background Paper: Public Perceptions of Biotechnology* (Washington, D.C.: U.S. Government Printing Office, 1987).

78. See Jeremy Rifkin, *Algeny* (New York: Viking, 1983). See also the more modest proposal and rationale offered by the Committee for Responsible Genetics in the *Federal Register,* Vol. 51, 122, June 25, 1986, pp. 23210–11.

79. Rescher, *Risk.*

80. For the controversy about valuing lives, see Steven E. Rhoads, ed., *Valuing Life: Public Policy Dilemmas* (Boulder, Colo.: Westview Press, 1980); and Rhoads, *The Economist's View of the World.* See also Rescher, *Risk.*

81. R. Thaler and S. Rosen, "The Value of Saving a Life: Evidence from the Labor Market," *Household Production and Consumption,* ed. N. Terlecky (New York: Columbia University Press, 1976). For a classic methodological statement, see Chauncey Starr, "Social Benefit vs. Technological Risk," *Science* 165 (1969): 1232–38.

82. Quoted in Steven E. Rhoads, "How Much Should We Spend to Save a Life?" in *Valuing Life,* ed. Rhoads, p. 293.

83. Barbara MacKinnon, "Pricing Human Life," *Science, Technology & Human Values* 11 (Spring 1986): 29–39.

84. Rescher, *Risk.*

85. On statistical lives, see Thomas Schelling, "The Life You Save May Be Your Own," in *Problems in Public Expenditure Analysis,* ed. Samuel B. Chase, Jr. (Washington, D.C.: Brookings Institution, 1966), pp. 127–66.

86. Richard Zeckhauser, "Procedures for Valuing Lives," *Public Policy* (Fall 1975): 447–48. Contrast Richard A. Rettig, "Valuing Lives: The Policy Debate on Patient

Care Financing for Victims of End-Stage Renal Disease,'' *The Rand Paper Series* (Santa Monica, Calif.: Rand Corporation, 1976).

87. John Moskop, "The Moral Limits to Federal Funding for Kidney Disease," *Hastings Center Report* 17 (April 1987): 11–15.

88. Steven Kelman, "Cost-Benefit Analysis: An Ethical Critique," *Regulation* (January–February 1981).

89. See Kristin Shrader-Frechette, "Values, Scientific Objectivity, and Risk Analysis: Five Dilemmas," and James Humber and Robert Almeder, "Quantitative Risk Assessment and the Notion of Acceptable Risk," both in *Quantitative Risk Assessment*, ed. James Humber and Robert Almeder (Clifton, N.J.: Humana Press, 1987), pp. 149–70, 239–62; and Harold Green, "Cost-Risk-Benefit Assessment and the Law: Introduction and Perspective," *George Washington Law Review* (August 1977): 908.

90. Herman B. Leonard and Richard J. Zeckhauser, "Cost-Benefit Analysis Applied to Risks: Its Philosophy and Legitimacy," in *Values at Risk*, ed. MacLean, p. 34.

91. Zeckhauser, "Procedures for Valuing Lives," p. 446.

92. U.S. Congress, Office of Technology Assessment, *The Role of Genetic Testing in the Prevention of Occupational Disease* (Washington, D.C.: U.S. Government Printing Office, 1983), p. 146.

93. U.S. Congress, Office of Technology Assessment, *Reproductive Hazards in the Workplace* (Washington, D.C.: U.S. Government Printing Office, 1985).

94. Eula Bingham, "Hypersusceptibility to Occupational Hazards," in National Academy of Engineering, *Hazards: Technology and Fairness*, p. 80.

95. Nicholas Ashford, *Crisis in the Workplace: Occupational Disease and Injury* (Cambridge, Mass.: MIT Press, 1976).

96. Roger E. Kasperon, "Hazardous Waste Facility Siting: Community, Firm, and Governmental Perspectives," in National Academy of Engineering, *Hazards: Technology and Fairness*, pp. 118–44.

97. Jerry Avorn, "Benefit and Cost Analysis in Geriatric Care: Turning Age Discrimination into Health Policy," *New England Journal of Medicine* 310 (1984): 1295.

98. U.S. Congress, Office of Technology Assessment, *The Implications of Cost-Effectiveness Analysis*, pp. 19–20.

99. Stuart Hampshire, "Morality and Pessimism," in *Public and Private Morality*, ed. Stuart Hampshire (Cambridge: Cambridge University Press, 1978), pp. 5–6.

100. See Rashi Fein, "What Is Wrong with the Language of Medicine?" *New England Journal of Medicine* 306 (1982): 863f.

101. For arguments that connect CBA and other analytic techniques to utilitarianism, see James C. Robinson, "Philosophical Origins of the Economic Valuation of Life," *Milbank Quarterly* 64 (1986): 133–55; Kelman, "Cost-Benefit Analysis"; and Alasdair MacIntyre, "Utilitarianism and Cost/Benefit Analysis: An Essay on the Relevance of Moral Philosophy to Bureaucratic Theory," in *Ethical Theory and Business*, ed. Tom L. Beauchamp and Norman Bowie (Englewood Cliffs, N.J.: Prentice-Hall, 1979), pp. 266–76. For a Kantian critique of these analytic techniques, see Alan Gewirth, "Human Rights and the Prevention of Cancer," in his *Human Rights: Essays on Justification and Applications* (Chicago: University of Chicago Press, 1982), chap. 7. See also K. S. Shrader-Frechette, *Science Policy, Ethics, and Economic Methodology: Some Problems of Technology Assessment and Environmental-Impact Analysis* (Dordrecht: D. Reidel, 1984).

6

The Principle of Justice

In a short story entitled "The Lottery in Babylon," Jorge Luis Borges depicts a society in which all social benefits and burdens are distributed solely on the basis of a periodic lottery.[1] Any given person, at the end of any lottery event, could be a slave, a factory owner, a priest, an executioner, a prisoner, and so on. The lottery takes no account of one's past achievements, one's training, or one's promise. It is a purely random selection system, without regard to merit, experience, contribution, need, or effort. Borges's story is compelling because of the jolting ethical and political oddity of such a system, which fails so noticeably to cohere with conventional standards. We evaluate the system as capricious and unfair, because we think there are valid principles of justice that determine how social burdens, benefits, and positions ought to be allocated.

However, if we attempt to state these principles with precision, they may seem as elusive as the lottery method seems capricious. It has proved an intractable problem to supply a single, unified theory of justice that brings together our diverse views. Indeed, many principles of justice do not seem distinct from and independent of the principles of respect for autonomy, nonmaleficence, and beneficence. We begin an examination of the nature of justice in this chapter by analyzing the terms *justice* and *distributive justice*. Later we examine a series of substantive problems about social justice, including problems in the allocation of biomedical resources, where a lottery or other impersonal mechanism may in some cases be warranted by justice.

Throughout this analysis we need to avoid a common confusion of justice

256

with justification. Appeals to "what is just" in the literature of biomedical ethics often use the term *just* in a broad and equivocal sense to refer to what is generally justified or morally right. For example, articles on research that uses double-blind techniques and deceives patients sometimes denounce the research as unjustly denying subjects information to which they have a right. Here the controlling moral principle is one not of justice but rather of respect for autonomy. (The argument could, of course, appeal to both principles.) Similarly, proponents of a physician's obligation to withhold potentially harmful information from patients for therapeutic reasons sometimes argue that it would be unjust for the physician to disclose the information. Here the moral concern is either nonmaleficence or beneficence rather than justice. Thus, many complaints of injustice are more properly categorized as alleged violations of some principle other than justice.

Some philosophers have also maintained that when the differences are clear between these principles and the principles come into conflict, justice must always be the overriding principle. By contrast, our argument about prima facie principles supports the conclusion that principles of justice do not always triumph over other principles. Hence a policy may be just but unjustified, or unjust but justified, when justice conflicts with other principles.

The concept of justice

Some moral philosophers, notably John Rawls, have argued that justice is best explicated in terms of fairness. Clearly there are close conceptual connections between these terms, but the concept of justice is also closely linked to desert: One acts justly toward a person when that person has been given what the person deserves. If a person deserves to be awarded an M.D. degree, for example, justice has been done if and only if that person receives the degree. Additionally, to use language introduced in Chapter 2, justice confers an entitlement whether deserved by the person or not. Justice is "giving to each his due," as it was put in some ancient accounts.[2] One who has a claim based in justice has a claim of entitlement and in this strong sense is due something. An injustice, in turn, involves a wrong where one has been denied that to which one is entitled.

What persons are entitled to or can legitimately claim is based on certain morally relevant properties they possess, such as being productive or being in need. It is wrong, as a matter of justice, to burden or to reward someone if the person does not possess the relevant property. For example, it is unjust to reward a superior for the work of his or her subordinates when the superior contributed nothing to their productivity. These examples show that both fairness and desert are central in our sense of justice but also that understanding justice in terms of entitlement is essential.

The term *distributive justice* helps narrow the scope of our inquiry. It refers to just distribution in society structured by various moral, legal, and cultural rules and principles that form the terms of cooperation for that society, that is, the implicit and explicit terms under which individuals are obligated to cooperate. A theory of distributive justice is an attempt to establish a connection between the properties or characteristics of persons and the morally correct distribution of benefits and burdens in society. The connection may be found, for example, in desert, in effort, or in misfortune. In the case of almost any set of rules of distribution, questions such as the following can be raised about the justice of the terms. What characteristics, if any, give one person or group of people an entitlement to more freedom or opportunities than others? What characteristics justify allowing one person to gain an economic advantage over another, if both are abiding by existing societal rules?

These challenging problems of distributive justice arise only under conditions of scarcity and competition. If there were ample fresh water for industries to use in dumping their waste materials and no subsequent problems of disease, then patterns of restricted use and entitlement would not be needed. Only if the supply of drinking water is endangered or public health problems are created by the pollutants do we need to set limits on the amounts of permissible discharge. Trade-offs are inherently involved. The goal of a pollution-free environment is directed at protecting the public health, but this goal also drains the economy of resources that might be used elsewhere. A trade-off is involved no less than in circumstances in which capital and labor are used to produce one commodity when they could have been used to produce another. Many contemporary discussions of just benefits in prepaid health maintenance programs, the justice of programs of care for the mentally retarded, the appropriate sources of funds for national health insurance, and the like inescapably involve trade-offs.

A compelling example of distributive justice and the necessity of trade-offs appears in the following case. An interdisciplinary panel of distinguished figures in medicine, ethics, and law was assembled in 1972 to consider the merits and demerits of using modern technology to produce an artificial heart—the so-called totally implantable artificial heart. The alternatives quickly narrowed to three possibilities: (1) produce no heart because it is too expensive, (2) produce a heart powered by nuclear energy, or (3) produce a heart with an electric motor and rechargeable batteries. The panel eventually decided that, on balance, the battery-powered heart would pose fewer risks to the recipient, to his or her family, and to other members of society than would the nuclear-powered heart. In assessing each alternative, the panel considered implications for the quality of life of recipients, the cost to society, and the relative expense of the technology by comparison with other medical needs that might be fulfilled instead. The panel concluded that despite the substantial costs, it would be an injustice not to allocate money for the provision of the artificial heart to those in need of it (on grounds that distributive justice requires it), and that the nuclear-powered heart would create more risk to society than could be justified.[3] (See also Case 32.)

This weighing of alternatives, especially involving risks or costs and benefits, is typical in circumstances of distributive justice, which concerns not only aggregate risks or costs and benefits of various alternatives but also their distribution throughout the society. Who should gain the benefits, and who should bear the risks or costs? The particular case of the artificial heart raises two separate problems of justice central to this chapter: whether to allocate money for the production of the heart, and how to allocate the hearts to individuals once the hearts are available. These two problems of distributive justice are distinguished later as the problems of macroallocation and microallocation (rationing).

Principles of justice

The principle of formal justice

Justice has been understood and analyzed in different ways in rival theories. The only principle common to all theories of justice is a minimal principle traditionally attributed to Aristotle: Equals must be treated equally, and unequals must be treated unequally. This elementary principle is referred to as the principle of formal justice, or sometimes as the principle of formal equality. It is formal because it states no particular respects in which equals ought to be treated the same and provides no criteria for determining whether two or more individuals are equals. It merely asserts that no matter which relevant respects are under consideration, persons equal in those respects should be treated equally. More fully stated in negative form, the principle says that no person should be treated unequally, despite all differences with other persons, until it has been shown that there is a difference between them relevant to the treatment at stake.

An abiding problem with the formal principle is its lack of substance. That equals ought to be treated equally is not likely to stir disagreement. But who is equal and who unequal? What respects are relevant for purposes of comparing which individuals in which range of cases? Presumably all citizens should be provided equal political rights, equal access to public services, and equal treatment under the law. But how far does equality reach? Can special groups receive special treatment? A typical problem is the following. Virtually all accounts of justice in health care hold that delivery programs and services designed to assist persons of a certain class, such as the poor and the elderly, should be made available to all members of that class. To deny access to some when others receive the benefits seems unjust. But is it unjust to deny access to equally needy persons outside of the delineated class, and, if so, why?

In a recent case a woman in labor, Hattie Mae Campbell, was denied access to an emergency room on grounds that she was at the wrong hospital and should have gone to a hospital where she had been provided with prenatal care. She and her sister retreated to their automobile in the hospital parking lot, where the woman gave birth to a son on the car's front seat. She then brought suit against the Marshall County Hospital, charging that its policy of not admitting patients who are not referred by local physicians is a capricious and arbitrary denial of the constitutional right to use of a government facility.[4] The hospital's policy clearly established a scheme by which patients were to be classified according to the criterion of referral by a local physician. This classification system resulted in the different treatment of individuals depending on the categories to which they belong; equals were treated equally, and unequals were treated unequally. The question, then, is not whether the hospital's classification system is just under the formal principle of justice—it is—but whether the criteria used by the hospital to establish the differences (inequalities) between people for purposes of the allocation of medical treatment are proper criteria. Some courts have affirmed that criteria such as those used by this hospital are proper under law.[5] But does the classification scheme employed by the Marshall County Hospital identify morally relevant differences between persons for differential access to health care? An answer to this question presupposes an account of justice that contains justified material principles in addition to the formal principle.

Material principles of justice

Many controversies about justice arise over the relevant characteristics for equal treatment. Principles that specify these relevant characteristics are said to be material principles because they alone put material content into a theory of justice by identifying relevant properties for distribution. Consider the principle of need, which declares that distribution based on need is just. In general, to say that a person needs something is to say that without it the person will be harmed (or at least detrimentally affected). However, we are not required to distribute all goods and services equally for all needs, such as needs for bedboards, athletic equipment, and antilock brakes (unless a radical form of egalitarianism is defensible). Presumably we are interested only in fundamental needs. To say that someone has a fundamental need for something is to say that the person will be harmed or detrimentally affected in a fundamental way if that thing is not obtained. For example, the person may be harmed through malnutrition, bodily injury, or nondisclosure of critical information. Without the proper nutrition, health care, and education, these harms could befall anyone; hence there is a fundamental need for these primary goods.

If we were to further analyze the notions of a fundamental need and primary goods, the material principle of need could be progressively fashioned into a policy for social distributions, perhaps into a full theory of justice. We will turn to such theories later. For the moment we are only emphasizing the significance of the first step in the argument, the acceptance of the principle of need as a valid material principle of justice. By contrast, if one accepts only a principle of free-market distribution, then one would be opposed to the use of a principle of need for developing public policy. All public and institutional policies based on distributive justice derive ultimately from the acceptance (or rejection) of some material principles and some procedures for applying and refining them. Many disputes over the right policy or form of distribution spring from rival, or at least alternative, starting points with their different material principles.

The following is a representative list of some major candidates for the position of valid material principles of distributive justice (though other lists have been proposed):[6]

1. To each person an equal share.
2. To each person according to need.
3. To each person according to effort.
4. To each person according to contribution.
5. To each person according to merit.
6. To each person according to free-market exchanges.

There is no obvious barrier to acceptance of more than one of these principles, and some theories of justice accept all six as valid. A plausible moral thesis is that each of these material principles specifies a prima facie obligation that, like obligations of respect for autonomy, nonmaleficence, and beneficence, cannot have its weight assessed independently of particular circumstances.

Most societies invoke more than one of these material principles in framing public policies, applying different principles in different contexts. In the United States, for example, unemployment subsidies, welfare payments, and many health-care programs are distributed on the basis of need (and to some extent on other bases such as previous length of employment); jobs and promotions in many sectors are awarded (distributed) on the basis of demonstrated achievement and merit; the higher incomes of some professionals are allowed and even encouraged (distributed) on the grounds of free-market wage scales, superior effort, merit, or potential social contribution; and, at least theoretically, the opportunity for elementary and secondary education is distributed equally to all citizens.

It seems attractive, then, to try to protect each of the above-listed principles in a theory of justice. But conflicts among them will still create a serious weighing or priority problem, another example of the problem of conflicts and dilemmas introduced in Chapter 1. Conflicts among the different material principles of justice, as well as their prima facie status, are illustrated by the case of Mark Dalton, a histology technician employed by a large chemical company.[7] Dalton was an excellent worker, but a week-long sick leave led a company nurse to discover that he had a chronic renal disease. It was determined that the permissible levels of chemical vapor exposure in Dalton's job might exacerbate his renal condition. The company management found another job, at the identical rate of pay, for which Dalton was qualified. However, it turned out that two other employees eligible for promotion were also interested in the job. Both employees had more seniority and better training than Dalton, and one was a woman. In this situation, each of the three employees could legitimately appeal to a different material principle of justice to support his or her claim to the available position. Dalton could cite the material principle of need, arguing that his medical condition required that he either be offered the new position or be dismissed from the company. With their superior experience and training, the other two employees could invoke material principles of merit, societal contribution, and perhaps individual effort in support of their claims to the position. In addition, considerations of equal opportunity could give the woman valid grounds for claiming that justice entitles her to the position.

Relevant properties

Material principles specify relevant properties that one must possess in order to qualify under a particular distributive principle. Several theoretical and practical difficulties plague the justification of alleged relevant properties. Moreover, ambivalence regarding which properties and ultimately which principles to emphasize in which contexts accounts in part for the patchwork character of federal regulation and health policy in the United States.

In some contexts relevant properties are firmly established, perhaps by tradition and perhaps by moral principle. For example, trophies are awarded (distributed) at the end of a tennis tournament on the basis of achievement; and achievement is determined by the tradition-bound rules of tournament tennis. Similarly, prison terms are distributed only to those found guilty of crimes; guilt is relevant to conviction and sentencing as a firm matter of law and morality. However, in many contexts, especially of social policy, it is appropriate either to institute a policy that establishes relevant properties where none previously existed or to develop a new policy that revises entrenched criteria. For example, the question has been raised whether nonresident aliens should be included on waiting lists in the United States for cadaveric kidney transplantation. The issue, which will be discussed later, is whether it is discriminatory to exclude nonresident aliens and whether being a citizen of a country is a relevant property to qualify a person for these lists.

In some cases it might be argued, "You ought to shift your operative set of 'relevant' properties to a better set of relevant properties." The argument is that certain properties accepted as relevant are actually irrelevant and that certain properties presumed irrelevant are actually relevant. A contemporary illustration of this problem occurs in Case 24, which involves an incompetent organ donor. In this case a forty-year-old woman's life depends on a kidney transplant, which her fourteen-year-old daughter offers to supply. The kidney is a fairly good match. However, the woman has a thirty-five-year-old mentally retarded brother who is a better match. (Some would say the brother is a far better match.) An informal survey of nurses, social workers, and physicians who work with such patients indicated that a majority would seek a court order to take the kidney from the thirty-five-year-old, institutionalized, mentally retarded brother.[8]

Here we have a straightforward dilemma regarding which criteria should be used to select between these two potential donors and regarding whether to wait for a cadaveric donor (an unlikely prospect at the time). The closeness of the match is seen to be a relevant property favoring use of the brother, but the impossibility of obtaining consent from the brother and the apparently knowledgeable consent of the minor introduces a reason favoring use of the child. There are also reasons against using either potential donor. The child may be overwhelmingly influenced by the fact that the recipient of her gift is her mother. The closeness of the relation and the emotion-laden situation undoubtedly exert pressure on the child, so heavy an influence that the quality of the consent becomes an issue.

In general, rules and laws are unjust when they make distinctions between classes of persons that are actually similar in relevant respects, or fail to make distinctions between classes that are actually different in relevant respects. One issue about justice and classes of persons concerns the selection of human subjects of research. There are two primary questions. First, should a particular class of subjects be used at all? For example, should prisoners, fetuses, children, and those institutionalized for reasons of mental disability be involved as subjects of research, and, if so, for what reasons and under what conditions? Second, if it is permissible to involve these subjects, should there be an order of selection of subjects within that class, based on relevantly different properties possessed by members of the class? For example, it seems morally relevant to distinguish within the class of children between older and younger children—or, better, between children who comprehend and report their feelings with clarity and those who have limited capacity to comprehend and describe. Typically, these distinctions have policy implications. For example, we might establish a national policy that adults, older children, and younger children be used in that order when doing biomedical research.

These considerations of justice are illustrated by Case 26, a case popularly known as Willowbrook. It took place at a state institution for mentally retarded children, some of whom were used as research subjects in order to develop an effective prophylactic agent against strains of hepatitis that were persistent in the institution. The research involved intentionally exposing children to the resident strain of hepatitis infection. Studies were carried out in a special unit that isolated the children and protected them from other infectious diseases. These studies precipitated a series of debates about the moral permissibility of this use of mentally retarded children and, more generally, about the moral permissibility of using the class of children, the class of the retarded, or the class of the ill and institutionalized in research. And if it is permissible to involve members of each of these three classes, is it permissible to use as subjects those who belong to all three classes, namely children who are institutionalized and retarded? If it is, under what conditions may they be used, and should there be an ordering, such as older children first or those most severely retarded last?

These cases and questions illustrate how abstract principles of justice may provide only rough guidelines when specific actions must be taken, so that further moral argument is needed to fix the specific relevant properties on the basis of which a reasoned judgment can be made. This problem frequently occurs when there are conflicting moral demands and no clearly preferable set of properties. As with the many cases of conflicts of principles and rules discussed previously, an assessment must be made concerning the weight of competing prima facie moral claims, and this assessment determines the acceptable relevant properties. The word *assessment* should not be taken to mean that the properties are arbitrary and without a principled basis. As we discussed when examining dilemmas in Chapter 1, there may be several conflicting good reasons for choosing different courses, and there may be no sufficient or determinative reason. Practical judgment and relevant experience will play a decisive role in such contexts.

Sometimes it is not unreasonable, unfair, or unjustified if the final assessment favors either of two or more competing positions, because they might carry equal weight in the circumstances. David Hume pointed out that if we could use a person's virtue as the criterion of distributive justice, justice would seem to be done when distribution of goods is proportional to virtue. But, he notes, "were mankind to execute such a law, so great is the uncertainty of merit, both from its natural obscurity, and from the self-conceit of each individual, that no determinate rule of conduct would ever result from it."[9] Personal merit and virtue are not the only obscure material principles of distributive justice; and, given this fact, we can expect perpetual, but not necessarily un-fruitful, debate over the fixing and interpreting of "the rules of justice."

Theories of justice

In the face of divergent and controversial appeals to justice, theories of justice are devoted to systemizing, simplifying, and ordering our diverse rules and judgments. Several well-reasoned and systematic theories have been advanced to determine how goods and services, including health-care goods and services, should be distributed—or, as some insist, redistributed. The theories largely differ according to the particular material criteria they emphasize.

The following are major types of theories: Egalitarian theories emphasize equal access to the goods in life that every rational person desires (often invok-ing the material criterion of need as well as equality); libertarian theories em-phasize rights to social and economic liberty (invoking fair procedures and systems rather than substantive outcomes); and utilitarian theories emphasize a mixture of criteria so that public utility is maximized, comparable to the way public health policy has often been formulated in Western nations. The accept-ability of any theory of justice is determined by the quality of its moral argu-ment that some one or more selected material criteria or principles ought to be given priority, or perhaps exclusive consideration, over others.

We can expect only partial success from the efforts to develop theories to bring consistency and comprehensiveness to our fragmented visions of social justice. Current policies for health-care distribution in many capitalist countries are indicative of the profound problems that confront any theory that would achieve an inclusive composite: We seek at once to provide the best possible health care for all citizens based on their needs, while simultaneously promot-ing the public interest through cost-containment programs. We also promote the ideal of equal access to health care for everyone, including care for indi-gents, while maintaining a free-market competitive environment in health care. Different visions of the just society underlie these competing objectives, and they cannot easily be brought into a stable balance. Theories of justice try either to achieve such equilibrium or to reduce some of our social objectives, while retaining others that are believed to reflect more important dimensions of justice.

Utilitarian theories

Utilitarian theories of justice follow the exact lines of utilitarianism presented in Chapter 2. These theories view distributive justice as one among several problems about maximizing value. Utilitarians argue that justice is not a principle independent of the principle of utility. Rather justice is the name for the most paramount and stringent forms of obligation created by the principle of utility. In the distribution of health care, utilitarians commonly see justice as involving trade-offs and balances. In devising a system of public funding for health care, the utilitarian believes we must balance public and private benefit, predicted cost savings, the probability of failure, the magnitude of risks, and so on. Many contemporary discussions of just benefits in prepaid health maintenance programs, the justice of programs of care for the mentally retarded, and the burden of payment for national health insurance inescapably involve such trade-offs from a utilitarian perspective. Utilitarians generally accept political planning to realize justice, including the redistribution of goods and wealth through taxation in order to benefit those who are genuinely needy, whenever redistribution would produce the greatest good for the greatest number.

Because utilitarianism as a general normative theory was thoroughly explored in Chapter 2, further consideration of theories of justice will be confined here to egalitarian and libertarian theories.

Libertarian theories

One of the most intense debates about distributive justice in recent years has focused on the scope and limits of national health policy. The United States has largely, though not exclusively, accepted the free-market rule that distributions of health-care services and goods are best left to the marketplace, which operates on the material principle of ability to pay and invokes some form of libertarian theory of justice as its justification. From this perspective, justice consists not in some distributed result, such as increasing public utility, but rather in the unhindered working of fair procedures. Events in a true free market should not be a matter of social planning but exclusively of individual choosing, and social intervention in the market in the name of justice perverts true justice by placing unwarranted constraints on individual liberty.

Even organs and babies, according to this theory, can be transferred for money by individuals in the free market. In one case a patient arrives at his physician's office accompanied by his cousin, who is willing to "donate" his kidney to the patient. As it turns out, the prospective "donor" is competent to make the decision but is motivated to do so by a sum of money offered by his cousin. The physician discusses with both parties whether the motive to provide a kidney is proper, but both are happy with the bargain they have struck.[10] Some libertarians have argued that current federal and state laws in the United States tend to create and then to perpetuate shortages of organs, babies available for adoption, and surrogate mothers because of our reluctance to leave availability up to the market. Economic efficiency as well as personal freedoms would be increased, they maintain, if qualified potential parents could purchase infants and qualified patients could purchase organs on the open market.[11]

In regarding free choice as central to justice in economic distribution, contemporary libertarian writers, as well as classical exponents such as John Locke and Adam Smith, assume an individualist conception of economic production and value: People should receive economic benefits in proportion to their free contributions to the production of those benefits. Libertarians reject the conclusion that utilitarian and egalitarian standards provide valid requirements of justice. Libertarians grant that people should be equal in various morally significant respects (e.g., in the right to vote), but they also believe that all other theories of justice inevitably entail practices of coercive and immoral expropriation of financial resources through taxation, which amounts to an unjust distribution of private property as if it were public property. Principles of equality and utility, from this libertarian perspective, sacrifice basic liberties to the larger public interest by coercively extracting financial resources from one set of individuals to benefit another set of individuals.

However, a libertarian is not opposed to utilitarian or egalitarian modes of distribution if they have been freely chosen by a group. What makes them right is precisely the free choice of the members of the group. Any distribution scheme for health care is justified if (and only if) it is freely chosen. Justice, in this theory, has nothing to do with redistribution unless the redistribution is contractually agreed to by those whose goods are redistributed. Obviously, in the complex modern state where agreement among individuals in a large group is virtually impossible, a libertarian generally prefers a system in which health-care insurance is privately and voluntarily purchased by individual initiative, because under this scheme no one has had personal property coercively extracted by the state in order to benefit someone else. In this system individuals may view the prices of available policies as too high, or as unaffordable, but the libertarian insists that in a true circumstance of free-market competition the price cannot be unfair. It is simply unfortunate, not unfair, if one cannot afford to pay for health insurance. The reason is the market-established nature of prices. To speak of unfair prices or trades is to express an opinion, but from a market perspective any price is fair, and no price is unfair. Individuals by themselves or in voluntary associations, such as religious organizations, may freely choose out of compassion or personal dedication to provide health care to meet others' unfortunate needs. But the society is not morally obligated to provide funds to cover such health care.

We earlier discussed a case in which Hattie Mae Campbell was denied admission to the Marshall County Hospital and gave birth to a baby in the front seat of a car. She had freely made an arrangement with another physician and health-care facility, had not made any arrangement with the county hospital, and therefore was denied admission to the latter facility. From the libertarian's point of view, a hospital might grant her admission as an act of charity and kindness, but unless she has a valid contractual entitlement she has no right of access; and therefore justice does not demand her admission, even if she is in a life-threatening circumstance. (The libertarian sees a stronger case if the hospital is private, which it was not in Campbell's case.)

The libertarian theory has been defended in an influential book by Robert Nozick, who refers to his social philosophy as an "entitlement theory" of justice.[12] Nozick promotes the minimal or "night-watchman" state, according to which government action is justified only if it protects the rights or entitlements of citizens. He argues that a theory of justice should affirm our rights not to be coerced rather than to create "patterns" of economic distribution such as those found in socialist and (impure) capitalist countries in which governments act to redistribute the wealth acquired by individuals in the free market. Here the wealthy are taxed at a progressively higher rate than those who are less wealthy, with the proceeds underwriting state support of the indigent through welfare payments and unemployment compensation.

Any proposal for health-care distribution that appeals to justice for social redistribution fallaciously substitutes, according to Nozick's theory, a utilitarian conception of what a majority prefers for a proper conception of what justice demands. His libertarian position rejects all material principles of justice that would impose distributional patterns on society and thus is committed to a form of procedural justice with three and only three principles: acquisition, transfer, and rectification. That is, for Nozick there is no pattern of just distribution independent of free-market procedures of acquiring property, legitimately transferring that property, and rectification for those who had property illegitimately extracted or otherwise were illegitimately obstructed in the free market.

The libertarian claim that there is no pattern of just distribution independent of these principles has been at the center of philosophical controversy, and many competing theories of justice reject the libertarian's uncompromising commitment to pure procedural justice. The leading competitor in recent years has been egalitarianism.

Egalitarian theories

Some idea of equality in the distribution of social benefits and burdens has had an important place in most influential moral theories. Political equality is a standard example. But egalitarian theories of justice propose that persons should be given an equal distribution of at least some goods and services, such as health care. In its radical form, egalitarianism holds that distributions of burdens and benefits in a society are just to the extent that they are equal, and that deviations from absolute equality in distribution are unjust. However, most prominent egalitarian accounts of justice are more guardedly formulated, so that mere membership in the human species does not entitle people to equal shares of all social benefits and so that desert does justify some differences in distribution. When structuring social arrangements, qualified egalitarianism points only to some basic equalities among individuals that take priority over their differences.

John Rawls's theory of justice, identified in Chapter 2 as a deontological theory, presents an egalitarian challenge to libertarian theories that has implications for a national health policy.[13] Rawls's central contention is that a social arrangement is a communal effort to advance the good of all who are part of the society. According to his moral viewpoint, inequalities of birth, natural endowment, and historical circumstance are undeserved, and thus persons in a cooperative society should make more equal the unequal situation of naturally disadvantaged members. Those who are naturally endowed with more advantageous properties or are more fortunate in their social position do not deserve those advantaging properties, and hence a just society would seek to nullify the advantages stemming from the accidents of biology and history. As Rawls puts it, these fortuitous advantaging properties seem arbitrary from the moral point of view. (See pp. 270–75 below on fair opportunity for amplification of this thesis.)

Rawls argues that we should distribute all vital economic goods and services equally, unless an unequal distribution would work to everyone's advantage. He uses an ahistorical, hypothetical social contract model in which valid principles of justice are those to which we would all agree if we could freely consider the social situation from a standpoint that he calls the "original position." Equality is built into that hypothetical position in the form of a free bargain among all parties, who are equally ignorant of all individual characteristics and advantages they have or will have in their daily lives.

According to one interpretation and extension of his views,[14] a follower of Rawls's theory of justice is committed to the following perspective on a national health policy. Rational agents behind the "veil of ignorance" would choose principles of justice that maximize the minimum level of primary goods in order to protect vital interests in potentially damaging or disastrous contexts. Social allocations to protect everyone's future health and to meet health needs would thus be elected by such agents (assuming that health is a primary good). This approach supplements the conventional marketplace system of distribution through a two-tiered conception of a minimal level of socially allocated goods and a second level of goods gained by individual initiative. This conception would rule out utilitarian systems (as attempts to produce the highest possible level of health care) as well as systems based on distribution of equal sums to be invested in any health commodity the individual wishes.

On another interpretation and extension of Rawls's theory, just distribution of health care is based centrally on a principle of needs and seeks to achieve "fair equality of opportunity," which we are required by justice to guarantee.[15] Needs are understood in this account as the means necessary to reach our goals, and disease and disability are viewed as undeserved restrictions on a person's opportunity to meet those goals. Health-care needs are determined by whatever is necessary to achieve, restore, or maintain adequate ("species-typical") levels of functioning or functional equivalents of these levels. Satisfaction of these needs should be designed in a health-care system to prevent disease, illness, or injury from reducing the range of opportunity open to the individual. Coverage in a reasonable social insurance package for health care, then, should be dictated by these determinants.

Both of these Rawls-inspired theories have far-reaching egalitarian implications for national health-care policies. Each member of society, irrespective of wealth or position, would be provided with equal access to an adequate (though not maximal) level of health care (contingent on social resources). The distribution would proceed on the basis of need, and needs would be met by equal access to services. Better services, such as luxury hospital rooms and expensive but optional dental work, would be made available for purchase at personal expense by those who are able to and wish to do so. Yet everyone's basic health needs would be met at an adequate level.[16]

The power of Rawls's theory of justice, together with the political significance of the decent-minimum proposal, have engendered support for the egalitarian theory. One of its most important achievements has been its encouragement of a discussion of fair opportunity.

Fair opportunity

The relevant properties and material principles that inform our judgments about distributive justice have thus far been our preoccupation. Consider now those properties that might and often do serve as bases of distribution but that nonetheless should not as a matter of justice be considered relevant. Sex, race, religion, IQ, accent, national origin, and social status are primary examples. In some limited, anomalous contexts these properties are relevant. For example, if a script calls for an actor in a male role, then females are properly excluded. But we do not acknowledge general rules such as "To each according to sex" or "To each according to IQ" as valid principles of justice.

The most widely accepted reason why we exclude such properties and often regard use of them as discriminatory is that they would allow us to treat people differently, sometimes with devastating effects, merely because of differences introduced by luck, for which the affected individual is not responsible and which he or she does not deserve. This fairness-based reason holds that differences between persons are relevant in distributional rules only if those persons are responsible for and deserve these differences (or if they would benefit everyone).

The fair opportunity rule

This account of unfairness in distribution can be formulated as a rule of just social distribution. The fair opportunity rule, as it may be called, says that no persons should be granted social benefits on the basis of undeserved advantaging properties (because no persons are responsible for having these properties) and that no persons should be denied social benefits on the basis of undeserved disadvantaging properties (because they also are not responsible for these properties). Properties distributed by the lottery of social and biological life are not grounds for morally acceptable discrimination between persons if they are not the sorts of properties that people have a fair chance to acquire or overcome. Although in many societies properties such as religion, accent, and social status can be altered and "overcome," race, sex, and IQ—those properties that bedevil fair treatment more than any other known to human species—are not easily altered. If IQ, for example, is something for which a person is not responsible, and if no one should be denied the benefits of a public distributional system on the basis of these morally irrelevant properties, then it would be unjust not to distribute to retarded persons the benefits generally conferred upon all who share in the system of benefits.

The example of supplying all citizens with a basic education illustrates why thorny policy problems are certain to arise. Imagine a community that offers a high-quality education to all students with basic abilities, regardless of sex, race or religion, but does not offer an education to students with reading difficulties or mental deficiencies. Intuitively this system seems unjust. The latter students lack basic abilities and need special training in order to overcome their problems and to receive what for them is a minimally adequate education. If these students were responsible for their retardation, we might believe that they are not entitled to special training. But if they are not responsible, they are entitled by justice to special consideration. Their claim in justice is conferred by the fair opportunity rule.

The equal distribution of economic resources is not here at stake. The mentally retarded or slow learners with special reading problems are not owed the same amount of money, training, or resources as other pupils. They should receive what for them is quality education. Even if it costs more, the fair opportunity rule requires that they receive these benefits in order to ameliorate the unfortunate effects (the disadvantaging incapacities) dispensed by the lottery of life (within, of course, limits of available resources, a distinct but closely related problem of justice).

This argument provides a justification of unequal (but larger) distributional shares to many classes of disadvantaged persons as well as a basis for numerous health policies. To determine a person's entitlement exclusively on the basis of material principles such as effort and personal merit would be morally wrong according to the fair opportunity rule. This rule systematically rejects the application of these material principles when disadvantageous properties are distributed by chance.

Many debates in health policy turn on an interpretation of the fair opportunity rule together with an assessment of relevant facts. If, for example, one believes that alcoholics are not responsible for their health problems, whereas smokers are, then one might argue that smokers should pay for their health care but that the state should pay for the care of alcoholics. The rule may also present a significant challenge to public programs of funding for the elderly. If people are not responsible for conditions introduced by the aging process, it would seem unjust to allocate so as to provide care for a younger person before an older person. We return to this problem of age discrimination below.

Despite the attractiveness of the fair opportunity rule, there will always be limits both to its use and to the goods and services that can be provided for the disadvantaged. Comparative justice demands a fair share, not an extremely large share. The problem of the nature of a fair share can be illustrated by children treated for myelomeningocele, a severe central nervous system anomaly. These children often receive partial treatment rather than total care, in the expectation that they will die. But some do not die, and over a period of years a series of expensive medical treatments for a variety of problems may then be required. These children may be afflicted by blindness, very low intelligence, and multiple medical problems in need of constant attention. It is perplexingly difficult to say what the fair opportunity rule demands for these children. Our society does not provide the exceptional medical care and training that such a child would need to receive a fair opportunity by comparison with other eight-year-olds. Nonetheless, the moral question endures: How much care discharges our obligations?

Ameliorating the effects of life's lotteries

If one accepts the fair opportunity rule in an account of distributive justice, as we do, it provides a startling and revisionary perspective on common practices of distribution. For the sake of moral consistency we must say that whenever persons are set back in the advancing of their interests by "disadvantageous" properties for which they are not responsible, they should not be denied important benefits because of those properties. Numerous properties might be disadvantaging—for example, a squeaky voice, an ugly face, a poor command of a language, or an inadequate early education. How far in life should we extend the range of undeserved properties that create a right in justice to some form of assistance in overcoming the handicap?

One hypothesis is that virtually all "abilities" and "disabilities" are a function of what John Rawls refers to as "the natural lottery" and "the social lottery." Here "natural lottery" refers to the distribution of advantageous and disadvantageous properties by birth, and "social lottery" refers to the distribution of social assets or deficits by such mechanisms as family, wealth accumulation, or school systems. Both have unpredictable outcomes, as all lotteries do. Suppose that all our talents and disabilities result from heredity, natural environment, and social contexts of family, education, and inheritance. From this perspective, even the ability to work long hours and the ability to compete are biologically, environmentally, and socially produced. If so, we are not responsible for our talents, abilities, and successes, just as genetic disease is acquired through no fault of the person having the disease. Advantageous properties are in many cases not something one deserves any more than are disadvantageous, handicapping properties (although it is controversial whether one deserves advantages that accrue from having such properties).[17]

If this theory of the causal origins of advantageous and disadvantageous properties were accepted, along with the fair opportunity rule, it would entail views about distributive justice radically different from the ones we now generally acknowledge. Rawls construes the fair opportunity principle as a broad principle of redress: In order to overcome handicapping conditions (whether they arise from biology or society) that are not deserved, his version of the principle compensates those with the handicaps. The goal is to redress the unequal distributions created by undeserved advantage in the direction of greater equality. Evening out handicaps in this way, Rawls claims, is a fundamental part of our shared conception of justice.

The full implications of this approach are uncertain, but the conclusions reached by Rawls are challenging:

[A free-market arrangement] permits the distribution of wealth and income to be determined by the natural distribution of abilities and talents. Within the limits allowed by the background arrangements, distributive shares are decided by the outcome of the natural lottery; and this outcome is *arbitrary from a moral perspective*. There is no more reason to permit the distribution of income and wealth to be settled by the distribution of natural assets than by historical and social fortune. Furthermore, the principle of fair opportunity can be only imperfectly carried out, at least as long as the institution of the family exists. The extent to which natural capacities develop and reach fruition is affected by *all kinds of social conditions and class attitudes*. Even the willingness to make an effort, to try, and so to be deserving in the ordinary sense is itself dependent upon happy family and social circumstances.[18]

At a minimum, we would view our system of distributing benefits and burdens from a revisionary perspective if this approach were accepted. Rather than allowing broad inequalities in social distribution based on effort, contribution, and merit, as practices in Western nations currently permit, we would tend to regard justice as achieved only if radical inequalities are diminished, so long as "disadvantaged" persons can be advantaged by the system of conferring benefits.

Nevertheless, this process of reducing inequalities introduced by the natural lottery will have to stop somewhere,[19] and many undeserved needs may not call for a social response. Libertarians have rightly (although we think too radically) pointed to the impossible dimensions of a program that carried the fair opportunity principle to conclusion without limits. Some disadvantages may properly be viewed as merely unfortunate, whereas others will be viewed as unfair (and therefore obligatory in justice to correct). From the lottery perspective, as Tristram Engelhardt has argued, society will need to call a halt to the demands of justice at the point of the distinction between the unfair and the merely unfortunate:

The sense of the duty to allocate resources to health care is different depending on which viewpoint one takes, for if the natural lottery is morally neutral, then providing inadequate health care is not prima facie unfair or unjust, though it may be indecent and unfeeling. However, if we view the world and the natural lottery's distribution of social goods as it should have been, were it to have been structured in order to support the moral order, such differences should, in justice and fairness, be obliterated as far as is reasonably possible. Where one draws the line between what is unfair and unfortunate will, as a result, have great consequences as to what allocations of health care resources are just or unfair as opposed to desirable or undesirable. If the natural lottery is neutral, in the sense of not creating an obligation to blunt its effects, one does not have [even] prima facie grounds for arguing for a right to health care on the basis of claims of fairness or justice.[20]

From this perspective, if needs are unfortunate they may still be ameliorated by benevolence or compassion; but only if they are unfair does the obligation of justice justify or require compensation through the use of state force required to tax and redistribute resources. Maleficently or negligently caused harms to health, then, warrant use of the term *unfair,* but other setbacks to health are matters of misfortune. In light of this problem of a criterion of unfairness, it remains uncertain what the full implications of the Rawlsian approach would be, and also whether the fair opportunity rule should have a revolutionary role in biomedical ethics or a role more like the one our society currently gives it in formulating health policies.

In the end, one's general theory of justice may be the most decisive consideration. Justice based on libertarianism, as in Engelhardt's approach, requires the consent of all parties to a distributive arrangement, and thus beneficence justifies specific allocations only if they have been autonomously chosen. However, justice based on egalitarianism, as in Rawls's approach, requires that obligations to benefit be fixed independent of autonomous choice.[21] We have concurred with Rawls on this point, but it would be inappropriate to pursue these theoretical problems farther. The point of exploring them as far as we have is to show that if one accepts a justification of unequal treatment based on the fair opportunity rule, then many areas of moral reflection and social policy will potentially be affected in significant ways. In what follows we will sketch some further implications of the fair opportunity rule for the distribution of health care.

The right to a decent minimum of health care

We have encountered several problems about justice that result from situations of limited social resources. We have seen, for example, that debates about a national health policy, unequal distributions of educational advantages to the disadvantaged, and whether to provide extensive therapies for those afflicted with myelomeningocele all turn on the question of who shall receive what share of society's resources, if any. Similar problems recur for the distribution of expensive medical equipment, artificial organs, and blood for the treatment of hemophilia. The issues are, in part, economic. How are these scarce resources to be most efficiently provided? Can more people be helped and costs be reduced? But the issues are at root ethical. What principles, policies, and procedures best ensure justice in the distribution of resources? Are we morally obligated to ensure access to some minimally adequate level of care for all citizens? Do they have a right to this or to some higher level of care?

The right to health care

The right to health care is a subject whose history has been characterized more by political rhetoric than by careful analysis. The primary question in these discussions has been, "Should the government be involved in health-care allocation and distribution at all, rather than leaving these matters to the marketplace?" Libertarians insist that all rights to social goods based on unconsented-to, enforced beneficence violate the principle of respect for autonomy.[22] Society has often allowed this libertarian-supported rule of ability to pay to determine the distribution of health goods and services, but is this rule consistent with justice?

More than one thousand dollars per person is spent annually for health care in the United States, yet the poor and the uninsured often cannot afford or find access to minimally adequate care. Many traditional proposals of social assistance to alleviate this situation have been based not on justice but on the virtues of charity, compassion, and benevolence toward sick persons. In former eras health care for the needy was primarily handled through social practices such as charity hospitals that had been founded on these aspirations of virtue. But in a new era of high technology and commensurately high costs, these older approaches have proved inadequate to the task of meeting many health-care needs. The older models of voluntary assistance based on virtue have gradually given way to the model that there is an enforceable right to health care based in justice.

An influential case (37) provides an example of various circumstances of modern health care that have prompted this shift of focus. In June 1985, an uninsured worker with third-degree burns was denied admission to several Dallas-area emergency rooms because he did not have the financial resources to qualify. After seven hours and seventy miles of travel in an automobile seeking admission to various hospitals, he gained admission to Parkland Memorial, a public teaching hospital, where he was given care for nineteen days at a cost of $22,189. Although several facilities to which he had sought admission declared him not an emergency case, Parkland considered him "definitely an emergency case." As a result of this and similar problems, a "Texas transfer law" was passed in April 1986 that became a model for national legislation regulating denials and transfers. In this same month the Comprehensive Omnibus Budget Reconciliation Act was passed as a federal law with provisions requiring both careful screening of such patients at hospitals and treatment for all patients who arrive under emergency conditions.[23]

However, to show that there is a moral right to health care requires more than an arrayal of desperate cases. It requires moral argument. We believe two arguments provide sufficient grounds for the claim that there is a right to health care. The two arguments are based on premises of (1) collective social protection and (2) the fair opportunity rule, as discussed above. We can here provide only a brief sketch of these two arguments.[24]

The first argument focuses on the similarities between health needs and other needs that have conventionally been protected by governments. Threats to health are relevantly similar to threats presented by crime, fire, and polluted environments. The latter threats are conventionally resisted by collective actions and resources. Consistency suggests that essential health-care assistance in response to threats to health should be a collective responsibility. However, there are also relevant dissimilarities between health care and the aforementioned collective goods and services.[25] In particular, these other goods and services pertain to what are generally considered social goods, such as the public health, whereas health care is largely a matter of the individual's private good.

This argument therefore needs supplementation. Additional premises are found in society's right to expect a decent return on the investment it has made in the education of physicians, the funding of biomedical research, and other parts of the medical system that pertain dominantly to health care as distinct from public health. The return we expect on this taxed investment is adequate individual health-care protection. We legitimately expect the scope of protection to extend beyond public health measures, because we fund even more training and research in medicine than in public health. However, any federal or state program will fall short of funding everything needed for health care, and we cannot expect a direct individual return on all collective investments. Some investments have as their purpose the discovery of cures or treatments rather than dispensing medicines or providing treatments once efficacious therapies have been discovered. The fact that the United States funds drug research at the National Institute of Health and drug regulation through the Food and Drug Administration does not indicate that we expect the federal government to subsidize or reimburse our drug purchases (although, in fact, it does reimburse for drugs in some cases). In the instance of physician education, it might be argued that the society's investment is in physician training and the protection of public health, but not in health-care services or distributional systems. This first argument, then, needs an account of a "decent return" that is not a "full refunding." We return to this subject of the decent minimum in the next section.

A second argument buttresses this first argument. From the perspective of the fair opportunity rule, the justice of social institutions is gauged by their tendency to counteract lack of opportunity caused by unpredictable bad luck and misfortune over which the person has no meaningful control. Insofar as injury or disease creates these profoundly significant disadvantages and disturbs our normal capacities to function properly, justice suggests that resources be used to counter the disadvantaging effects.[26] Moreover, the need for health care is far greater among the seriously diseased and injured, because—unlike fundamental needs for food, shelter, and the like—the costs of health care are unpredictable and can be uncontrollable and overwhelming, particularly as health status worsens. In the case of catastrophic illness, and often in the instance of the chronically ill and elderly, adequate private funding is unavailable. By this argument, a lack of access to health care is unjust whenever health-care needs have a powerful and even controlling effect on opportunity and functional capacity.

These two arguments for the right to health care are more suggestive and programmatic than complete. But jointly they suggest that using only material principles of merit, contribution, and effort for health care allocations is inappropriate, at least for some range of health-care needs.

This conclusion has been challenged as a proper account of justice by libertarians, who defend a material principle based on free-market arrangements. For example, we noted above Engelhardt's libertarian views, which he summarizes as follows: "It may very well be unfeeling or unsympathetic not to provide [health care to those in need], but it is another thing to show that one owes others such help in a way that would morally authorize state force to redistribute resources, as one would collect funds owed in a debt."[27] We believe this statement tends to blur a worthwhile distinction between what is morally optional and what should be done from the moral point of view. However, there may be an acceptable way to accommodate the libertarian, or at least to bring the two positions into some measure of agreement. If the libertarian holds that it is virtuous and ideal from the moral point of view to provide collective plans of health care, but not strictly a matter of justice, there may in the end be no dispute over which health policies and social programs we should adopt.

The primary dispute seems to concern how far to extend the language of enforceable obligation. Libertarians can insist on our right to retain our property free of social compulsion and at the same time assert that morally we should be generous and provide health-care services for the indigent. Both Nozick and Engelhardt propose that we should not coercively redistribute goods (through enforced beneficence or justice) but that we should attempt to bring about the same objectives by voluntary contributions. That is, they deny an enforceable obligation in justice (or in beneficence) to provide such goods and services but do not deny an unenforceable obligation. This is why Engelhardt can consistently say both that "a basic human right to the delivery of health care, even to the delivery of a decent minimum of health care, does not exist" and that his "analyses of the principles of beneficence and autonomy support a two-tiered system of health care."

Although we depart from libertarianism on these issues of enforceable social obligation, we retain a respect nonetheless for this tradition's foundations of respect for autonomy. It is again advisable, as we cautioned in Chapter 2, to consider whether certain levels of moral disagreement ultimately make a difference in normative viewpoint or proposed policy. If Nozick and Engelhardt endorse a morally good outcome identical to the one we envision, then the fact that we disagree over the enforceability of beneficence or the precise contours of justice may not be as large a barrier in biomedical ethics as first appearances might suggest. In this case it turns out that the differences are minimal, because we fully agree with Engelhardt (and perhaps other libertarians) that the principles of beneficence and autonomy give support to a two-tiered system of health care.

The right to a decent minimum

Quite apart from the contest between libertarian and nonlibertarian views of justice, the most intractable—and we think ultimately the most important—problem has been how to specify the exact commitments of a right to health care. Two major contemporary views have attracted the most support: that there is a right to equal access to medical care and that there is a right to a decent minimum of medical care.[28] Access to health care takes on several meanings in these discussions. Sometimes it means only that no one may be prevented from obtaining health care, not that any health care must be provided by others. This interpretation is favored by libertarians. More commonly, however, equal access means an equal right to certain goods and services. An expansive view of equal access requires that everyone should have equal access to any treatment that is available to anyone. A more limited view of equal access asserts that every citizen has a right to a decent minimum, but this rule leaves open the question of where to set limits on expansive and expensive health care.

The right to a decent minimum of health care suggests, but need not entail, a government obligation to meet certain basic health needs of all citizens, at least as a last resort. (None of the above arguments is, as presented, powerful enough to prove a national or any particular jurisdictional responsibility for funding or administration.) This approach accepts the two-tiered system of health care mentioned above: social coverage for basic and castastrophic health needs (tier 1), together with private coverage for other health needs and desires (tier 2). On the first tier, distribution is based on need, and needs are met by equal access to basic services. Better services might be made available for purchase at personal expense, but everyone's health needs would be met at the first tier.

This proposal offers a compromise along libertarians, utilitarians, and egalitarians. It provides a modicum of health care for all on a premise of equal access, while also allowing unequal additional purchase by individual initiative and contract. It is a mixture of private and public forms of distribution, an affirmation of collective as well as free-market methods of delivering health care. Theories such as utilitarianism may find the compromise attractive because it serves to minimize public dissatisfaction and to maximize social utility, without demanding a burdensome taxation of resources. The egalitarian finds an opportunity to use an equal access principle and to see the principle of fair opportunity ensconced at the basis of the distributional system. And the libertarian is left with an opportunity for free-market production and distribution of health care. The model also provides indigents with choices for health care that would otherwise not be available to them.

This approach also avoids the straitjacket of a one-tiered, equal-access-for-all health-delivery system. We do not propose an equal right to health care that would entitle people to health-care goods and services needed "to provide an opportunity for a level of health equal as far as possible to the health of other people."[29] This application of the principle of justice to health care would result in a health-care delivery system with only one class of services available, an approach rejected by the decent-minimum theory.

Despite its attractions, this proposal of a decent minimum has proved difficult to explicate and implement. It raises problems of whether society can fairly, consistently, and unambiguously structure a public policy that recognizes a right to care for primary needs without creating a right to exotic and expensive forms of treatment, such as liver transplants. More importantly, the model is purely programmatic unless one is able to define what ''decent minimum'' means in concrete, operational terms. This task is, we believe, the major problem confronting health policy in the United States today. It is here, however, that moral philosophy tends to run out of answers, turning the task over to the appropriate channels of decision making in a procedurally just political system.

The cautions we introduced in Chapter 2 about the language of rights deserve reiteration here. Some writers have maintained that the language of rights is appropriate exclusively for claims that are not subject to political or social trade-offs. Ronald Dworkin, for example, has depicted rights as ''trumps''[30] against the state's utilitarian goals, and John Rawls has maintained that ''the rights secured by justice are not subject to political bargaining or to the calculus of social interests.''[31] It is true that the rights cannot be bargained away. However, these ideals, like certain legal claims to absolute freedoms springing from the American Bill of Rights, can be as misleading as they are illuminating if they are applied without qualification to policies that implement the right to health care, particularly in the setting of allocational responsibilities and policies. Innumerable trade-offs are involved in establishing precise entitlements, and no right to health care will trump all competing claims of social utility when the larger circumstance of macroallocation is considered.

We have argued in this section for a right to health care not as a trump but rather as a claim correlative to obligations based on justice and established in final form through macroallocation decisions. Only through such decisions can the abstract right to health care become a living social entitlement. Macroallocation is the enterprise of calculating the respective weights of social obligations, rights, and interests. It is the task of moral theory to explore arguments for the right to health care and its proper boundaries, but moral theory cannot work out the concrete nature of the entitlement, a task that partially depends on society's structure, technology, financial resources, and competing objectives. Although we cannot here fix such an entitlement or a comprehensive public policy needed for allocation decisions, we can further explore some of the moral problems inherent in any effort to do so.

Can individuals forfeit the right to health care?

If we assume the right to a decent minimum of health care, can individuals forfeit, in contrast to voluntarily surrendering, that right? Here the idea is not that a person yields the general right to health care, but only that the person could forfeit the right to certain forms of care. The relevant sense of *forfeit* is the loss of a claim as a result of one's personal neglect or misdeed. These questions of forfeiture have emerged about the societal coverage of health care for patients whose diseases may be the result of their personal life-styles or individual actions. Examples include patients with AIDS as a result of sexual activities or intravenous drug use, patients with lung cancer as a result of smoking cigarettes, and patients with liver disease as a result of heavy consumption of alcohol. When people engage in actions that result in their ill health and medical needs, does society have the same obligation to provide health care to them as it does to patients who are "victims" of the natural, social, and environmental lotteries?

A person may forfeit his or her right to liberty by criminal actions that violate basic social responsibilities, and, some argue, a person similarly may forfeit his or her right to health care by failing to act responsibly. It is unfair, they charge, for individuals to pay higher premiums or taxes to support people who voluntarily engage in risky actions, counting on the health-care system for rescue. Using an appeal to the formal principle of justice, Robert Veatch contends that "it is just, if persons in need of health services resulting from true, voluntary risks are treated differently from those in need of the same services for other reasons. In fact it would be unfair if the two groups were treated equally."[32] It is not unfair, as some now put it, to withhold societal funds from health needs that result from voluntary risk-taking.

From the perspective of our use of the rule of fair opportunity, these arguments seem defensible because of the shift of responsibility to the patient. However, we will argue that even if principles of justice, strictly conceived, do not entail that individual risk-takers continue to have a justified claim to a decent minimum of health-care resources, several principles set limits on policies of exclusion of individual risk-takers from societal funds for health care. A policy of withholding societal funds from such patients cannot be justified unless it meets several additional conditions, set by the principle of justice in conjunction with other moral principles. First, it must be possible to identify and differentiate various causal factors in morbidity, such as the natural lottery, the social environment, and personal activities, and to confirm that a pertinent disease or illness is the result of personal activities. Second, it must be possible to show that the personal activities in question were autonomous, in the sense that the actors were aware of the risks and voluntarily accepted them.

Regarding the first condition, it is virtually impossible to isolate causal factors for many of the most critical cases of ill health because of the complexity of causal links and the limitations of our knowledge. Medical needs often result from the conjunction of genetic predispositions, personal actions, and environmental and social conditions. The respective roles of these different factors will often be impossible to establish with sufficient evidence. Whereas it may be possible to determine responsibility for an injury in mountain climbing or skiing, it is not possible to determine with certainty whether a particular individual's lung cancer resulted from cigarette smoking, environmental pollution, work conditions, or heredity (or some combination of these causal conditions), even though there is clear evidence that cigarette smoking can cause lung cancer.

And if, as many argue, ill health is broadly rooted in socially induced causes such as environmental pollutants and infant feeding practices, then the class of diseases covered by the right to a decent minimum would expand as evidence concerning the causal role of these factors increases. In the meantime, social policy may rest more on ignorance of causal factors than on real knowledge.

Individuals also may not be fully responsible for some of their risky actions, even if they are partially responsible. Some individual risk-taking may have genetic roots or sociocultural roots. A denial of a person's right to health care would be unfair if the person could not have acted otherwise or could have acted otherwise only with the utmost difficulty. This point holds if a contributing condition of a harmful behavior is beyond the person's control. As in the area of criminal justice, denial of individual responsibility on the basis of genetic or environmental factors can be overplayed, but there are legitimate questions about whether particular life-styles or behavioral patterns are substantially involuntary in at least some important cases. If they are, then it would not be fair to exclude risk-takers from the social system of health care. They are victims (at least partially victims) rather than free riders taking advantage of the distributive system.

In addition, as we stressed in Chapter 3, autonomous choice presupposes relevant knowledge about the risks that are inherent in life-styles and behavioral patterns. Some of the risks of disease, injury, and ill health are not known at all or are not known by particular individuals. If the risks are generally unknown at the time of action, individuals cannot be justly held responsible for them. If an individual does not know a particular risk that is generally known, then there will be additional questions about whether it is fair to use the standard of what a reasonable person should have known. (Furthermore, the individual needs to know the rules of the system of health care—e.g., if it has established rules to exclude patients with medical problems as a result of their life-styles and conduct.)

Other constraints on the forfeiture of rights to health care are also relevant. Even if it were possible to determine with accuracy the causal conditions of particular health problems, society would at some points have to compromise the principle of respect for autonomy and derivative rules of privacy and confidentiality. A system that excluded risk-takers would in many instances need "health police" in order to ensure fairness; and, in the worst-case scenario, these officials would be authorized to invade privacy, break confidentiality, keep detailed records, and so on, in order to document health abuses that could result in a forfeiture of the right to health care. Such enforcement would also be costly.

A major reason for the current debates about forfeiture of rights to health care is the rising cost of health care. Prevention, especially through alterations in life-style and conduct, has been touted as the major hope for controlling health-care costs.[33] If this is true, then the forms of cost-benefit analysis (CBA) studied in Chapter 5 might justify the exclusion of risk-takers when they develop medical problems. However, careful attention to the facts is indispensable, and results are often tricky and counterintuitive in the use of CBA. Some risk-taking may require less rather than more medical care, because it results in earlier and quicker deaths than might occur if the individual lived longer and developed a chronic debilitating condition. In addition, from the standpoint of utility, it is not sufficient to limit CBA to the system of health care. When it is extended to include other programs developed to support the elderly, the case for denying care to individual risk-takers may disappear altogether. As Howard Leichter argues, "over the long run, under public or private health and retirement systems, one can expect an increase rather than decrease in social expenditures as a result of avoiding health risks."[34]

It would not be unfair, however, to require individuals who engage in certain risky actions that result in costly medical needs to pay higher premiums or taxes, even if those needs do not cost the society more money when all social programs are considered. Risk-takers might be required to contribute more to particular pools such as insurance schemes or to pay a tax on their risky conduct—such as an increased tax on cigarettes. These requirements may fairly redistribute the burdens of the costs of health care, and they may deter risky conduct without unduly compromising the principle of respect for autonomy.

Priorities in the allocation of health-care resources

Macroallocation and the limits of ethical theory

Detailed specification of the right to a decent minimum or adequate level of health care encounters both theoretical and practical difficulties, some of which again point to the limits of ethical theory. One specification in particular requires further attention, namely how to establish priorities in the allocation of resources for and within health care. In this section we will examine these questions of macroallocation, reserving microallocation for the following section on rationing health care. The line between macroallocation and microallocation is not distinct and absolute, but in general, macroallocation decisions determine how much should be expended and what kinds of goods will be made available in society, as well as how it is to be distributed. These decisions are made by Congress, state legislatures, health organizations, private foundations, and health insurance companies. Microallocation decisions determine who will obtain available resources.

As Norman Daniels put it, "the macro level concerns the scope and design of *basic health-care institutions,* the central institutions and social practices which form a health-care system." Daniels has rightly argued that these macro decisions determine "(1) what kinds of health-care services will exist in a society, (2) who will get them and on what basis, (3) who will deliver them, (4) how the burdens of financing them will be distributed, and (5) how the power and control of those services will be distributed."[35] Therefore, major macro decisions concern the societal allocation of funds to determine how much health care, what kind of health care, for what sorts of problems, will be made available.

Limitations of ethical theories have been evident in the discussion of other ethical principles in this volume, but they are particularly prominent in debates about what the principle of justice implies for macroallocation decisions. In Chapter 1, we dealt with some of the generic problems that arise in applying ethical principles to policies. Earlier in this chapter we discussed problems of the meaning and weight of the principle of justice that make application less clear and definite than theorists and practitioners might desire. In general, theories of justice differ according to which material rules or principles they emphasize. In particular, there are debates about how much weight the selected rules or principles should have in the design and structure of the institutions, practices, and policies of particular societies in their own historical circumstances, faced with conflicting moral principles and practical constraints. Because of these conflicts, public policies sometimes move in cycles as society tries to reaffirm the principles it has previously compromised.[36]

Questions of justice arise within social systems that themselves realize principles of justice only in partial and fragmentary ways. When the overall social system is only relatively just, and no system appears to be perfectly just, questions about just health policy may seem somewhat misplaced. For instance, health and disease are seriously affected by numerous aspects of the social system in addition to personal medical care. Some of these other aspects may be subsumed under health policy, but many of them—such as those having to do with income, food, and shelter—would not ordinarily be considered under health policy, even though they contribute to health status. Some commentators have rightly pointed out that "equalizing medical care is probably not the most effective stategy" to equalize health in a society.[37] Studies from Britain indicate that the National Health Service has neither significantly improved health indices nor reduced the inequalities in health indices among the social classes.[38] These studies may only indicate that medical care is not as statistically significant for health as some other conditions in the society, such as the standard of living. Nevertheless, as long as medical care is important for some needs and serves to increase the sense of personal security (e.g., by providing reassurance), just access to medical care will remain a central ethical question.

Whether the social system is relatively just or relatively unjust in civil, political, and economic matters, there will be disputes about just health policies, because policymakers must determine the allocation of funds for and within health care. Elizabeth Telfer's typology of health-care systems accommodates their wide range: free market, liberal humanitarian, liberal socialist, and pure socialist.[39] These systems vary largely according to the weight assigned to the liberty rights of citizens, consumers, and providers (based on respect for autonomy) and the weight assigned to rights of equality (based on justice). The United States can, in Telfer's scheme, be best characterized as liberal humanitarian, with its emphasis on liberty combined with its recognition of the need for a safety net. Within this context debates about health policy largely concern how high and how tight the safety net should be—for example, in determining whether to fund organ transplants, provide catastrophic health insurance, or contain costs through diagnosis-related groups (DRGs).

Macroallocation and the debate about heart transplants

When these questions of macroallocation arise, what directions and constraints are set by justice and other moral principles? Or, to put the question differently, what is the content and scope of the right to health care, and what does it require in the allocation of resources for and within health care? We can begin to identify the lineaments of a framework of health policy by considering the debates over the last several years about whether society should fund heart transplants. Techniques of transplantations have become increasingly effective in the 1980s, as a result of various improvements, especially in immunosuppressant medication. In 1980, in the United States there were only thirty-six heart transplants, but those numbers have increased dramatically each year so that by 1987, there were more than fifteen hundred heart transplants. Major policy questions have arisen because the average cost for heart transplants is more than one hundred thousand dollars, well beyond the means of most citizens (although some insurance policies do cover heart transplants).[40]

As Case 33 indicates, on February 1, 1980, the twelve lay trustees of the Massachusetts General Hospital announced their decision not to permit heart transplants at that institution "at the present time." They noted that it was difficult to turn away even one patient in need of a heart transplant, but they underlined the importance of making such decisions "in terms of the greatest good for the greatest number." In June of that same year, Patricia Harris, then secretary of the Department of Health and Human Services (DHHS), withdrew an earlier tentative authorization for Medicare to pay for heart transplants because of the need to evaluate the technology's "social consequences," including its costs. In 1987, legislators in Oregon made an equally dramatic change in the Oregon Medicaid program (the state/federal program that provides funds to cover medical needs for financially needy citizens in the state). They decided not to pay for most transplants in order to use their limited budget for other purposes. In particular, they noted that the money that would have covered approximately thirty heart, liver, bone marrow, and pancreas transplants would instead be used to provide regular prenatal care for fifteen hundred pregnant women. The altered allocation was justified by its proponents because it would save more lives.

In each situation, changing medical and political circumstances led to at least partial alterations of previously announced policies.[41] These kinds of decisions reveal tensions between utility and equality in determining just access, often in the form of disagreements about the use of utility to specify the content and scope of a right to health care. Within a two-tiered system, in which the normative standard is that of a right to a minimum, there will inevitably be debate about how trade-offs between utility and equality are to be made, about how much money should be available for health care, and about where it should be allocated within health care. These debates will leave islands of uncertainty. For example, it is not clear that under the decent-minimum rule justice requires society to provide funds to cover heart transplants (or any massively expensive form of health care) under present circumstances.

The federal Task Force on Organ Transplantation recommended in 1986 that "a public program should be set up to cover the costs of people who are medically eligible for organ transplants but who are not covered by private insurance, Medicare, or Medicaid and who are unable to obtain an organ transplant due to the lack of funds."[42] This recommendation was limited, for the foreseeable future, to the nonexperimental transplants of hearts and livers. By contrast to the federal program that ensures coverage for kidney transplants, the task force limited its proposed policy to the financially needy.

The task force's recommendation was based on two arguments from justice. The first emphasizes the continuity between heart and liver transplants on the one hand and other forms of medical care (including kidney transplants), on the other hand, that are already accepted as part of the decent minimum or adequate level of health care that the society is committed to provide. The task force argued that these transplants are comparable to other funded procedures in terms of their effectiveness in saving lives and enhancing their quality. According to the National Heart Transplantation Study, eighty percent of the recipients of heart transplants survive for one year, and fifty percent are alive at the end of five years, with a good quality of life according to both objective and subjective criteria.[43] In response to the charge that heart and liver transplants are too costly and that the costs of health care must be contained, the task force argued that the burden of saving public health funds should be distributed equitably rather than imposed on particular groups of patients, such as those suffering from end-stage heart or liver failure. Thus, the task force contended, when the society is committed to providing funds to meet a wide variety of health-care needs, "it is arbitrary to exclude one life-saving procedure while funding others of equal life-saving potential and cost."[44]

The task force offered a second argument for the federal government's role in guaranteeing equitable access to organ transplants, without regard for ability to pay. Whereas the first argument focuses on the similarity between organ transplantation and other procedures, the second argument focuses on the distinctiveness of organ transplantation, especially the social practice of organ procurement and donation. Various public officials, including the president of the United States, participate in efforts to increase the supply of donated organs by appealing to all citizens to donate their own and their dead relatives' organs. This appeal is aimed at all segments of society. However, the task force argued, it is unfair and even exploitative for the society to solicit people, rich and poor alike, to donate organs if those organs are then distributed on the basis of ability to pay. Implicit in this argument is a claim based on the society's efforts to avoid commercialization in the transfer of organs. It is inconsistent for a society to prohibit the sale of organs, as U.S. Federal law does, and then distribute them according to ability to pay. It is difficult to distinguish buying an organ for transplantation from buying an organ transplant procedure, when the organ is provided with the procedure.[45]

The task force made these arguments in the context of advocating a public policy of governmental funding of heart and liver transplants as a last resort. Although it did not address larger societal questions about trade-offs between transplants and other medical procedures and goods in the context of limited resources, these questions, too, have to be addressed. Recommendations about funding heart transplants must be placed in a larger context with more general questions, which mix normative, conceptual, and empirical considerations.

Problems of macroallocation

The most general question for a society committed to providing a decent minimum of health care to all citizens is how much of its budget should be allocated for health care and how much for other social goods, such as housing, education, culture, and recreation. Health is not our only value, and expenditures for other goods inevitably compete with health care for limited resources. Some commentators argue that this question is basically political rather than moral and that it should be resolved through the political process, which can best reflect the values, preferences, and priorities of the entire society.[46] According to this argument, a citizen may not be able to complain of injustice if the society puts more money into space programs or defense than into health care. Nevertheless, there would be grounds for complaint if the society did not allocate enough funds to provide the decent minimum of health care.

Once society, through the government as the last-resort funder, has determined its budget for health care, it still has to allocate funds within health care. A vital question is whether priority should go to prevention or to critical care.[47]

For example, the government might choose to concentrate on prevention of heart disease rather than on rescuing individuals by heart transplants or artificial hearts. Prevention may in some cases be more effective and efficient than crisis medicine in saving lives, saving money, and raising health levels. How society might mix preventive and rescue strategies will depend in part on knowledge of causal links, such as those between environmental or behavioral factors and disease. Polio vaccine and preventive dentistry are staple examples of success in prevention, but these models may not work for kidney failure and heart failure. The latter complications are not the result of single disease factors, and prevention is only a speculative possibility.

Even for illnesses and injuries in which prevention is more effective and efficient than critical care, concentration on prevention might neglect needy persons who could directly benefit from critical care. Most prevention reduces morbidity and premature mortality for "statistical persons," but critical interventions concentrate on "identified persons."[48] Society has typically been more likely to favor identified persons and to allocate resources for critical care, even if there is evidence that prevention would be more effective and efficient. It has been argued that this social preference in part led the U.S. Congress to provide funds for the treatment of end-stage renal disease. As a rough rule, general principles of justice will be of little help in resolving these issues, because these principles neither require that we concentrate on the critical care of "identified persons" nor preclude such an allocation.

Utilitarian principles require opting for the preferability of preventive strategies if they would maximize social utility (so long as no utilitarian moral rule would thereby be violated). Sometimes evidence points to a particular strategy as maximal. For example, it has been argued on the basis of reasonable evidence that every public health dollar targeted at poorer communities for preventive measures in prenatal care saves many times that amount in later care. However, there is no evidence of cost-effectiveness for all useful programs of prevention. And, as we saw above, it has been argued in recent health policy literature that preventive medicine often only prolongs health-care costs to a later age and, in the long run, may be more rather than less costly. Here the motivation and justification for emphasizing preventive medicine is not cost-effectiveness but quantity and quality of life. Thus, we may choose to pay for prevention over other approaches because it allows us to live longer with increased health, presumably the same justification for funding crisis medicine.

It is also necessary to determine which categories of injury, illness, or disease (if any) should receive priority in the allocation of public resources if it is not possible to fund maximal research and therapy in all areas. For example, should heart disease have priority over cancer? When we discuss equal access or a decent minimum of medical care, we most often consider need, in contrast to geography, finances, and the like, as the relevant property justifying similar treatment. But, from the standpoint of public policy, it may be necessary to give certain categories of medical need priority in research and therapy.

Gene Outka has argued that it is more "just to discriminate by virtue of categories of illness . . . rather than rich ill and poor ill."[49] For purposes of justice, according to this line of argument, the relevant similarity between persons under conditions of scarcity is the type of medical need rather than medical need as such. In trying to determine priorities among medical needs, policy-makers could take into account such factors as the communicability, frequency, cost, pain and suffering, and prospects for rehabilitation of various diseases. It might be appropriate, for instance, to concentrate less on killer diseases, such as some forms of cancer, and more on pervasively present disabling diseases, such as arthritis.

Finally, which technologies or procedures should be funded within categories of medical need and for what reasons? For example, within the category of heart disease, should cardiac transplantation be supported? In order to answer this particular question, former DHHS secretary Patricia Harris once argued that it is essential to have a technology assessment—that is, an examination of all the direct and indirect impacts of cardiac transplantation, arrayed roughly in the form of the cost-benefit studies we examined in Chapter 5. But several problems of justice are involved other than the probable costs and medical benefits of a technology, including vital issues of fair access to new technologies. For example, once the U.S. government provided equal access to costly medical treatments for victims of end-stage renal disease, the composition of the patient population changed dramatically, as measured by such criteria as sex, race, age, education, marital status, and employment status. In the late 1960s, the patients were largely white, married, male high-school graduates between twenty-five and forty-five, and more than forty percent were employed. Ability to pay and judgments of social contribution had served as primary factors in their selection. But by the late 1970s, the patient population more closely reflected the actual incidence of end-stage renal failure among various groups.[50]

Hence, the process of determining whether, on grounds of justice and the decent minimum of health care, a society should provide funds to cover heart transplants is vastly complicated. There are several levels of analysis and deliberation, all within a social system that itself is only relatively just. In addition, as we have seen, considerations of utility play an important role in shaping the content and scope of the right to a decent minimum of health care (assuming a level of wealth in the society that would support the policy and assuming that supplying other goods besides those of health care would not be an overriding consideration).

Where it is difficult to resolve disputes about substantive standards, such as an adequate level of health care to satisfy the minimum required, it is usually necessary to revert to procedural rules. As the President's Commission for the Study of Ethical Problems in Medicine and Biomedical and Behavioral Research concludes, "It is reasonable for a society to turn to fair, democratic political procedures to make a choice among just alternatives. Given the great imprecision in the notion of adequate health care, however, it is especially important that the procedures used to define that level be—and be perceived to be—fair."[51]

Rationing health care

The language and practice of rationing health care

Health-care professionals often must decide which persons will receive some available but scarce medical resource that cannot be provided to everyone who needs it. These decisions are variously characterized as microallocation, rationing, selection, or triage. The variations in language are not unimportant, because each term has a different history and suggests a different degree of urgency. As two policy analysts note:

Earlier, policymakers spoke of the general problem of *allocating* scarce medical resources, a formulation that implied hard but generally manageable choices of a largely pragmatic nature. Now the discussion increasingly is of *rationing* scarce medical resources, a harsher term that connotes emergency—even war-time—circumstances requiring some *societal triage mechanism.*[52]

In this discussion we will use the terms *microallocation* and *rationing* interchangeably to refer to these decisions about the selection of patients. Later we will turn to an analysis of *triage*.

Whatever language is used, the necessity of selecting patients under conditions of scarcity is common. Dramatic examples include penicillin, insulin, dialysis, cardiac transplantation, and the availability of intensive care units. Rationing decisions are more difficult when the illness is life-threatening and the scarce resource offers the possibility of saving life. The question can escalate to, "Who shall live when not everyone can live?" Unlike many contractual arrangements between patients and physicians, this question cannot be resolved by the principle of respect for autonomy, because it is not answerable by the patient. Rather, it is largely decided for the patient by others, who must consider the claims of a group of patients.

Rationing is a problem within various health-care systems. Because health needs and desires are virtually limitless, any system must face relative if not absolute scarcity. Unless it puts more of its resources into health care than any society currently does, not everyone who needs a particular form of health care can gain access to it. In the United Kingdom, rationing occurs by several means, including queuing and the use of restrictive criteria for services.[53] In the United States, health care has often been rationed by ability to pay for health care or health insurance, and this pattern continues along with other forms of rationing. Because we earlier discussed ability to pay, we concentrate on other modes of rationing in this section.

Macroallocation and microallocation decisions interact. On the one hand, macroallocation decisions determine the extent of rationing by determining how much of a good will be made available. On the other hand, a society's distress at making tragic choices through explicit rationing may lead it to modify its macroallocation policies in order to increase the supply of the resource and thus to eliminate the need for rationing. One plausible explanation for the decision in the United States to provide universal access to kidney dialysis and kidney transplantation without regard for ability to pay is that the society could not tolerate the explicit rationing that resulted in the deaths of identified persons.[54]

We will here assess actual and proposed policies of rationing (beyond ability to pay) according to the criteria of justice and the right to health care proposed earlier in this chapter, emphasizing that it is impossible to apply these criteria independently of other moral principles. We will seek to determine which policies are just or unjust but also which policies satisfy or violate other principles. Most theories of justice permit rationing under conditions of scarcity, but they also rule out criteria of selection that reflect morally irrelevant characteristics, such as race or sex. The major debates focus on which characteristics are morally relevant and which are morally irrelevant in the selection of patients.

Substantive standards and procedural rules

We begin our investigation of what principles of justice imply for rationing by recalling the distinction developed in Chapter 4 between just procedures and just outcomes. Sometimes it is impossible to guarantee a just outcome by any feasible procedure, yet we remain interested in the justice of the procedures by which outcomes are determined. We may feel more secure in our judgments about the justice of procedures than in our judgments about just outcomes.[55] For example, we may be more confident in our judgment about the justice of democracy as a procedure than in our judgment about the justice of the decisions reached by that procedure. The common-law tradition also encourages this attitude by concentrating on the procedural rules of justice. For example, no party may be condemned without a hearing; the parties in a dispute are entitled to know the reasons for the decision; and no one may judge his or her own case.

Both procedures and outcomes need attention in rationing health care. "Who should make the decisions?" is a procedure-oriented question, whereas "What should the criteria be for decision making?'' is a substance-oriented question. Although distinct and in need of different answers, these questions are interrelated. For example, if criteria of medical acceptability are used, medical experts will play a central role in formulating and applying them. A lay committee would similarly have a role to play in judgments of social worth but none in a system of queuing or a lottery (unless the system admits exceptions).

Two sets of substantive standards and procedural rules are required for rationing many scarce medical resources, such as organs for transplantation. First it is necessary to formulate standards and procedures for determining the relevant pool of potential recipients, such as patients eligible for heart transplantation. Then it is necessary to develop standards and procedures for final selection of recipients, such as the patient to receive a particular heart. Although these two sets of standards and procedures may overlap, it is useful to distinguish them and to consider them separately.

It is generally easier to secure agreement about initial eligibility than about final selection, in part because selecting the initial pool of potential recipients appears to involve medical criteria that can be objectively formulated and applied by medical professionals. Nevertheless, as we will see, so-called medical criteria may incorporate arbitrary distinctions and unfounded claims, such as the value-laden judgment that only people below or above a certain age can benefit from a particular treatment. These criteria need to be subjected to careful scrutiny rather than accepted at face value.

Screening potential recipients

Criteria for screening potential recipients can be arranged in three basic categories, as suggested by Nicholas Rescher: constituency, progress of science, and prospect of success.[56] It is appropriate to raise questions about all three factors from the standpoint of justice.

THE CONSTITUENCY FACTOR. The first criterion is determined by clientele boundaries (e.g., veterans are served by veterans' hospitals), geographic or jurisdictional boundaries (e.g., citizens of a state are served by a state-funded hospital), and ability to pay. We have already discussed ability to pay, stressing the limits principles of distributive justice set on this factor. Case 28 illustrates how this criterion led to a controversial system for the distribution of AZT (or Retrovir), a drug that slows the progress of the AIDS virus and that was the only approved treatment for AIDS. The manufacturing company had limited quantities and was free to set its price for the drug. The initial cost was established as ten thousand dollars per year per patient, a price high enough to exclude some patients. However, a sufficient number of patients could afford the drug so that the limited supply required Burroughs Wellcome to use further criteria of allocation. It chose to allocate first to the sickest patients. The company was heavily criticized on grounds that the price was unreasonably high, creating a potential hardship for patients who lack any real treatment alternative, and on grounds that the less sick patients could return more easily to productive lives than the sickest patients. Many physicians and consumer advocates insisted that Burroughs Wellcome publicly justify its pricing and allocation scheme.

Even though clientele boundaries are often acceptable, they are sometimes controversial. For example, in the United States the distribution of organs donated for transplantation has raised questions about the accidents of geography. Should donated organs be given to patients in communities where they were donated or given to the patients in the national system (or even international network) who most need and could most benefit from those particular organs? Problems of logistics and preservation of donated organs obviously are significant, and local use may offer an incentive to organ procurement and donation. However, the Task Force on Organ Transplantation proposed that donated organs be considered public resources to be distributed, within limits, according to both the needs of patients and the probability of successful transplantation.[57]

In its most debated recommendation, the task force acknowledged that foreign nationals do not have the same moral claim on organs donated in the United States as its own citizens and residents do. Case 34 presents some of the moral difficulties in this conclusion. Luiza Magardician, a twenty-eighty-year old Rumanian citizen, came to New York City in June 1985 in the hope that she would be able to obtain a kidney transplant because all available methods of treatment in her country had failed. However, because there were not enough donated kidneys in 1985 (or now) to meet the needs of all U. S. citizens and residents, her chances of obtaining a transplant were considered slight, particularly since she had exhausted her financial resources.[58]

In conceding that national citizenship and residency are morally relevant properties for distribution, the task force nevertheless stressed that compassion should lead to the admission of some nonresident aliens. It recommended in a split vote that nonresident aliens comprise no more than ten percent of the waiting list for cadaver kidneys donated for transplantation and that all patients on the waiting list, including nonresident aliens, have access to organs according to the same criteria of need, probability of success, and time on the waiting list.[59]

PROGRESS OF SCIENCE. The second criterion, advancement of scientific knowledge, may be relevant during the experimental phase of the development of a treatment such as cardiac transplantation. For example, it may be important to exclude patients who have other complicating diseases in order to determine whether an experimental treatment is effective and how it can be improved.

(See our discussion of clinical trials in Chapter 7.) The medical criteria that are relevant to and acceptable for selection of patients for participation in clinical research will, however, need to be reassessed and perhaps modified or eliminated when a treatment becomes accepted.

PROSPECT OF SUCCESS. Whether a treatment is experimental or routine, the criterion of likelihood of success is relevant because a scarce medical resource should only be distributed to patients who have a reasonable chance of benefiting from it. Ignoring this factor would be unjust, because it would result in a waste of resources, as in the case of organs that can be transplanted only once. This factor is usually analyzed in terms of medical acceptability. Although medical acceptability can only be formulated by medical experts, the public has a strong interest in ensuring that the formulation does not covertly incorporate irrelevant or at least undefended criteria. For example, in Case 33, the U.S. government in 1980 withheld funding for heart transplants in part because the operative screening criteria appeared to include "social" along with "medical" criteria. At that time the criteria at the major heart transplant center excluded patients with "a history of alcoholism, job instability, antisocial behavior, or psychiatric illness," while requiring "a stable, rewarding family and/or vocational environment to return to post transplant." Critics held that these "social" criteria are inappropriate for use in programs receiving public funds.

Medical utility and social utility

The debate about the criteria for screening and selecting heart transplant recipients has focused to a great extent on whether those criteria represent medical utility or social utility. In judgments of medical utility, physicians and others try to maximize the welfare of patients, whereas in judgments of social utility, they try to maximize the welfare of society.[60] For example, in distributing scarce organs for transplantation, medical utility would require that the organs be used in the most effective and efficient way to maximize the welfare of patients suffering from end-stage organ failure. Relevant factors would include urgency of need and prospect of success. By contrast, in judgments of social utility, decision makers consider which recipient of health care would probably contribute the most to the society. Medical utility considers the differential value of a treatment for different patients, whereas social utility considers the differential value of patients for society. Judgments of medical utility are consistent with the equal social value of lives, whereas judgments of social utility may distinguish between the greater and lesser social worth of lives.

There is ongoing controversy about whether specific operational criteria are designed to realize medical utility or social utility. The Task Force on Organ Transplantation ruled out criteria such as race and sex as unjust, but it did not rule out several other criteria that could be medical or social, holding that these criteria require constant public scrutiny through a fair and open process.[61] The debate about such criteria is evident in three examples: age, life-style, and social network of support.

In the United Kingdom, elderly victims of end-stage kidney failure have been excluded from dialysis and transplantation because they are considered too old.[62] On the one hand, age may be a rough indicator of the probability of surviving a major operation and thus may be medically relevant. In addition, determining the probability of success may include the length of time that the recipient of an organ may be expected to survive. But the major medical concern is physiological age rather than chronological age, and each case must be assessed individually. On the other hand, the use of age as a criterion may reflect unjust discrimination against the elderly by an ageist society, parallel to a racist or sexist society.

Nevertheless, age itself is different from race and sex in several ways. People generally remain in the same race and sex throughout their lives (apart from sex-change operations), but they pass through all ages if they live long enough. Hence in a discussion of rationing it is fair to consider how much health care persons deserve over the course of a life span and even to concentrate health care in the earlier rather than the later years in order to ensure maximal opportunity for living a full life span.[63] This argument justifies age discrimination in certain circumstances on grounds of both fairness and limited resources. However, in practice, this argument would encounter serious difficulties because the elderly person now in need of a heart transplant did not have access to current biomedical technologies in his or her earlier years and would regard a negative decision as unjustified age discrimination. These difficulties would be magnified in a society in which access hinges on ability to pay.

Life-style is another controversial criterion in patient selection. It has been argued that it is just to assign low priority to transplant candidates whose life-styles (in contrast to bad luck in the lottery of life) contributed significantly to their end-stage organ failure. An example is end-stage liver failure as a result of alcohol and drug abuse. Even if it is not unjust to consider the patient's responsibility for his or her illness—a debated matter—it would be morally difficult to apply this criterion, as we argued above when we considered whether voluntary risk-taking constituted a forfeiture of the right to health care. Nevertheless, life-style itself may be medically relevant in predicting the probability of a successful transplantation. For example, a patient's continued heavy use of alcohol and drugs may greatly reduce the probability that a liver transplant will be successful, and neither medical utility nor justice requires that such a patient receive a transplant under conditions of scarcity.

A social network of support has also been used as a criterion in heart transplant programs. For example, it was invoked in the initial decision to deny

Baby Jesse a heart transplant at Loma Linda University, a case in which the baby's parents were unmarried. Such a social network of support, including the family, may indicate the patient's social value to others, but it may also be medically important in the overall success of the transplantation, particularly in posttransplant care, and thus may have an impact on medical utility in the sense of an effective and efficient use of a donated organ. Of course, justice may require the society to seek alternative support systems rather than using the absence of such a social network as a reason for excluding a patient from transplantation.[64] Here again, medical utility and social utility need to be distinguished carefully, and both must be constrained by principles of justice.

Because judgments about medical need and probability of success are value-laden, the operational criteria for patient screening and selection will require constant medical and public scrutiny. For instance, there is debate about what will count as success—length of graft survival, length of patient survival, quality of life, or rehabilitation—and about the factors that influence the probability of success. In view of these disputes, judgments of medical utility can often mask deeper judgments of social utility. A just process, one that is fair and open with public input, may be the most that can be expected in view of the ongoing uncertainties and the evolution of organ transplantation. Furthermore, specifically within organ transplantation, public confidence that the criteria of allocation are morally acceptable and fairly applied is important for the maintenance of the trust that is essential to organ donation. These points hold for final selection as well as for preliminary screening.

Final selection of patients for particular treatments

The standards and procedures of final selection from screened candidates have been even more controversial than those for the initial screening of potential recipients. Debate has centered on the place of judgments of relative medical utility and relative social utility and on the role of such impersonal mechanisms as a lottery and queuing. All of these approaches have been used in the selection of patients. For example, in the days of scarce dialysis equipment, centers providing dialysis made judgments of medical suitability, but some centers also made judgments of social worth; some use queuing ("first come, first served"), and at least one used a lottery.[65] In effect, however, all centers used one form of the rule of "first come, first-served": They did not drop patients from dialysis or refuse a second or third transplant because someone of superior social worth subsequently appeared.

MEDICAL UTILITY. We assume, as an unargued premise, that in rationing scarce medical resources it is morally imperative to consider medical utility, understood as the maximization of the welfare of patients in need of treatment. The differences in patients' urgency of need and prospects of successful treatment are both relevant considerations. If the resource is not reusable, as in the case of transplanted organs, it is especially important not to waste it. Selection should also try to save as many lives as possible through the available resources. Hence, in patient selection, medical utility requires attention to the effective and efficient uses of scarce medical resources.

Although this approach does not violate principles of justice, there are difficulties. Both need and prospect of success are value-laden concepts, and there is uncertainty both about the factors that contribute to success and about probabilities. To take another example from kidney transplantation, transplant surgeons dispute whether it is now important to have a good tissue match because cyclosporine is such an effective medication in reducing the body's tendency to reject transplanted organs. In addition, medical need and prospect of success may come into conflict. For example, a patient's urgent condition may make him or her a less likely candidate for a successful heart transplant. And in intensive care units, trying to save a patient whose medical need is greatest may consume resources that could be used to save more people.[66]

In ICUs the emergency demand can exceed the available resources, and physicians sometimes can provide intensive care to some patients only by denying it to others. If an ICU reaches capacity, and other patients need admission, decision makers face a dilemmatic choice to raise the census and thereby lower the standard of care or to look carefully at the claims of all.[67] The *Von Stetina* case indicates that the choice to raise the census and lower the standard of care may have legal risks. In this case the plaintiff, who had been severely injured in an automobile accident, was accidentally disconnected from her ventilator for a prolonged period and became permanently comatose as a result. The suit contended that the ICU nurses were too busy with new admissions to meet the standard of care for the plaintiff, that one patient in the ICU was already close to meeting brain-death criteria (and was declared dead thirty-six hours later), and that two others were discharged the following morning. The jury ruled in favor of the plaintiff.[68]

Although judgments of medical utility are complex and frequently involve uncertainties about probable outcomes, they are indispensable in rationing health care and are consistent with the demands of justice. But further problems of justice arise when medical utility is roughly equal among candidates for scarce medical resources. Here justice needs additional criteria, the search for which takes us to the subject of chance and queuing.

IMPERSONAL MECHANISMS OF CHANCE AND QUEUING. The use of chance and queuing in rationing is based on justice as equality and fair opportunity. We began this chapter by noting the oddity of using a lottery, as in Borges's short story, to distribute all social goods and branches. However, when medical resources are scarce and there are no major disparities in medical utility—and particularly when selection may determine life or death—fair opportunity, equal respect, and equal evaluation of lives may require queuing, a lottery, or randomization (whichever procedure is the most appropriate and feasible in the circumstances). This conclusion was reached by the Artificial Heart Assessment Panel of the National Heart Institute:

In the event artificial heart resources are in scarce supply, decisions as to the selection of candidates for implantation of the artificial heart should be made by the physicians and medical institutions on the basis of medical criteria. If the pool of patients with equal medical needs exceeds supply, procedures should be devised for some form of random selection. Social worth criteria should not be used, and every effort should be exerted to minimize the possibility that social worth may implicitly be taken into account.[69]

Some critics of this policy contend that the use of impersonal mechanisms is an irresponsible refusal to make a decision, but we believe the decision to use such impersonal mechanisms can be justified by either deontological or rule-utilitarian perspectives. Both can be ways to express fair opportunity when patients are roughly equal in medical utility.

However, there are both theoretical and practical problems to be overcome. One difficult question concerns the weight of the rule of "first come, first served" when a patient already receiving a particular treatment has a severely limited chance of survival, while other patients who also need the treatment have a much greater chance of survival. ICU staffs often experience conflicts between claims of "early arrivers," who have already gained access, and "newcomers."[70] Does "first come, first served" imply that those already receiving treatment have absolute priority over those who arrive later but have either more urgent needs or better prospects of success?

In Chapter 4, we argued against a sharp distinction between withholding and withdrawing treatment, on the grounds that it is often necessary to begin a treatment in order to determine a patient's diagnosis and prognosis. That argument was focused on the patient's best interests. In the context of competition for intensive care as a scarce lifesaving medical resource, there is a conflict of interests. Admission to the ICU establishes a presumption in favor of continued treatment in that setting, but it does not give a person a permanent absolute claim for priority over others, regardless of the person's changing medical circumstances. Requirements of medical utility may dictate early discharge in order to make room for others who have a more urgent need or a higher probability of benefit. Such displacement from the ICU is not tantamount to abandonment, if other levels and forms of care are provided.

This argument for the use of chance or queuing in rationing health care applies only if there are no major disparities in medical utility. Again, a similar position was taken by the Task Force on Organ Transplantation: "If two or more patients are equally good candidates for a particular organ according to the medical criteria of need and probability of success, the principle of justice suggests that length of time on the waiting list is the fairest way to make the final selection."[71] Which mechanism, queuing or chance, is preferable will depend largely on practical considerations, but queuing appears to be more feasible in most health-care settings, including in organ transplantation, emergency medicine, and ICUs. A complicating consideration is that some people may not enter the queue or the lottery in time because of such factors as slowness in seeking help, inadequate or incompetent medical attention, delay in referral, or overt discrimination. For example, a person's limited funds may have prevented a search for medical care until it was too late to benefit from a particular therapy. The principle of justice will in some cases require efforts to correct such blockage of access in order to provide fair opportunity.

SOCIAL UTILITY. Whatever the difficulties of application—and they are considerable—medical utility is important in the selection of recipients of scarce medical resources. More controversial is social utility. Can the comparative value of potential recipients to a community ever be a relevant and decisive criterion? An analogy often used is giving priority to some sailors on a crowded lifeboat in order to increase the chances of saving more people than would otherwise be saved. Another familiar example is taken from World War II, when the scarce resource of penicillin was distributed to U.S. soldiers suffering from veneral disease rather than those suffering from battle wounds. The rationale was military need: The soldiers suffering from venereal disease could be quickly restored to battle.[72]

One argument in favor of social-utilitarian selection is that medical institutions and personnel are trustees of society and thus should consider the probable future contributions of patients in need of scarce lifesaving resources. After all, Nicholas Rescher contends, "in its allocation . . . society 'invests' a scarce resource in one person as against another and is thus entitled to look to the probable prospective 'return' on its investment."[73] This argument can be sharply criticized from rule-utilitarian as well as deontological perspectives. For example, both may resist these utilitarian judgments in order to protect the relationship of personal care and trust between patients and physicians, which would be threatened if physicians routinely looked beyond their patients' needs to society's needs. Numerous moral and practical problems also confront such direct appeals to social utility in this context, including difficulties of developing acceptable criteria of social worth in a pluralistic society with many different conceptions of the valuable life, reduction of persons to their social roles and functions, violation of equal respect for persons and equal evaluation of their lives, and denial of fair equality of opportunity.[74]

TRIAGE. Defenders of social-utilitarian calculations in rationing health care sometimes invoke the model of triage, which has become increasingly common in medicine and health care. The French term *triage* means "sorting," "picking," or "choosing." It has been applied to sorting such items as wool and coffee beans according to their quality. In the delivery of health care, triage has been practiced in war, in community disasters, and in emergency rooms where injured persons have been sorted for medical attention according to their needs and prospects. Decisions to admit and to discharge patients from ICUs often involve some form of triage. In all case of triage in health care the objective is to use available medical resources as effectively and as efficiently as possible. The traditional and contemporary rationale for triage is "Do the greatest good for the greatest number."[75]

Triage decisions often involve medical utility rather than social utility in determining the greatest good for the greatest number. In one type of situation, victims are sorted according to their medical needs: those who will die without immediate help, those whose treatment may be delayed without immediate danger, those with minor injuries, and those for whom no treatment will be efficacious. Such a medical utilitarian classification scheme may legitimately be used to establish priorities of treatment, but it does not involve judgments about individuals' comparative social worth.

However, judgments of social worth may be inescapable in some situations. Suppose, for example, that after an earthquake some injured persons are medical personnel with minor injuries. These persons may, and in some contexts should, be given priority of treatment so that they can be restored to help others. Similarly, in an outbreak of disease, it seems justifiable to inoculate physicians first so that they can care for others. In such emergencies communities and individuals have an immediate need of protection against disaster, sometimes even to survive. Under these emergency conditions, a person may be given priority for treatment on grounds of social utility if and only if his or her contribution is indispensable to attaining a major social goal or function—for example, the president of a country in wartime would be given priority. In such contexts, as in the analogous lifeboat cases, our judgments about comparative social value should be limited to the specific qualities and skills that are essential to the community's maintenance, security, or protection. These judgments should not attempt to assess the general social worth of persons. So stated, rule deontologists and rule utilitarians alike can support this position.

If such exceptions based on social utility are limited to genuine emergencies involving necessity, they do not threaten the normal moral universe. Accepting social-utilitarian judgments in emergencies does not imply the general acceptability of social-utilitarian calculations in distributing health care. The structure of justification in such exceptional cases follows our usual pattern: Presumptions are set by important principles that are prima facie binding, but in some cases of conflict it is possible to rebut those presumptions. Arguments to rebut these presumptions need to show that the competing principle is stronger in the circumstances, that it would probably be realized through infringing another principle, that it cannot be realized without infringing another principle, and that the infringement is the least required by the circumstances.

Our contention, then, is that justice, in conjunction with other principles, mandates attention to medical utility followed by the use of chance or queuing for scarce resources when medical utility is roughly equal for eligible patients. Justified departures from this system for reasons of social utility are possible but require the usual burden of argument when vital moral rules are to be overridden. Our approach does not demand equality of opportunity regardless of the consequences. Nevertheless, the contrast with a system such as Rescher's is significant: His system relies on calculations of social utility until there are no major disparities in social value among the candidates for a scarce resource; at this point, he resorts to chance. After attending to medical utility, our system, based on fairness and equality, uses chance and queuing until there are major disparities in potential recipients' social responsibilities and probable social contributions in an emergency. These emergencies are rare, but when they do occur, difficult choices will have to be made.

Conclusion

In this chapter we have examined several alternative approaches to justice, including egalitarian, libertarian, and utilitarian theories. We have not maintained that a single theory of justice must be adopted in order to reflect constructively on these problems or to develop health policies. Each influential general theory of justice has developed from a distinct perspective on the moral life that only partially captures the diversity of that life. The richness of our moral traditions, practices, and theories helps explain why egalitarian theories, libertarian theories, and utilitarian theories of justice have all been skillfully defended in recent philosophy. This conclusion is consistent with the conclusions reached in Chapter 2 about the types of ethical theory discussed in that chapter.

A widely accepted thesis is that these theories of justice are irreconcilably opposed, springing from rival starting points and eventuating in intractable and interminable disagreements. Although we have no available theory at the present time to bring these diverse accounts into systematic unity, skepticism about the theory of justice should be kept in proper perspective. Each of the theories we have discussed highlights a material principle that is important for moral reflection on issues of justice and health policy. Absent a social consensus about these competing theories of justice, it is to be expected that public policies will shift ground, now emphasizing one theory, later emphasizing another.

This unsteady territory may reflect a certain hesitancy and ambivalence but does not necessarily amount to injustice.

Notes

1. Jorge Luis Borges, *Labyrinths* (New York: New Directions, 1962), pp. 30–35.
2. See Martin Golding's "Justice and Rights: A Study in Relationship," in *Justice and Health Care,* ed. Earl E. Shelp (Boston: D. Reidel, 1981). The connections to certain ancient theories, including Ulpian's famous third-century definition, are treated by Golding; see pp. 23–35. See also Allen Buchanan, "Justice: A Philosophical Review," in the same volume, pp. 3–21.
3. *The Totally Implantable Artificial Heart: A Report of the Artificial Heart Assessment Panel of the National Heart and Lung Institute* (June 1973), DHEW Publication No. NIH 74-191. See also Albert R. Jonsen, "The Artificial Heart's Threat to Others," *Hastings Center Report* 16 (February 1986): 9–11.
4. *Campbell* v. *Mincey,* 413 F. Supp. 16 (1975), 16–23.
5. *Goesaert* v. *Cleary,* 335 U.S. 464, 69 S.Ct. 198, 93 L.Ed. 163 (1948); *Campbell* v. *Mincey,* at 22; *Whitney* v. *State Tax Commission,* 309 U.S. 530, 542, 60 S.Ct. 635, 64041, 84 L.Ed. 909, at 915 (1940). But see Public Law 99-272, in note 23 below.
6. See, e.g., Nicholas Rescher, *Distributive Justice* (Indianapolis: Bobbs-Merrill, 1966), chap. 4.
7. This case was reported by Robert E. Stevenson in the *Hastings Center Report* 10 (December 1980): 25.
8. Audience Survey, Symposium on Death and Dying, Southeastern Dialysis and Transplantation Association Meetings, Miami, August 1977 (unpublished).
9. David Hume, *An Enquiry Concerning the Principles of Morals* (London: Andrew Millar, 1772), p. 257.
10. See M. O. Basson, ed., *Ethics, Humanism, and Medicine* (New York: Alan R. Liss, 1980).
11. Richard Posner, for example, uses this argument, which he refers to as "the market solution." See "The Legal Protection of Children and the Case for Legalizing Baby Sales," in his *Economic Analysis of Law* (Boston: Little, Brown, 1986).
12. Robert Nozick, *Anarchy, State, and Utopia* (New York: Basic Books, 1974), esp. pp. 149–82.
13. John Rawls, *A Theory of Justice* (Cambridge, Mass.: Harvard University Press, 1971). For applications or extensions to health care, see Norman Daniels, *Just Health Care* (New York: Cambridge University Press, 1985), esp. pp. 37–58; and John Moskop, "Rawlsian Justice and a Human Right to Health Care," *Journal of Medicine and Philosophy* 8 (November 1983): 329–38. We do not deal in this chapter with what have been called communitarian theories of justice, which have been developed in recent years to counter the individualism of liberal and libertarian theories. Their criticisms have at times been penetrating, but their constructive proposals remain sketchy. They tend to emphasize a substantive theory of the good toward which human beings as social beings, and hence human institutions and policies, should be directed. For an instructive communitarian criticism of Rawls's theory of justice, see Michael Sandel, *Liberalism and the Limits of Justice* (Cambridge: Cambridge University Press, 1982). See also Alasdair MacIntyre, *After Virtue,* 2d ed. (Notre Dame, Ind.: University of Notre Dame Press, 1984), esp. chap.

17; and Alasdair MacIntyre, *Whose Justice? Which Rationality?* (Notre Dame, Ind.: University of Notre Dame Press, 1988). For an application of a communitarian (and egalitarian) perspective to health care, see Larry Churchill, *Rationing Health Care in America* (Notre Dame, Ind.: University of Notre Dame Press, 1987).

14. See Ronald M. Green, "Health Care and Justice in Contract Perspective," in *Ethics and Health Policy,* ed. Robert M. Veatch and Roy Branson (Cambridge, Mass.: Ballinger, 1976), pp. 111–26. Green's extension of Rawls occurs largely by adding health to the list of primary social goods that can be affected through the social structure of distribution and allocation. Rawls himself does not have health on the list and does not discuss the distribution of health care. Whereas Green's approach utilizes Rawls's difference principle, Norman Daniels utilizes Rawls's principle of fair equality of opportunity.

15. Daniels, *Just Health Care;* Norman Daniels, "A Reply to Some Stern Criticisms and a Remark on Health Care Rights," *Journal of Medicine and Philosophy* 8 (November 1983): 363–71; and Norman Daniels, "Why Saying No to Patients in the United States Is So Hard: Cost Containment, Justice, and Provider Autonomy," *New England Journal of Medicine* 314 (1986): 1380–83.

16. See Charles Fried, "Equality and Rights in Medical Care," *Hastings Center Report* 6 (February 1976): 29–34.

17. Both Thomas Nagel and Robert Nozick have provided theoretical reasons to show that, as Nagel puts it, "yet one probably does deserve the punishments or rewards that flow from these undeserved qualities." From "Equal Treatment and Compensatory Discrimination," *Philosophy and Public Affairs* 2 (1973), n. 5. Nozick questions much of what we have argued above, but neither Nagel nor Nozick destroys the validity of the point we are making in this section. See Nozick, *Anarchy, State, and Utopia,* chap. 7 and the first two sections of chap. 8.

18. Rawls, *A Theory of Justice,* pp. 73f (italics added).

19. See Bernard Williams, "The Idea of Equality," as reprinted in Hugo Bedau, *Justice and Equality* (Englewood Cliffs, N.J.: Prentice-Hall, 1971), p. 135.

20. H. Tristram Engelhardt, Jr., "Health Care Allocations: Responses to the Unjust, the Unfortunate, and the Undesirable," in *Justice and Health Care,* ed. Shelp, pp. 126–27. See also Engelhardt's *The Foundations of Bioethics* (New York: Oxford University Press, 1986), pp. 339–43.

21. See Engelhardt, *The Foundations of Bioethics,* esp. p. 353. For the commitments of strong egalitarianism, see Robert M. Veatch, *The Foundations of Justice* (New York: Oxford University Press, 1986), esp. chaps. 4–6, and his *A Theory of Medical Ethics* (New York: Basic Books, 1981), chap. 11.

22. Engelhardt, *The Foundations of Bioethics,* chap. 8.

23. Public Law 99-272 (April 7, 1986), sec. 9121.

24. For more detail regarding these and other arguments, see Tom L. Beauchamp, "The Right to Health Care in a Capitalistic Democracy," in *The Right to Health Care,* ed. William Bondeson, H. Tristram Engelhardt, Jr., and Stuart Spicker (Boston: D. Reidel, 1989); and James F. Childress, "Rights to Health Care in a Democratic Society," in *Biomedical Ethics Reviews 1984,* ed. James Humber and Robert Almeder (Clifton, N.J.: Humana Press, 1984), pp. 47–70.

25. See Loren E. Lomasky, "Medical Progress and National Health Care," *Philosophy and Public Affairs* 10 (1980): 72–73; and Gary E. Jones, "The Right to Health Care and the State," *Philosophical Quarterly* 33 (1983): 278–87.

26. See Daniels, *Just Health Care,* chaps. 3 and 4.

27. Engelhardt, *The Foundations of Bioethics*, p. 340.
28. For issues of equal access, see President's Commission for the Study of Ethical Problems in Medicine and Biomedical and Behavioral Research, *Securing Access to Health Care: The Ethical Implications of Differences in the Availability of Health Services, Vol. I: Report* (Washington, D.C.: U.S. Government Printing Office, 1983), and *Securing Access to Health Care: The Ethical Implications of Differences in the Availability of Health Services, Vol. 2: Appendices, Sociocultural and Philosophical Studies* (Washington, D.C.: U.S. Government Printing Office, 1983). See esp. Allen Buchanan, "The Right to a Decent Minimum of Health Care," in Vol. II, pp. 207–38.
29. Veatch, *A Theory of Medical Ethics*, p. 275. See also his *The Foundations of Justice*. Veatch's theory is another extension of Rawls's theory, in the direction of strong egalitarianism. He uses the contractarian model rather than Rawls's substantive principles of justice and contends that this model generates a theory requiring equal distribution. In a Rawlsian spirit, this analysis concentrates health-care resources on the worst off.
30. Ronald Dworkin, *Taking Rights Seriously* (Cambridge, Mass.: Harvard University Press, 1977), p. xi.
31. Rawls, *A Theory of Justice*, p. 4.
32. Robert M. Veatch, "Voluntary Risks to Health: The Ethical Issues," *Journal of the American Medical Association* 243 (1980): 50–55. For other influential discussions, see Dan E. Beauchamp, "Public Health and Individual Liberty," *Annual Review of Public Health* 1 (1980): 121–36; and Daniel Wikler, "Persuasion and Coercion for Health: Ethical Issues in Government Efforts to Change Lifestyles," *Milbank Memorial Fund Quarterly/Health and Society* 56 (Summer 1978): 303–17. See also James F. Childress, *Who Should Decide? Paternalism in Health Care* (New York: Oxford University Press, 1982), chap. 8.
33. Several commentators contend that interest in containing the spiraling costs of health care was primary in the attention to prevention. See, for example, Howard Leichter, "Public Policy and the British Experience," *Hastings Center Report* 11 (October 1981): 32–39.
34. Ibid., p. 38.
35. Daniels, *Just Health Care*, p. 2.
36. Guido Calabresi and Philip Bobbitt, *Tragic Choices* (New York: W. W. Norton, 1978), pp. 196 et passim.
37. Paul Starr, "The Politics of Therapeutic Nihilism," *Hastings Center Report* 6 (October 1976): 23–30.
38. See Howard M. Leichter, *A Comparative Approach to Policy Analysis: Health Care Policy in Four Nations* (Cambridge: Cambridge University Press, 1979), chap. 6.
39. Elizabeth Telfer, "Justice, Welfare, and Health Care," *Journal of Medical Ethics* 2 (1976): 107–11.
40. For an overview and developments into 1986, see Task Force on Organ Transplantation, *Organ Transplantation: Issues and Recommendations*, April 1986, U.S. Department of Health and Human Services.
41. See the references provided in Case 33.
42. Task Force, *Organ Transplantation*, pp. 105, 11.
43. Roger W. Evans et al., *The National Health Transplantation Study* (Seattle: Battelle Human Affairs Research Centers, 1984). Vols. I–V.
44. Task Force, *Organ Transplantation*, p. 104.

45. Ibid., chap. 6.
46. See Paul Ramsey, *The Patient as Person* (New Haven, Conn.: Yale University Press, 1970), chap. 7.
47. In order to simplify matters, we do not consider chronic care at this point.
48. See Thomas Schelling, "The Life You Save May Be Your Own," in *Problems in Public Expenditure Analysis*, ed. Samuel B. Chase, Jr. (Washington: Brookings Institution, 1966), pp. 127–66.
49. Gene Outka, "Social Justice and Equal Access to Health Care," *Journal of Religious Ethics* 2 (Spring 1974): 24.
50. Roger W. Evans, Christopher R. Blagg, and Fred A. Bryan, Jr., "Implications for Health Policy: A Social and Demographic Profile of Hemodialysis Patients in the United States," *Journal of the American Medical Association* 245 (1981): 478–91.
51. President's Commission, *Securing Access to Health Care*, Vol. I, p. 42.
52. Richard Rettig and Kathleen Lohr, "Ethical Dimensions of Allocating Scarce Resources in Medicine: A Cross-National Case Study of End-stage Renal Disease" (draft proposal).
53. Henry J. Aaron and William B. Schwartz, *The Painful Prescription: Rationing Hospital Care* (Washington, D.C.: Brookings Institution, 1984); and William B. Schwartz and Henry J. Aaron, "Rationing Hospital Care: Lessons from Britain," *New England Journal of Medicine* 310 (1984): 52–56. For a critical response to their interpretation of the situation in Great Britain, see Frances H. Miller and Graham A. H. Miller, *"The Painful Prescription:* A Procrustean Perspective?" *New England Journal of Medicine* 314 (1986): 1383–86.
54. See Richard Zeckhauser, "Procedures for Valuing Lives," *Public Policy* 23 (Fall 1975): 447–48. Contrast Richard A. Rettig, "Valuing Lives: The Policy Debate on Patient Care Financing for Victims of End-Stage Renal Disease," *The Rand Paper Series* (Santa Monica, Calif: Rand Corporation, 1976).
55. Rawls, *A Theory of Justice.*
56. Nicholas Rescher, "The Allocation of Exotic Medical Lifesaving Therapy," *Ethics* 79 (1969): 173–86.
57. Task Force, *Organ Transplantation.*
58. For another case, see Andrew Schneider and Mary Pat Flaherty, "Woman Passed Over after 3-Year Wait," *Pittsburgh Press*, May 12, 1985, p. A10.
59. Task Force, *Organ Transplantation*, p. 95. The task force recommended that hearts and livers not be allocated to nonimmigrant aliens unless it was clear that no U.S. citizen or resident could use the organs. The different recommendations for renal and for extrarenal organs were based in part on the fact that there is no alternative or backup treatment for heart or liver failure in contrast to the availability of dialysis for most cases of end-stage kidney failure.
60. See James Childress, "Triage in Neonatal Intensive Care: The Limitations of a Metaphor," *Virginia Law Review* 69 (1983): 547–61.
61. Task Force, *Organ Transplantation*, chap. 5.
62. See A. J. Wing, "Why Don't the British Treat More Patients with Kidney Failure?" *British Medical Journal* 287 (1983): 1157; V. Parsons and P. Lock, "Triage and the Patient with Renal Failure," *Journal of Medical Ethics* 6 (1980): 173–76.
63. See Daniels, *Just Health Care.* For a full discussion and defense, within limits, of age as a criterion in rationing health care, see Daniel Callahan, *Setting Limits: Medical Goals in an Aging Society* (New York: Simon and Schuster, 1987). See

also James F. Childress, "Ensuring Care, Respect, and Fairness for the Elderly," *Hastings Center Report* 14 (October 1984): 27–31.

64. See *Report of the Massachusetts Task Force on Organ Transplantation* (October 1984).

65. See "Scarce Medical Resources," *Columbia Law Review* 69 (1969).

66. While holding that nonconsequentialist principles should generally not be balanced against consequentialist principles, Robert M. Veatch does concede that such a balancing might be necessary in order to avoid the conclusion that "a medically hopeless patient has a claim that exhausts all resources." Robert M. Veatch, "The Ethics of Resource Allocation in Critical Care," *Critical Care Clinics* 2 (January 1986): 73–89. Gerald Winslow offers a principle of "conservation" and John Kilner a principle of "disproportionate resources" to override in some cases the egalitarian principle of medical neediness. See Gerald Winslow, *Triage and Justice: The Ethics of Rationing Life-Saving Medical Resources* (Berkeley: University of California Press, 1982); and John Kilner, "A Moral Allocation of Scarce Lifesaving Medical Resources," *Journal of Religious Ethics* 9 (Fall 1981): 264.

67. H. Tristram Engelhardt, Jr., and Michael A. Rie, "Intensive Care Units, Scarce Resources, and Conflicting Principles of Justice," *Journal of the American Medical Association* 255 (1986): 1159–64. For other discussions of rationing intensive care, see Michael J. Strauss et al., "Rationing of Intensive Care Unit Services," and William A. Knaus, "Rationing, Justice, and the American Physician," both in *Journal of the American Medical Association* 255 (1986): 1143–46, 1176–77.

68. The amount of the award was more than twelve million dollars, and the supreme court of Florida returned the case for retrial because four million dollars of the award had been for pain and suffering. *Von Stetina* v. *Florida Medical Center*, 2 Fla. Supp. 2d 55 (Fla. 17th Cir 1982), 436 So. Rptr. 2d 1022 (1983), *Florida Law Weekly* 10 (May 24, 1985): 286. This case is discussed by Engelhardt and Rie, "Intensive Care Units."

69. *The Totally Implantable Artificial Heart*, p. 198.

70. Engelhardt and Rie, "Intensive Care Units."

71. Task Force, *Organ Transplantation*, p. 89.

72. See Ramsey, *The Patient as Person*, pp. 257–58.

73. Rescher, "The Allocation of Exotic Medical Lifesaving Therapy," p. 178.

74. See James F. Childress, "Who Shall Live When Not All Can Live?" *Soundings* 53 (1970): 339–55; James F. Childress, "Rationing of Medical Treatment," in *The Encyclopedia of Bioethics*, ed. Warren T. Reich (New York: Macmillan/Free Press, 1978); George J. Annas, "Allocation of Artificial Hearts in the Year 2002: 'Minerva v. National Health Agency,' " *American Journal of Law and Medicine* 3 (Spring 1977): 59–76; Kilner, "A Moral Allocation of Scarce Lifesaving Medical Resources"; Ramsey, *The Patient as Person;* and Winslow, *Triage and Justice.*

75. See Winslow, *Triage and Justice.*

7

Professional-Patient Relationships

In the previous four chapters we developed four moral principles applicable to scientific research, medicine, and health care. In this chapter we apply these principles to establish rules of veracity, privacy, confidentiality, and fidelity. We then use these rules to analyze various relationships between health-care professionals or researchers on the one hand and their patients or subjects on the other. Some of these rules are grounded in a single principle, while others are grounded in several principles.[1]

Rules of veracity

Surprisingly, codes of medical ethics generally ignore rules of veracity. The Hippocratic oath does not impose obligations of veracity, nor does the Declaration of Geneva of the World Medical Association. The Principles of Medical Ethics of the American Medical Association in effect from 1957 to 1980 made no mention of an obligation of veracity; presumably a member physician had unlimited discretion about what to divulge to patients. In its 1980 revision of the Principles of Medical Ethics, the AMA held that the physician should "deal honestly with patients and colleagues." The uncertainties and ambiguities in these guidelines lead to questions about the content and weight of general rules of veracity.

In contrast to the codes, it is commonly agreed that we have an obligation of veracity, an obligation to tell the truth and not to lie or to deceive others.

But, as Henry Sidgwick observed many years ago, "It does not seem clearly agreed whether Veracity is an absolute and independent obligation, or a special application of some higher principle."[2] One contemporary philosopher, G. J. Warnock, includes veracity as an independent principle ranking with beneficence, nonmaleficence, and justice.[3] Others have held that rules of veracity are derived from the principles of respect for autonomy, fidelity, or utility. We maintain, in Sidgwick's language, that obligations of veracity involve a special application of several principles.

Arguments for rules of veracity

Three arguments for the obligation of veracity are applicable to relationships between health-care professionals and patients. The first argument is that the obligation of veracity is part of the respect we owe to others. As we saw in Chapter 3, this respect is commonly expressed in biomedical ethics through the principle of respect for autonomy, which is the foundation of rules of disclosure and consent. An act of consent cannot express autonomy unless it is informed, and it therefore depends on truthful communication. Even if informed consent is not an issue, the obligation of veracity may be derived from the principle of respect for autonomy. As Alan Donagan writes (in discussing respect for persons):

Relations between human beings are largely carried on by means of language; and much of what is communicated in language consists of expressions of opinion about what is the case. Unless it is required by a specific moral precept, nobody has a right to know another's opinion. The respect owed to other human beings includes respect for their liberty to withhold their thoughts when it is not their duty to divulge them; but, if anybody chooses to divulge his thoughts, the respect he owes to his audience requires that the thoughts he communicates must really be his.[4]

Second, the obligation of veracity also derives from obligations of fidelity or promise keeping.[5] When we communicate with others, we implicitly promise that we will speak truthfully, that we will not lie by misrepresenting our opinions, and that we will not deceive our listeners. Our willing participation in these conventions, governed as they are by a social contract, engenders an obligation of veracity. In biomedical contexts, it is sometimes possible to point to a specific, although implicit, contract or promise. By entering into a relationship in therapy or research, the patient or subject enters into a contract, thereby gaining a special right to the truth regarding diagnosis, prognosis, procedures, and the like—just as the professional gains a right to truthful disclosures from patients. We will later discuss several implications of this argument when we examine rules of fidelity.

Third, relationships of trust between persons are necessary for fruitful interaction and cooperation. At the core of these relationships is confidence in and reliance on others to respect rules of veracity. Relationships between health-care professionals and their patients or between researchers and their subjects ultimately depend on trust, and adherence to rules of veracity is essential to maintain this trust.

Lying and failures of adequate disclosure, then, fail to show respect for persons and their autonomy, violate implicit contracts, and also threaten relationships based on trust.[6] But like other obligations in this volume, veracity is prima facie, not absolute. Nondisclosure, deception, and lying will occasionally be justified when veracity conflicts with other obligations.

Conceptual problems

These moral debates about veracity involve conceptual problems as well as problems of moral justification. Some of these conceptual problems are definitional, whereas others concern the scope of the term *veracity*.

Consider, for example, the meaning of *lying* (as an extension of our analysis in Chapter 2). We define lying as telling another person what one believes to be false in order to deceive that person. So understood, lying is prima facie wrong and can be justified in some circumstances. If, however, lying is defined as intentionally withholding the truth from a person who has an absolute right to it, then lying is absolutely wrong. The latter definition "resolves" moral dilemmas by redefining them, because some statements that would be described as lies according to our definition would not be lies according to this definition.

Rules of veracity include the obligation not to deceive others as well as the obligation not to lie. Forms of deception that stand to violate obligations of truth telling include giving placebos, intentionally deceiving patients for their own benefit, and the manipulation of information, as described in Chapter 3. Although the weight of various obligations of veracity is difficult to determine outside specific contexts, some generalizations may be tendered. Deception that does not involve lying is generally less difficult to justify than lying, because it does not as deeply threaten the relationship of trust between deceiver and deceived as does lying. Underdisclosure and nondisclosure are still less difficult to justify in many contexts. By contrast to the obligation not to lie and the obligation not to deceive, the obligation to disclose (as examined in Chapter 3) usually depends on special relationships between the parties involved. For example, the patient entrusts care to the clinician and thereby obtains a right to information that the clinician would not otherwise be obligated to provide. It is, we suggest, advisable not to conflate these various obligations to disclose information, not to lie, and not to deceive, although much of the literature treats them as a single obligation.

Many subtleties about the nature of veracity are present in discussions of these obligations. As with informed consent, courts of law have typically assimilated obligations of veracity to obligations of disclosure. Generally the obligation of veracity in law is an obligation to disclose that applies to procedures to which patients consent. But this conception is clearly too narrow for biomedical ethics. Veracity refers to the comprehensiveness, accuracy, and objectivity with which information is handled, as well as the manner in which understanding is fostered in the relationship. Consent may not be a factor.

In at least one important case—*Truman* v. *Thomas*[7]—an influential court permitted the children of a woman who died from cervical cancer to sue her doctor for failing to disclose the risks of not undergoing the Pap smear test, which she had reportedly refused. The court held that the patient must be apprised of risks of "a decision *not* to undergo the treatment," as well as the "risks inherent in the procedure." This obligation of veracity to disclose the risks of no treatment resembles the well-established obligation to disclose alternatives to a proposed procedure. In many instances, no treatment is an alternative to the procedure proposed. Thus, the risks of doing nothing are likely to fall within the scope of the physician's obligation to disclose information about any proffered procedure.

If one accepts this obligation as fixed in routine practice—as we do, at least from the moral point of view—*Truman* said nothing new. What was new in this case was the application of a disclosure obligation even if the patient refuses a physician's recommendation and there has been no bodily intrusion. The court held that the importance of the right to make decisions about one's body is not diminished by the kind of decision one makes, reasoning that no other result is consistent with the fiduciary nature of the physician's obligation to present the proper information. We can generalize this conclusion in the moral context by noting that veracity in medical practice can pertain to any truthful and honest management of information that stands to affect a patient's understanding or decision making. It is not limited to situations in which informed consent is sought.

Arguments for limited disclosure and deception

In Chapter 3, we considered some conditions that must be satisfied in order to justify deception and incomplete disclosure in research. Those conditions were so narrowly drawn that most biomedical and social-science research involving intentional deception would be unjustified. Nevertheless, we held that some low-risk research involving minor deception or incomplete disclosure could be justified if the undisclosed information would have invalidated the research had it been disclosed. (See pp. 96–99). We also considered when the "therapeutic privilege" is applicable, as well as when other paternalistic deception or incomplete disclosure is justifiable, all in the context of consent to and refusal of medical procedures.

Issues of veracity, limited disclosure, and deception are not limited to these contexts of consent and refusal. For example, provision of information regarding diagnosis and prognosis may have no role in a process of consent or refusal. The most widely discussed cases of disclosing or withholding information involve the diagnosis of cancer and the prognosis of imminent death where no further procedures are available. In Case 4 a fifty-four-year-old male patient consented to surgery for probable malignant cell transformation in his thyroid gland. After the surgery, Mr. X was told that the diagnosis had been confirmed and that the tumor had been successfully removed, but he was not informed that there was a likelihood of lung metastases and death within a few months. Although his wife, son, and daughter-in-law were well informed by the physician, they and the physician agreed to conceal the diagnosis and prognosis from Mr. X. He was told only that he needed "preventive" treatment, and he consented to irradiation and chemotherapy. He was not informed of the probable cause of his subsequent shortness of breath and back pain. And he was not given a chance to discuss his impending death, because everyone pretended that he would soon recover. He died three months later.[8]

Over the last thirty years, there has been a dramatic shift in physicians' stated policies of disclosure of the diagnosis of cancer to patients. In 1961, eighty-eight percent of the physicians surveyed had a policy of not disclosing a diagnosis of cancer to the patient, while in 1979 ninety-eight percent of those surveyed had a policy of telling the cancer patient.[9] Although it is more difficult to determine actual practices of disclosure, changes in physicians' stated policies of disclosure of a diagnosis of cancer are well documented. The reasons for the changes include the availability of more treatment options for cancer (including experimental treatments), improved rates of survival from some forms of cancer, fear of malpractice suits, involvement of several professionals in health care in hospitals, altered societal attitudes about cancer, and increased attention to patients' rights, including rights to information.[10]

Sometimes it is unclear whether the physicians believe that the obligation of disclosure is directed at the patient or at the family. The 1979 study reveals a significant ambiguity about the role of the patient's wishes and of the family's wishes in withholding information about cancer. According to the physicians surveyed, the four factors "most frequently believed to be of special importance" in deciding whether to tell the cancer patient were the patient's expressed wish to be told (fifty-two percent), emotional stability (twenty-one percent), age (eleven percent), and intelligence (ten percent). The first poses no problem, because acting on the competent patient's wishes is prima facie required by the principle of respect for autonomy. The other three factors could be relevant in determining whether the patient is autonomous or nonautonomous, and thus whether nondisclosure or partial disclosure would be inconsistent with the principle of respect for autonomy. However, in the same survey, physicians identified the "four most frequent factors considered in the decision to tell the patient as age (fifty-six percent), a relative's wishes regarding disclosure to the patient (fifty-one percent), emotional stability (forty-seven percent), and intelligence (forty-four percent).[11]

Three of the four factors on each list are identical, but one list has the patient's wishes while the other includes the family's wishes. From our standpoint, familial preferences tend to be unjustifiably influential in clinicians' decisions about disclosure of diagnosis and prognosis to patients. For an example, see Case 7, in which a patient's daughters demanded that the nurse provide false reassurance when the patient inquired whether everything was all right after an operation for a cancerous tumor that had metastasized (and about which she knew nothing). Critics of our position may contend that the family can help the physician determine whether the patient is autonomous, can receive information about serious risk, and really wants the information. But this response begs an important question: By what right did the physician initially disclose information to the family without the patient's consent? The family provides important and desired care and support for many patients, but the autonomous patient—and the adult patient should be presumed to be autonomous in the absence of conflicting evidence—has the moral right to veto familial involvement. The best policy is to ask the patient both at the outset and as the illness progresses about the extent to which he or she wants to share information and to involve others in the disclosure or decision-making process.

In the literature on the justification of limited disclosure and deception in therapeutic settings, three arguments have emerged. These arguments are particularly (although not exclusively) directed at contexts in which consent or refusal is not at issue.[12] These arguments all assume that although breaches of rules of veracity are prima facie wrong, they can sometimes be justified.

The first argument for nondisclosure of some diagnoses and prognoses in the therapeutic setting represents what Henry Sidgwick calls "benevolent deception." It holds that disclosure of a diagnosis of cancer, for example, might violate the obligations of beneficence and nonmaleficence by causing the patient anxiety, by leading the patient to commit suicide, and the like. This general line of argument—"What you don't know can't hurt and may help you"—is consequentialist and previously appeared in our discussion of paternalism in Chapter 5. One objection to his argument is based on the uncertainty of predicting consequences. As Samuel Johnson put it:

I deny the lawfulness of telling a lie to a sick man for fear of alarming him. You have no business with consequences; you are to tell the truth. Besides, you are not sure what effects your telling him that he is in danger may have. It may bring his distemper to a crisis, and that may cure him. Of all lying, I have the greatest abhorrence of this, because I believe it has been frequently practised on myself.[13]

Objections to benevolent deception often stress violations of the principles of respect for autonomy and rules of fidelity, as well as the long-term threat to the relationship of trust between physicians and patients. These are strong reasons for caution. Whereas it is sometimes sufficient to justify the use of deceptive means by the end of the health of the patient, alternative nondeceptive means are generally more satisfactory, and blanket appeals to benevolent deception are clearly inexcusable. The prima facie obligation of veracity demands a search for alternatives even if they sometimes require more time, energy, and financial resources. Furthermore, on utilitarian grounds deception may have long-term negative effects on the patient's self-image and may threaten trust in health-care professionals. Thus, although we accept benevolent deception in a narrow range of cases, its invocation should be infrequent. Similar constraints apply to deception intended to protect parties other than the one deceived.

A second argument for nondisclosure and deception is that health-care professionals cannot know, let alone communicate, the "whole truth," and if they could, many patients and subjects would not be able to comprehend and understand the "whole truth." This argument, however, should not be allowed to undermine the obligation of veracity, understood as the obligation to be truthful.[14] The "whole truth" is a useful concept only in the way infinity is useful in mathematics. Disclosing the whole truth is an ideal against which health-care professionals can measure their performance. But it can only be approximated, never reached; and we can best use this ideal to help formulate a standard of substantial completeness that is both realistic and binding for health-care professionals. As discussed in Chapter 3, the obligation of truthful disclosure requires that health-care professionals disclose as fully as possible what a reasonable patient would want to know and what particular patients want to know.

A third argument for nondisclosure and deception is that some patients, particularly the very sick and the dying, do not want to know the truth about their condition, despite the conclusions of opinion surveys that they do want to know. According to this argument, neither the obligation of fidelity nor the obligation of respect for autonomy requires truth telling, because patients indicate by various signals—if not by actual words—that they do not want the truth. To the rejoinder that many, and perhaps most, patients say they want disclosure of relevant information, proponents of this third argument hold that the patients they have in mind really do not want to know when they say they do.

Claims about what patients really want when they contradict the patients' own reports are inherently dubious, and this third argument sets dangerous precedents for paternalistic actions under the guise of respect for autonomy. However, occasionally there is good evidence (not fragile inference) that patients do not want to know. For example, patients who suspect that they might have cancer explicitly ask not to be informed of the diagnosis and prognosis, and some patients with a high risk of developing Huntington's disease, an incurable, debilitating, and fatal genetic disease, indicate that they would not be interested in a simple, safe, and reliable predictive test. In one sample, twenty-three percent of the high-risk respondents indicated that they might not take such a test.[15] Although studies generally indicate that the majority of people at risk would want to undergo a similar test,[16] in the early phases of a clinical trial of presymptomatic predictive test for Huntington's disease, only twelve percent of the at-risk individuals who were contacted were willing to participate in a trial of a test that was shown to be ninety-five percent accurate in preclinical studies.[17] Various reasons may account for these discrepancies. For example, individuals at risk may view a predictive test with ninety-five percent probability as insufficiently accurate and may not want to involve other family members who would be required for this genetic linkage test.

Disclosure of unwanted or unrequested information

Some writers go so far as to suggest that a patient has an obligation to seek and appropriate the truth, not merely a right to the truth.[18] This claim may be sustainable, but it does not follow that we have a right to force unwanted information on a patient for his or her benefit, an act that may violate that patient's autonomy rights and may constitute an act of disrespect. Coercion of information on an unreceptive patient can on occasion be justified—as when a person is acting on false beliefs—but only rarely. Persons generally should be free to exercise the right not to know when they are adequately informed about the risks of doing so, are acting autonomously, and are not putting others at risk.

In the debate about screening for Huntington's disease, Margery Shaw stresses that at-risk patients have a right to know and a correlative right not to know, but she also contends that the at-risk individual has "an ethical duty to know whether or not he or she is a carrier" in circumstances where a third party might be harmed by the lack of knowledge.[19] These circumstances include contemplating or not preventing reproduction because of the moral obligation to spouse and offspring. In addition, because the current test involves the need to test other relatives, including siblings, aunts, uncles, and cousins, it is possible to argue that relatives also have a moral obligation to participate, based on the principle of beneficence. However, these moral obligations should not be translated into legal obligations under current technologies and risks.

Another good test case for the right to impose information has arisen from the AIDS epidemic. The right not to know has appropriately been challenged when people, such as those donating blood, have tested antibody-positive for HIV (human immunodeficiency virus), the retrovirus that causes AIDS. Those who have positive test results should be told about their status, even if they do not want to know and seek to avoid disclosure. Although persons with positive test results might not benefit because there is no known effective treatment for the prevention of AIDS-related complex (ARC) or for AIDS itself after infection with the virus (it is now believed that virtually all who are antibody-positive will go on to develop ARC or AIDS), it is argued that they should be told so that they can avoid imposing the risk of AIDS on others.[20] We concur with this argument on grounds of the obligation of nonmaleficence.

In one case a thirty-five-year-old man who had engaged in homosexual activities went to a physician because of symptoms consistent with infection with HIV, and he consented to have his blood tested for HIV antibodies. However, the next day the patient called to say that he had changed his mind and wanted to cancel the test. But the test had already been completed, and the physician, who had been notified that the patient did not want to know the results, decided to tell the patient that he had been infected with HIV in order to reduce the risks for others who could be infected through sexual contact.[21]

A further problem concerns a health-care professional's responsibility when a test undertaken for a specific purpose reveals information not specifically requested by the testee, who might, however, be interested in receiving the information. In one case a forty-one-year-old woman had unexpectedly become pregnant and was referred by her physician to the human genetics unit in order to determine whether her fetus might have Down syndrome.[22] Because of her age, she was considered at increased risk of having a child with Down syndrome. The woman underwent amniocentesis, a procedure in which a sample of amniotic fluid surrounding the fetus is withdrawn by a needle for purposes of a biochemical or chromosomal analysis. The test showed that the fetus did not have Down syndrome; there was no extra twenty-first chromosome. But the sex chromosomes were abnormal. They were XYY rather than the normal patterns of XX for female or XY for male. There is debate about the significance of the extra Y chromosome. Although some studies show that XYY males tend to commit more violent crimes, other studies reject those findings. What should the genetic counselor do? Would the counselor fulfill the obligations of fidelity and veracity if he or she reported only that the fetus did not suffer from Down syndrome? Or is the counselor also morally required to report the other findings? Does the woman have a right to this information if she did not specifically request it? That the causal connection between the XYY chromosomes and antisocial behavior is disputed makes this disclosure more risky, because it could lead the woman to choose an abortion or could be a self-fulfilling prophecy if the woman did not abort and the parents and others subsequently treated the child as potentially antisocial. The fundamental question is whether the pregnant woman should have the right to make her own decision about the significance of this information.

If the obligation of veracity is based on respect for persons and their autonomy, as we believe it is, a strong case can be made for disclosure, although the woman did not specifically request this information. The counselor should also indicate the uncertainty about the significance of the extra Y chromosome while conveying the information carefully and sensitively. Attitudes toward abortion may also affect the counselor's response. However, if a woman has a legal right to have an abortion within the first two trimesters whatever her reasons, it would seem unfair to deprive her of information that she might consider relevant.

Disclosures about colleagues and patients

Another problem of veracity and disclosure is presented by incompetent or un-scrupulous health-care professionals. The current AMA Principles of Medical Ethics require disclosure of information in order to preserve trust between the public and the medical profession: "A physician shall deal honestly with pa-tients and colleagues, and strive to expose those physicians deficient in char-acter or competence, or who engage in fraud or deception." Exposés by fellow physicians are, however, uncommon. The bond of loyalty to the profession, so accented in the Hippocratic and "gentlemanly" traditions of medical ethics, presents a formidable barrier. On the basis of studies of professional ethics and competence, it is difficult to believe that all or most cases of deficiency in character or competence are disclosed to the proper bodies or to the public.

Another important area is the "wall of silence" surrounding medical mal-practice, particularly in situations where the patient may be unaware that he or she is the victim of malpractice but members of the treatment team or consul-tants are aware of the problem. A physician may make a mistake, such as a technical or judgmental error, in a particular case, without being deficient in character or competence.[23] Even if there is a situation of further treatment, and hence the need for information for decision making, it might be argued that this information about the cause of part of the medical problem is unnecessary. But this argument takes an indefensibly narrow view of respect for autonomy in the physician-patient relationship, inasmuch as people have to make other sorts of decisions including whether to sue for malpractice. Justice in the dis-tribution of benefits and burdens (the subject of Chapter 6) may also require disclosure so that the injured patient can claim his or her due.

In one case a boy, age three and a half, was taken by his parents to a medical center for treatment of a respiratory problem. After being placed in the adult intensive care unit, he was given ten times the normal dosage of muscle relax-ant, and the respirator tube slipped and pumped oxygen into his stomach for several minutes. He suffered cardiac arrest and permanent brain damage. The parents accidentally overheard a conversation that mentioned the overdose. The physician involved explained that he had decided not to inform the parents of the mistake because they "had enough on [their] minds already."[24] Some commentators have even suggested a legally imposed obligation on both the primary physician and observing members of the treatment team to report malpractice to the victim, not simply to organizations that examine physician competence.[25]

In addition to loyalty to colleagues, which may conflict with the obligation to disclose information about colleagues, the physician may also experience a conflict between the obligation of confidentiality and the obligation of veracity. This form of conflict is evident in Case 3. After tests have shown that he is histocompatible, a father decides that he does not want to donate a kidney to his five-year-old daughter who needs a transplant. Because he fears that the truth might shatter his family, he asks the physician to lie by telling the members of his family that he is not histocompatible. The physician then tells the family that, "for medical reasons," the father should not donate a kidney. It is possible to analyze this case in utilitarian terms of maximizing good and minimizing harm, but it is also reasonable to maintain that the father's relationship with the physician was confidential and that the obligation to respect confidentiality outweighed the obligation of veracity. Some would argue that in this case the obligation of confidentiality justifies nondisclosure and even deception but does not justify lying if the wife were to press the physician for an explanation of "medical reasons." We will return to these problems of confidentiality after analyzing the closely related topic of privacy.

Rules of privacy

When syndicated columnist Jack Anderson reported that Roy Cohn, a lawyer, was being treated for AIDS in an experimental trial of the drug AZT (azidothymidine) at the National Institutes of Health, critics of the report accused Anderson of violations of the right of privacy and the right of confidentiality.[26] They argued that some health-care professionals, perhaps with legitimate access to medical records at NIH, had violated Cohn's rights of privacy and confidentiality by releasing information to Anderson, who again violated Cohn's right of privacy by publishing the report.

Debates about the basis and limits of rules of privacy and confidentiality pervade controversies about control of the spread of AIDS. On the one hand, proposals to screen individuals to determine whether they are antibody-positive for HIV threaten their privacy. On the other hand, physicians ponder the limits and applicability of rules of confidentiality when AIDS patients refuse to inform their spouses or lovers of their condition. An example of the latter conflict—analogous in several respects to the Tarasoff case—is Case 2, in which a patient who is antibody-positive for HIV infection refuses to warn his wife.

Questions of rights of privacy and confidentiality (or, correlatively, obligations to respect privacy and confidentiality) have appeared in many areas of biomedicine—for example, in screening employees in the workplace for genetic diseases and for use of illicit drugs. Privacy and confidentiality are often discussed together, as in federal regulations that require protection of privacy and confidentiality in research involving human subjects and in the American Nursing Association Code of Ethics, which requires nurses to safeguard ''the client's right to privacy by judiciously protecting information of a confidential nature.'' Despite this common association, privacy and confidentiality are distinct concepts that only partially overlap. We begin with privacy.

In the history of moral and legal theory, privacy received little explicit attention until late in the nineteenth century, when J. F. Stephen defended a sphere of privacy against state interventions, and two legal scholars argued for a right of privacy in an influential article in the *Harvard Law Review*.[27] The U.S. Supreme Court early in the 1920s employed an expansive ''liberty'' interest to protect family decision making about various issues, including child rearing and education.[28] The Court later switched to the term *privacy* and expanded the individual's and the family's protected interest in family life, child rearing, and other areas of personal choice.[29] The clearest and most modern expression of this privacy right has come in the Court's family-planning decisions. *Griswold* v. *Connecticut* (1965), a case dealing with contraception, was the first to discuss the right of privacy as not merely shielding information from others but as creating a zone of protected activity within which the individual is free from governmental interference. According to this modern legal inerpretation, the right to privacy protects liberty by delineating a zone of private life—including, for example, family-planning decisions—within which the individual is free to choose and act. The Court's decision in this case overturned state legislation that prohibited the use or dissemination of contraceptives, and in 1973 the Court invoked this right to overturn restrictive abortion laws.[30]

Although not explicitly enumerated in the Bill of Rights, the right of privacy is now generally thought by the Supreme Court to arise from the ''penumbra' of the first, ninth, and fourteenth amendments to the Constitution. But an individual holds the right, like other constitutional rights, only against the state and against parties acting on behalf of the state—not against other individuals or nongovernmental entities. It may seem inapposite to make this personal right one of privacy rather than liberty or autonomy, but it can be understood as a right to maintain certain activities as private in the sense that they are not subject to governmental oversight or intrusion. The constitutional right of privacy shields certain personal information, choices, and activities from governmental imposition. This right is still an inchoate notion, no doubt in process of further development in the law.[31] Of special relevance to biomedical ethics is the appeal to the right to privacy since the mid-1970s as a legal and constitutional basis for termination of life-sustaining treatments (see the *Quinlan* case in Chapter 4).

However, frequent invocation in law, ethics, or public discourse does not guarantee clarity, and the issues are complicated by several competing conceptions of privacy. At the same time, there are disagreements regarding the grounds, limits, and weight of a right to privacy. In this section we discuss first the conceptual problems and then the justification and limits of rules of privacy.

The concept of privacy

For our purposes, *privacy* may be defined as "a state or condition of limited access to a person."[32] A person has privacy if others do not have or do not use access to him or her. Several definitions (including our own in the second edition of this book) focus on the agent's control or rightful control over access to himself or herself. These definitions confuse privacy, which is a state or condition, with either control over privacy or the right to privacy, which involves the agent's rightful control over access. A person may have privacy without having any control over access, as occurs when others ignore the person. In modern society the condition of privacy often results from sheer indifference.

The criterion of limited access to a person needs further specification. Discussions of privacy often focus on limited or restricted access to information about a person, but privacy should not be defined in terms of limited access to information. A loss of privacy occurs if others use various forms of access to a person, including intervening in zones of intimacy, secrecy, anonymity, or solitude.[33] These and many other forms of access are included when we speak of limited access. The person in our definition includes the body and its associated parts—including the voice and bodily products and objects intimately associated with the person. Privacy as limited access to a person also extends to the person's intimate relationships with friends, lovers, spouses, physicians, and the like.

A person's privacy (or loss of privacy) should not be confused with a person's sense of privacy (or sense of loss of privacy). A person may have privacy while wrongly believing that someone is eavesdropping, or a person may unknowingly have lost some measure of privacy when someone discovers a personal diary and discloses its contents to others. What counts as a loss of privacy and affects an individual's sense of loss of privacy can also vary from society to society and individual to individual. One reason is that no particular item is intrinsically private.[34] The value we place on a condition of limited access explains how it comes to be categorized as private. A loss of privacy may also depend not only on the kind or amount of access but also on who has access through what means to which aspect of the person. As Charles Fried notes:

We may not mind that a person knows a general fact about us, and yet feel our privacy invaded if he knows the details. For instance, a casual acquaintance may comfortably know that I am sick, but it would violate my privacy if he knew the nature of the illness. Or a good friend may know what particular illness I am suffering from, but it would violate my privacy if he were actually to witness my suffering from some symptom which he must know is associated with the disease.[35]

The justification and limits of rules of privacy

In their celebrated article on "The Right to Privacy,"[36] Warren and Brandeis argue that a legal right to privacy can be derived from the fundamental rights to life, liberty, and property. Rather than basing it on rights of liberty and property, they derive it largely from the right to life, using an extended sense to include "the right to enjoy life—the right to be let alone." They also view this right as reflecting the principle of "an inviolate personality." In recent discussions several other types of justification of the right to privacy have been prominent, three of which deserve our attention.

One approach reduces the right to privacy to a cluster of other rights. Judith Thomson contends that the right to privacy is "derivative" in this sense: It is possible to explain each right in the cluster without at any point mentioning the right to privacy and to explain the wrongness of every violation of the right to privacy without mentioning it.[37] This cluster of personal and property rights includes rights not to be looked at, not to be listened to, not to be caused distress (e.g., by the publication of certain information), not to be tortured (e.g., to get certain information), and so on. Although it is plausible to hold that the right to privacy overlaps other rights and that it is rarely claimed unless other interests and values are at stake, Thomson's argument rests on several allegedly foundational rights that have an uncertain status, such as the right not to be looked at. We are not convinced that each of these alleged rights is a right, but, more importantly, some of these rights may have the right to privacy as their basis, rather than the converse.

Another and more promising approach emphasizes the instrumental value of privacy and the right to privacy by identifying various ends that are served by rules of privacy. Different consequentialist theories, including utilitarianism, justify rules of privacy according to their instrumental value for ends that include individual development and intimate social relations. Charles Fried argues that privacy is a necessary condition—"the necessary atmosphere"—for intimate relationships: "It is my thesis that privacy is not just one possible means among others to insure some other value, but that it is necessarily related to ends and relations of the most fundamental sort: respect, love, friendship and trust. . . . Privacy is not merely a good technique for furthering these fundamental relations; rather without privacy they are simply inconceivable.''[38]

There can be little doubt that privacy has an instrumental value. We grant others access to ourselves in order to have and maintain such relationships as love, friendship, trust, and the variety of intimate social relationships with others that we desire. Whether some aspect of our lives is someone else's prerogative to know thus will depend on the relationships we permit in order to realize our goals. For example, we allow physicians to gain access in order to protect our health.

But does the instrumental value of privacy express its only value? Is this value the only justification of rules of privacy? Although both of the above rationales for rules of privacy are important, we believe the primary justification resides in the principle of respect for autonomy. For example, we often respect persons by respecting their autonomous wishes not to be observed or touched. Rights of privacy, then, are protections against unauthorized access to and reports about the person. Joel Feinberg has observed that the language of autonomy has a history as a political metaphor referring to a domain or territory in which a state is sovereign. Personal autonomy carries over the idea of having a domain or territory of sovereignty for the self and a right to protect it—an idea closely linked to the ideas of privacy and the right to privacy. The personal domain includes its spatial dimensions—the persons's body. Thus, the principle of respect for autonomy includes the right to decide insofar as possible what may happen to one's body. By emphasizing the spatial and territorial model, Feinberg is able to enlarge the conception of the personal domain to include ''a certain amount of 'breathing space' around one's body.'' Other metaphors expressing privacy in the personal domain include zones and spheres of privacy that express and protect autonomy.[39]

One possible objection to our use of respect for autonomy as the justificatory basis of rules of privacy is the following. Suppose that a patient in a hospital leaves a sealed note for a night nurse. A physician who suspects a conspiracy between the two not to follow a prescribed regimen opens and reads the note while the patient is asleep. The patient's privacy has been violated, but where is the violation of autonomy? If there is no disrespect for autonomy, then it would seem that the right to privacy is not based on respect for autonomy. But there is a violation. Respect for the patient's autonomy requires that no one reads the note without being autonomously authorized to do so by the patient. Reading the note without consent is as much a violation of autonomy as proceeding to surgery without consent. In this way, any such violation of a right of privacy is a violation of a right of autonomy.

A second possible objection to an autonomy-based derivation of rules of privacy focuses on the incompetent patient who cannot exercise autonomy, such as the patient in a permanent vegetative state.[40] The nonautonomous patient has not lost the right of privacy. We can view some dimensions of the right to privacy as flowing from a person's previous exercise of autonomy, but even patients who have never been autonomous have rights of privacy, such as the rights not to be needlessly viewed or touched by others. It seems intuitively correct to say that it is a violation of privacy to leave a comatose person undraped on a cart in the hospital corridor, not merely a tasteless act of negligence.

Yet it is difficult to explicate, on our theory or any available theory, why the offense is a violation of rules of privacy rather than rules of tastelessness. One argument is based on beneficence and nonmaleficence to others, including the family. Failure to protect such patients' "privacy" would offend these parties. This justification invokes instrumentalist reasons in support of rules of privacy. An alternative (although not one that we pursue or defend here) is to emphasize a broader view of respect for persons than respect for their autonomy and to assign derivative rights of privacy to nonautonomous persons through a general standard of respect for human dignity.

When a person voluntarily grants others access to himself or herself, it is preferable to see the act as an exercise of the right to privacy rather than as a waiver of the right. Consider, for example, a patient's decision to grant the physician access for diagnostic, prognostic, and therapeutic procedures. The decision to grant access is an exercise of a right to control access that parallels a decision to exclude access. The different kinds of access do not alter this conclusion. For example, a physician may need to take a personal history involving our private activities, touch our bodies, observe our bodies directly or through various instruments, listen to our bodies, run tests on our blood, and so on. With a psychotherapist we may have to expose our innermost thoughts, emotions, dreams, and fantasies. Here we exercise the right to privacy by reducing privacy with the intention of gaining other important goals through the health-care system.

Granting others access to oneself may involve implicit as well as explicit consent. By entering the public realm—for example, by walking down a public street—a person implicitly consents to some access by others. Upon voluntary admission to a hospital, a patient gives both explicit and implicit consent to limited losses of privacy, although the patient's decision to enter the hospital does not grant or imply unlimited access. Unfortunately, the limits of access are often not well understood by the different parties. For example, few patients understand the extent of their potential loss of privacy when they enter a teaching hospital, where professionals in training may seek access to them for reasons that have nothing to do with their care. In order to protect autonomy and privacy, it is advisable to disclose information about teaching hospitals to entering patients as part of the consent process, and in such contexts patients should also have the right to restrict some access of professionals and students not involved in their care. (These issues are examined later in this chapter, on pp. 346–47.)

Indefensible paternalism

We are occasionally justified in overriding rules of privacy in order to protect other moral objectives, although it is usually possible for society to handle conflicts by protecting zones of privacy that cannot be invaded, while distinguishing other zones where conduct that would offend in a public setting is prohibited. Some reasons that have been offered for overriding the right of privacy in medicine are indefensibly paternalistic. An example is found in H. J. McCloskey's argument that

respect for privacy would seem to be dictated by respect for persons only in that persons commonly wish their privacy to be respected, hence in so far as we ignore such wishes, without good reason, to that extent we show lack of respect. If we have good reason to ignore a person's wishes, for example, if we suspect that he is concealing a tumor which is now operable but will soon become inoperable and fatal, we are showing no lack of respect in intruding on his privacy in this matter.[41]

This intrusion does, in our judgment, infringe rules of privacy as well as the principle of respect for autonomy (in the autonomous patient). We argued in Chapter 5 that it is difficult but not impossible to justify paternalistic infringements of a person's right to privacy. In the sort of case envisioned by McCloskey, it may sometimes be justified to override the person's right of privacy, at least temporarily, in order to make a better diagnosis or to determine whether the person is autonomous. But we invoke the wrong premises and argument if we act as if there is no infringement of privacy and no disrespect for autonomy.

To justifiably override rights of privacy, it is necessary to show that it is more important in the circumstances to abide by other moral principles and rules, that these other principles and rules could probably be successfully followed by infringing the right of privacy, that they could not be realized or expressed without an invasion of privacy, and that the infringement is the least intrusive option. In addition to these conditions of proportionality, effectiveness, last resort, and least infringement, there is another moral condition: Respect for autonomy may require that we inform the person whose right of privacy has been infringed, although he or she may not be aware of the loss of privacy. In some contexts secret or deceptive actions are more disrespectful and destructive of trust than coercive actions.[42] Disclosure to the person of the act and objective indicates that the person is not a mere means to other ends but an end in himself or herself. Proper disclosure at least mitigates the intrusion on privacy.

Finally, to affirm a right of privacy, as we have, does not rule out moral criticism of various ways people exercise this right. For instance, a person may choose to lose privacy in a degrading or cheapening manner or to maintain privacy for foolish reasons. These criticisms may be appropriate but still not sufficient grounds for paternalistic or moralistic intervention. (See Chapter 5, pp. 209–22.)

Selected applications

Two examples will indicate how we propose to apply rules of privacy so as to respect rights of privacy while also allowing some justified intrusions on privacy. These examples are concerned with privacy in computerized information and in public screening programs.

TAPPING COMPUTER DATA BANKS. The first example involves the use of data banks. William Head, a twenty-seven-year-old leukemia patient from Louisiana, was at risk of dying without a bone marrow transplant.[43] He decided to call medical centers involved in research on bone marrow transplantation with nonrelated donors to see if there might be a suitable donor. At the University of Iowa, a technician, without authority to do so, told Head that their computer files identified a possible matching donor. At this point the potential donor— Mrs. X from California—had already had her right to privacy violated at least twice. First, she had been tissue-typed at the University of Iowa because she wanted to see whether she could donate bone marrow to her three-year-old son, who later died from leukemia. Her name and records were subsequently entered into the bone marrow registry without her consent, an unjustified breach of her right of privacy. Second, the technician violated her rights of privacy and confidentiality by disclosing this information (without mentioning her name) to Head.

Head then asked the Institutional Review Board (IRB), which is charged with protecting human subjects in research, to contact Mrs. X. After careful consideration, the IRB sent her a letter describing the nonrelated bone marrow transplant program and asked her if she would be willing to participate. The chair of the IRB called her after she failed to respond to the letter, and Mrs. X indicated that she was not willing to be a donor unless "it was for my family." The letter and telephone call from the IRB were further intrusions on privacy, although they might have conceivably been justified intrusions if the IRB had merely asked whether she was willing to be included in a registry that already (without her consent) had her name and records.

Head once again asked the IRB to request Mrs. X's help, this time by disclosing to her that a specific patient was in need of a bone marrow transplant. When the IRB refused, Head sought a court order to compel the university to disclose Mrs. X's identity so that he could try to persuade her to donate. He again proposed that a letter be written to inform her of his specific need and her potential suitability as a donor. After a district court ruled in favor of the letter but against the disclosure of Mrs. X's identity, the Iowa supreme court rejected the letter, holding that Mrs. X's record was confidential and that her privacy should remain protected.

On the one hand, this protection of privacy seems to us both morally and legally appropriate, however tragic for Head. On the other hand, we have argued that a person's right of autonomy may sometimes be overriden in order to protect others. Why was protection of Head not in order? Morally and legally, the case for overriding privacy is particularly strong when one's actions or inactions will cause harm to others (in violation of the obligation of nonmaleficence). The case is less strong, but still sometimes strong enough, when one fails to prevent or remove harm or provide benefit (in violation of the obligation of beneficence). The obligation to rescue is not widely recognized in law, apart from special circumstances (see Chapter 5), and those circumstances were not present in the case of Head and Mrs. X. The conditions for a moral obligation to rescue, as an expression of the principle of beneficence, are absent in this case. Even when word of Head's need penetrated the thin shield of privacy at Iowa and was transmitted to Mrs. X, it would have been charitable and supererogatory, rather than obligatory, for her to act on his behalf. (See Case 25 and our discussion in Chapter 5.)

One philosopher has argued that it would be wrong to approach Mrs. X again, not because manipulation or coercion would be involved but "only because in this case the probable benefits do not outweigh the probable harms."[44] However, we should also focus on the extent and seriousness of the moral violations. The violation of Mrs. X's right to privacy by discussing her identity with Head or anyone else would have compounded the earlier violations without any compensating hope of a positive outcome for Head. And even if Head's life could have been saved, the system of rules of privacy would not have justified further manipulation of Mrs. X.

COMPULSORY AND VOLUNTARY SCREENING. A second privacy issue has been widely discussed in recent years: screening or testing to determine whether persons are positive for antibodies to the human immunodeficiency virus (HIV). This virus is considered a necessary condition for the development of AIDS, a disease that is usually, perhaps universally, fatal. It is not necessary to belabor why the control of AIDS is a legitimate public health concern, not merely a private matter: AIDS is an infectious disease; people may be infectious for many years before they are aware that they are infectious; there is a wide clinical spectrum after exposure to HIV; there is no known cure for AIDS; the death rate from AIDS is very high, perhaps one hundred percent over time; the suffering of AIDS patients and others is tremendous; and, finally, the care of AIDS patients is expensive.

The goal of controlling the spread of AIDS is a moral imperative for societies and individuals in view of the principles we have discussed. But there are limits to the intrusions on privacy that can be justified, in accordance with the best current scientific evidence about the spread of AIDS.[45] For example, intrusions would not be warranted unless there existed a reasonable probability of preventing spread of the infection. Because policies of screening may infringe autonomy, privacy, and confidentiality, we need to examine why society wants and what it plans to do with information about a person who is antibody-positive for exposure to HIV. This question is vital because there is no evidence that the virus is spread through casual contact. It must be assumed that anyone who is antibody-positive for HIV can transmit the virus to others, but the evidence indicates that transmission occurs only through the transfer of bodily fluids, as in sexual activities, sharing intravenous drug needles, and blood transfusions. Most transmission occurs between parties in consensual, intimate relations that are paradigmatic of zones of protected privacy.

The enzyme-linked immunosorbent assay (ELISA) test, which became available in March 1985, made possible the detection of antibodies to HIV. A positive result usually leads to the use of the Western Blot test, which is more accurate. It is customary to distinguish between testing individuals and screening groups for antibodies to HIV, but we will use the term *screening* to cover both. Screening that retains identifiers necessarily involves some loss of privacy, because some persons gain access to private information about another person that they would not otherwise have. If the individual takes the test and receives the information anonymously, such as by number, so that the results cannot be traced to him or her, there is no such loss of privacy.

The following is a chart of the scope of possible policies toward screening for exposure to HIV. (We assume that identifiers are used as part of the screening process. Anonymous programs raise different and usually less complex issues. We note also that the issues below reach far beyond privacy questions.)

		Form of Authorization	
		Voluntary	*Compulsory*
Extent of Screening	*Universal*	1	2
	Selective	3	4

There appears to be no justification for either of the first two types of screening policy: voluntary-universal or compulsory-universal. Voluntary-universal screening, which would involve encouragement rather than coercion, does not violate any moral rules, including the rights of privacy and autonomy. However, it is not justified by current evidence, which, admittedly, may change in upcoming years; and it does not pass cost-benefit analysis. It also is not nec-essary, would produce many false positives outside groups engaging in risky activities, and has a potential stigmatizing effect that would outweigh any known potential benefit.[46] These objections to policy 1 also apply to policy 2, which is subject to the additional charge that it would infringe rights of autonomy and privacy without sufficient compensating benefit. If policy 2 were proposed in order to inform people of their antibody status so that those who are infectious will avoid exposing others, this goal can probably be realized by other means that will infringe less on the principle of respect for autonomy and the rule of privacy. If it is proposed in order to quarantine (more correctly, isolate) people who are antibody-positive, it is unjustified because such restrictions on liberty are not at present essential to protect the public health.

Our arguments against politics 1 and 2 are, however, subject to reversal if various conditions change. For example, the disease could spread so that it becomes much more difficult to identify classes of persons at risk; the false positive and false negative rates in testing might be substantially reduced by improved techniques; if an anti-AIDS drug is developed, there would be a critical need to contact affected parties; many more people might be harmed by the failure of their partners to inform them of their infection; and the cost-effectiveness of screening programs could improve substantially. Hence, our position is not opposed in principle to universal testing, whether voluntary or mandatory.

Policy 3, voluntary-selective screening, can be justified, especially for peo-ple engaging in unsafe sexual practices and sharing needles in intravenous drug use, but the policy is not free of problems. On the one hand, people who want to take the antibody test should be able to do so, and a case can be made that societal funds should be available for those who cannot afford the test. On the other hand, there is legitimate debate about whether people at risk should be urged to undergo such tests. Recommendations regarding conduct for those potentially affected will, in the absence of effective therapy, be the same whether the test results are positive or negative. Some commentators have therefore argued that it is not appropriate to urge screening, particularly in view of risks to privacy and confidentiality. However, others argue that those who test posi-tive for antibodies to HIV will be more likely to accept and act on the recom-mended precautions. The debate about the value of policy 3 thus hinges in part on different predictions about human behavior, in particular on predictions re-garding whether people will be more likely to avoid risky actions if they know that they are antibody-positive than if they do not know.

One major question about voluntary screening is whether it should be man-datory to report the test results to the public health department, as some juris-dictions require.[47] Mandatory reporting of the results of voluntary screening may prove to be counterproductive, because many people will probably choose not to undergo such tests if their names are recorded and positive results are reported to public health officials.

Regarding policy 4, several specific policies of compulsory-selective screening have already been adopted, and others can be expected. It may appear to be inappropriate to call some of these practices compulsory, insofar as individuals often can choose whether to enter situations or institutions where screening is mandatory, such as military service without conscription. However, screening is mandatory for individuals who enter those situations or institutions and thus is situationally compulsory.

There is no moral difficulty in justifying mandatory screening whenever persons are engaged in actions or involved in procedures that impose risks on others without their consent. Examples include blood donation, sperm donation, and organ donation. Compulsory screening of all surgical candidates in an institution may also be justified in order to protect health-care workers in the institution. However, it may be possible and sufficient to take adequate precautions in the care of all patients without knowing their antibody status. More careful examination is needed in order to determine whether screening should be required for marriage licenses. Such screening is not now cost-effective but could become justified in order to protect the spouse or offspring.[48]

Complex issues arise in several institutional settings, which differ in the extent to which individuals are free to enter and leave and to control risky contacts within the institutions. For example, it is doubtful that the policy of mandatory screening for entry into military service can be morally justified. Many suspect that the military in the United States instituted such screening in order to identify homosexuals, but the Defense Department's stated reasons for mandatory screening include the military's use of live-virus vaccinations and blood transfusions on the battlefield from other soldiers. The justification is still weaker for the U.S. government's policies of screening foreign service applicants, officers, and their dependents and of screening young people entering the Job Corps. However, screening prospective immigrants could be morally justified on the grounds of protection of citizens and avoidance of additional financial burdens.

Other institutions pose special problems because of lack of freedom of choice about entry and exit and about some forms of intimate contact within an institution. Especially significant are prisons and institutions for the mentally ill and mentally retarded. Compulsory screening, followed by isolation, can be justified in such settings only after careful consideration of alternative ways to prevent involuntary sexual contact. Compulsory screening for employment also does not generally appear to be warranted, including for people involved in health care, the preparation of food, and the like. However, if evidence emerges that HIV can be transmitted through such activities, compulsory screening could meet the conditions for justification identified earlier.

Some legal jurisdictions permit authorities to screen convicted prostitutes for antibodies to HIV, and in one state a prostitute with AIDS was restricted to her home and required to wear an electronic monitor that would enable the police to know if she moved more than two hundred feet from her telephone. Prostitution constitutes a serious public health threat inasmuch as several thousand males may become infected with the AIDS virus every year through contact with female prostitutes. These men, in turn, have sexual relations with other partners, who themselves have relations with others. There is also an enormously high exposure risk in the community of male and female prostitutes. One study of prostitutes in Newark, New Jersey, indicated that 51.7 percent tested positive for antibody to HIV.[49]

Once information has been generated that a person is antibody-positive or had AIDS, there remain important questions about the limits of disclosure of that information, as in tracing and informing past sexual contacts or in warning current sexual partners. However, those limits are best examined under rules of confidentiality, which are designed to protect information that emerges in special relationships.

Rules of confidentiality

Even though we necessarily lose some of our privacy when we grant access to our personal histories or to our bodies, we generally retain some measure of control over any information generated about us, at least in diagnostic and therapeutic contexts and in research. For example, our physician may not grant an insurance company or a prospective employer access to that information without our authorization.

When others gain access to such protected information without our consent, we sometimes describe their access as an infringement of confidentiality and at other times as an infringement of privacy. The difference is this: An infringement of X's confidentiality occurs only if the person to whom X disclosed the information in confidence fails to protect that information or deliberately discloses it to someone without X's consent. A person who sneaks into a hospital record room or breaks into a hospital computer data bank, despite appropriate protections, would be accused of a violation of privacy rather than a violation of confidentiality. Thus, only the person (or institution) to whom a patient grants information in a confidential relationship can be charged with violating confidentiality. If a patient or subject authorizes a professional to disclose that same information to others, there is no infringement of confidentiality, although there is a loss of both confidentiality and privacy.

Traditional rules and contemporary practices in health care

Rules of confidentiality are widespread, and it would be difficult to find other rules that are so common in codes of medical ethics over time and across different cultures and societies. Practitioners and others who have thought about relations between physicians and patients have usually considered confidentiality to be of paramount importance, perhaps subordinate only to the main goal of the relationship, namely health benefits for the patient.

In Western codes of medical ethics, the requirement of confidentiality appears as early as the Hippocratic oath, which contains this vow: "What I may see or hear in the course of the treatment or even outside of the treatment in regard to the life of men, which on no account one must spread abroad, I will keep to myself holding such things shameful to be spoken about." It persists in the Code of Ethics of the American Medical Association. For example, the code adopted in 1957 included this rule: "A physician may not reveal the confidences entrusted to him in the course of medical attendance, or the deficiencies he may observe in the character of patients, unless he is required to do so by law or unless it becomes necessary in order to protect the welfare of the individual or of the community." In 1980, the AMA revised this rule to hold that a physician "shall safeguard patient confidences within the constraints of the law." The World Medical Association has likewise affirmed rules of confidentiality. Its Declaration of Geneva (1948, as revised in 1968) has the following pledge: "I will respect the secrets which are confided in me, even after the patient has died." And its International Code of Medical Ethics (1949) has the most stringent requirement of all: "A doctor shall preserve absolute secrecy on all he knows about his patient because of the confidence entrusted to him."

Beyond professional codes, rules of confidentiality have also been developed from the standpoint of patients. In "A Patient's Bill of Rights" adopted in 1973 by the American Hospital Association, one rule is "The patient has the right to every consideration of privacy concerning his own medical care program. Case discussion, consultation, examination, and treatment are confidential and should be conducted discreetly. Those not directly involved in his care must have the permission of the patient to be present. The patient has the right to expect that all communications and records pertaining to his care should be treated as confidential."[50]

Even though some rule of confidentiality appears in virtually every code of medical ethics, some commentators have suspected that the rule is at present little more than a ritualistic formula or convenient fiction, publicly acknowledged by professionals but widely ignored and violated in practice. For instance, Mark Siegler has argued that "confidentiality in medicine" is a "decrepit concept," because what both physicians and patients have traditionally understood as medical confidentiality no longer exists. It is "compromised systematically in the course of routine medical care." To make his point graphic, Siegler presents the case of a patient who became concerned about the number of people who appeared to have access to his record and threatened to leave the hospital prematurely unless the hospital would guarantee confidentiality.

Upon inquiry, Siegler discovered that many more people than he had suspected had legitimate needs and responsibilities to examine the patient's chart. When he informed the patient of the number—approximately seventy-five—he assured the patient that "these people were all involved in providing or supporting his health-care services." The patient retorted, "I always believed that medical confidentiality was part of the doctors' code of ethics. Perhaps you should tell me just what you people mean by 'confidentiality.' "[51]

In a survey of patients, medical students, and house staff about expectations and practices of confidentiality, Barry D. Weiss reports that "patients expect a more rigorous standard of confidentiality than actually exists." According to one Harris poll, only seventeen percent of the patients surveyed were dissatisfied with the way physicians handled confidential information, but, according to Weiss's study, more would be dissatisfied if they knew what actually occurs. Virtually all patients (ninety-six percent) recognized the common practice of informally discussing patients' cases for second opinions; most (sixty-nine percent) expected cases to be discussed openly in professional settings in order to receive other opinions; and a majority (fifty-one percent) expected cases to be discussed in professional settings simply because they were medically interesting. Half of the patients expected cases to be discussed with office nursing staff, but they generally did not expect cases to be discussed in other settings, such as in medical journals, at parties, or with spouses or friends. Yet, to take two actual examples, house staff and medical students reported that cases were frequently discussed with physicians' spouses (fifty-seven percent) and at parties (seventy percent). Weiss comments: "If this practice [regarding confidentiality] does not change, and if patients were to become aware of it, they might become increasingly reluctant to divulge sensitive information even if it is pertinent to their medical problem."[52]

It may be possible to alter current practices in the delivery of care to approximate more closely the traditional ideal of confidentiality, but a gulf will remain because of the need for information in medicine. Weiss's study indicates that patients understand some—though by no means all—of the institutional and societal constraints that limit confidentiality. Under these conditions it is important to inform patients about what is meant by medical confidentiality in the modern hospital with its large and diversified health-care team, its bureaucracy, and third-party payers. Whatever the needs for information in order to provide the best possible medical care, they do not justify many of the violations of confidentiality that Weiss's study identified, such as the casual and unnecessary discussion of cases at parties.

The nature of medical confidentiality

Confidentiality is present when one person discloses information to another, whether through words or an examination, and the person to whom the information is disclosed does not divulge that information without the other person's permission. In schematic terms, information I is confidential if and only if A discloses to B, and B refrains from disclosing I to C without A's consent. Party A is the one who controls access to the information, disclosing it to B, while continuing to determine who has access.

A rule of confidentiality prohibits (some) disclosures of (some) information gained in certain relationships to (some) third parties without the consent of the original source of the information. The limits to retaining and sharing the information, and the process of protection, should all be governed by the relevant rules.[53] The limits determine who may disclose what to whom; the process concerns how the information should be protected. Because rights and obligations are correlated, the rules can be stated either in terms of a person's right to have information treated confidentially or in terms of another's obligation to treat information confidentially (i.e., not to disclose it to third parties without the patient's permission).

Rules of confidentiality can be violated or infringed in several different ways. Such rules prohibit deliberate disclosure, and they also require that agents in special relations take precautions to protect information. Therefore, B may violate the rule by deliberately disclosing confidential information to their parties without A's permission; or B may violate the rule by carelessly or negligently handling the information. There may be moral negligence even if there is no legal negligence. However, there is disagreement about the precise scope of affirmative obligations to protect information.

Rules of confidentiality exist in the context of other social practices that limit rights and legitimate expectations. Often there are acknowledged exceptions to the kind of information that can be considered confidential. For example, external limits to confidentiality may be set by legal obligations, as when practitioners are required to report gunshot wounds and venereal diseases. These limits are expressed in many codes of medical ethics, which may also recognize that the line between private and public information is often difficult to draw and varies from society to society.

Some disclosures of information to third parties may not be breaches of confidentiality because of the context of the original disclosure. For example, in one case, an IBM physician, Dr. Martha Nugent, informs her employer about her belief that an employee, Robert Bratt, has a problem of paranoia relevant to behavior on the job.[54] Bratt knew that Nugent was retained by IBM to conduct the examination but expected nonetheless that conventional medical confidentiality would obtain. The company held that the facts disclosed by Nugent were necessary for evaluating Bratt's request for transfer and, under law, were a legitimate business communication. In our view it is a reasonable conclusion that Nugent is not bound by the rule of confidentiality in the same way as a private physician. This is not to say that a physician employed by a corporation is free to disclose everything to the corporation, but there may be a valid contract for at least limited disclosures. A similar point applies to military physicians who have a dual responsibility—to the soldier as patient and to the military. Nevertheless, the company and the military, along with the physicians in each context, do have a moral responsibility to ensure that employee-patients and soldier-patients understand at the outset that the traditional rule of confidentiality does not apply.

Foundations of rules of confidentiality

One person's disclosure of information received from another in a special relationship is not inherently or intrinsically wrong, that is, wrong in and of itself. We can easily imagine a society that did not recognize any rules of confidentiality. Many of the important goods of medicine—and perhaps research—could also be realized without rules of confidentiality. Why, then, should we have the rules of confidentiality that have been so widely adopted? We construe this question as an inquiry into the normative grounds of confidentiality, rather than an inquiry into the historical origins and development of rules of confidentiality. In terms of our levels or tiers of moral justification, the question is, "Which moral principles and arguments justify which rule of confidentiality?"

A rule of confidentiality may be justified either by the principles it expresses or by the consequences it produces. Consider first the consequences. A rule of confidentiality enables physicians to meet the needs of patients to have information both transmitted and protected.[55] If patients could not trust physicians not to reveal some information to third parties, they would be reluctant to disclose full and forthright information in the first place. Without that information, physicians would not be able to make accurate diagnoses and prognoses or to recommend the best course of treatment. This point has special force in psychotherapeutic relations. According to Justice Clark's dissent in the *Tarasoff* case (Case 1), assurance of confidentiality is indispensable for psychotherapy because it enables people to seek help without the stigma that would result from disclosure to others. It encourages full disclosure essential for effective treatment, and it is necessary for trust, "the very means by which treatment is effected."[56]

Consequentialist arguments establish a need for some rule of confidentiality, but consequentialists disagree about which construal of the rule of confidentiality should be adopted and about its scope and application. In *Tarasoff*, both the majority opinion, which affirmed an obligation on the part of professionals in psychotherapeutic relationships to warn intended victims, and the dissenting opinion, which denied such an obligation, used utilitarian principles to justify their interpretation of the rule of confidentiality and its exceptions. Their debate hinged on different predictions and assessments of the consequences of (1) a rule that required therapists to abandon confidentiality and warn intended victims when there is a public peril, and (2) a rule that allowed therapists to exercise their discretion and to maintain confidentiality in the face of some peril to a member of the public. The majority opinion pointed to the victims who would be saved—such as the young woman, Tatiana Tarasoff, who had been killed by Prosenjit Poddar in this case—and contended that a professional's obligation to disclose information to third parties could be justified by the greatest good for the greatest number. By contrast, the minority opinion contended that if it were common practice to break rules of confidentiality, the fiduciary relation between the patient and the doctor would soon erode and collapse. Patients would lose confidence in psychotherapists and would refrain from disclosing information important to effective therapy. As a result, violent assaults would increase because dangerous persons would refuse to seek psychiatric aid or would be reluctant to disclose important information, such as their violent fantasies.[57] Hence a difficult moral question from the consequentialist perspective is whether one rule of confidentiality is better than another rule of confidentiality in achieving the desired objectives.

Consequentialist arguments for a strict rule of confidentiality depend on the claim that the absence of confidentiality will prevent people who need medical and especially psychiatric treatment from seeking and fully participating in it. Another version of this claim is that people who suspect they may have been exposed to the virus that causes AIDS may not seek testing unless they can expect positive test results to remain confidential. Although these claims are empirical, they have not been adequately tested. Of the few available empirical studies, one supports the consequentialist approach by examining the responses of thirty psychiatric inpatients to hypothetical questions about confidentiality. Eighty percent of those surveyed indicated that an assurance of confidentiality improved their relationship with the staff; sixty-seven percent said they would be upset or angry at the release of verbal information without their permission; seventeen percent indicated that they would leave treatment if verbal information were released without their permission; and ninety-five percent said they would be upset if their charts were shared without their consent.[58] A subsequent study focused on fifty-eight outpatients. These patients indicated that they would take vigorous actions, such as complaints or legal suits, in cases of breaches of confidentiality.[59]

Even though these studies support the consequentialist argument for a rule of confidentiality, they do not support a rule of absolute nondisclosure. In addition, they do not deal with the question of whether the absence of an explicit or implicit promise of confidentiality would deter people from seeking treatment at the outset. They also suffer from the methodological flaw of using hypothetical questions to gauge probable responses in practice.

The second major approach to rules of confidentiality grounds them not in goals or consequences (or at least not exclusively in them) but rather in the moral principles or rules they express. Two relevant moral principles or rules are (1) respect for personal autonomy (and privacy) and (2) fidelity, especially to implicit or explicit promises. To respect persons properly involves respecting their zone of privacy and their decisions to grant and to limit access to that zone. The argument for privacy in the previous section thus extends to confidentiality.

Often the binding force of confidentiality derives from an implicit or explicit promise by the professional to the patient seeking help. For example, if the public oath taken by the professional or the accepted code of professional ethics pledges confidentiality, and if the professional does not expressly disavow confidentiality, the patient has a right to expect it. An implicit promise is valid even if the professional has said nothing about it. In the absence of an express disavowal, the professional can reasonably be expected to affirm the public stance of the profession.

Justified infringements of rules of confidentiality

In addition to requiring rules of confidentiality and shaping their content, both utilitarian and deontological considerations can help determine the stringency or the weight of these rules. Should the rules of confidentiality be viewed merely as rules of thumb? Are they absolute rules, as in the requirement of absolute secrecy in the International Code of Medical Ethics? Or should they be regarded as establishing prima facie obligations? Parts of the majority decision in the *Tarasoff* case can be read as holding that confidentiality is only a rule of thumb. The decision as a whole, however, indicates that maintaining confidentiality is a prima facie obligation. Even the minority dissent does not claim that confidentiality is absolute. In both opinions, an act is prima facie wrong if it breaches confidentiality, but the conditions under which it is actually wrong vary in the two opinions.

Our view follows from the discussion of rules in Chapter 2. A rule of confidentiality states a prima facie obligation, and anyone who makes an exception bears the burden of proving that some other moral obligation outweighs the obligation of confidentiality in the circumstances. Furthermore, it is not adequate to hold that health-care professionals have a right to disclose confidential information in some circumstances but no obligation to do so. From this perspective disclosure is permitted but is not obligatory. However, we believe there are clear legal and moral obligations to divulge confidential information when necessary to report certain contagious diseases, gunshot wounds, child abuse, and the like. We thus concur with the court's holding in *Tarasoff* that psychiatrists may have a duty, not merely an option, to warn of their patient's intention to kill or harm.

An AMA code in effect until 1980 held that the physician should not infringe the rule of confidentiality "unless he is required to do so by law or unless it becomes necessary in order to protect the welfare of the individual or of the society." Although some have interpreted this statement as permitting but not requiring the physician to break confidences, we interpret it differently. One may not break a confidence except to fulfill another and more stringent obligation—either an obligation to obey the law or an obligation to protect the welfare of the patient or the community. There is no right or privilege to infringe confidences in such cases unless there is also an obligation to do so. The health-care professional's breach of confidentiality thus cannot be justified unless it is necessary to meet a strong conflicting obligation, such as an epidemiologist's obligation to protect the public's health. This conclusion does not entail, of course, that some moral rules require one to break confidences. It means, rather, that rules protecting confidences must sometimes yield to other principles and rules.

But which obligations legitimately override confidentiality? The previously discussed AMA code mentioned both legal obligations and actions necessary to protect patients or society as legitimate grounds for overriding confidentiality. Most instances of disclosing confidential information to protect the patient (rather than others) are not legally required. Some legal obligations, such as the requirement to report epileptic seizures to the division of motor vehicles, may be enacted to protect the patient in some cases but society in others. Legal obligations to break confidentiality in order to protect others sometimes pose difficult conflicts of obligation for the health-care professional. On the one hand, he or she is obligated to protect a patient; on the other hand, he or she is legally obligated to act to protect the society, even if the law is unwise or unjust.

In a sufficiently just political system there is a moral obligation to obey the law, but this obligation, too, is prima facie.[60] Sometimes it may be morally justified for the health-care professional to infringe the obligation to obey the law in order to fulfill a responsibility to his or her patient. He or she may sometimes justifiably reason that obedience to law will result in inadequate treatment for a patient, as in complicated circumstances where there is a legal obligation to report venereal disease. The point is that difficult moral dilemmas cannot be resolved merely because a law requires disclosure. If a code of medical ethics were formulated only by reference to legal rules, the code would be inadequtae.

Infringing rules of confidentiality by disclosures to the family rather than to the patient raises another set of issues. As we have seen, physicians sometimes consult a patient's family members in order to determine whether they should tell the patient that he or she has terminal cancer. In Case 4 the attending physician discussed Mr. X's terminal cancer with the family, and the family wanted to conceal the diagnosis and prognosis from him. The physician accepted their decision. Ethical analyses of such cases often focus on and criticize the apparently paternalistic decision by the family and physician to withhold information from the patient. If a family can offer evidence about a patient's inability to make autonomous choices (e.g., evidence of emotional instability), this evidence may form part of a justification for withholding information from a patient or for overriding his or her choices. There is generally no moral justification, however, for acceding to the family's request to withhold information from a competent patient such as Mr. X when there is no evidence that he does not want such information and does not want to make decisions about treatment. There is a still more fundamental question about why the family, rather than the competent patient, was given the information in the first place. The physician should not have disclosed information to the family without Mr. X's prior permission. Both actions—the breach of confidentiality and the subsequent deception of the patient—violated Mr. X's right of autonomy.[61]

Several considerations about justified infringements of confidentiality turn on prevention or removal of harms and the provision or promotion of benefits, as we analyzed these notions in Chapters 4 and 5. One question concerns which risks to others, if any, outweigh the rule of confidentiality—such as risks to life, physical health, mental health, property, or reputation. The number of individuals at risk is also pertinent. Because risks are probable rather than certain harms, another issue is how probable a harm must be in order to justify or require a breach of confidentiality. In general, it is necessary to consider both the probability and the magnitude of harm and to balance both against the rule of confidentiality. We can analyze these considerations by the chart of risk assessment introduced in Chapter 5:

		Magnitude of Harm	
		Major	*Minor*
Probability	*High*	1	2
of Harm	*Low*	3	4

As the health professionals' assessment of the situation approaches 1 in the above chart, where there is a high probability of a major harm—including both the numbers affected and the magnitude of harm for particular individuals—the weight of the obligation to breach confidentiality increases. As the situation approaches 4, the weight decreases. If there is a low probability of a minor harm, there is generally no moral obligation to breach confidentiality, and it would usually be wrong to do so. Obviously, 2 and 3 are more complicated. If there is a high probability of minor harm, there is generally no moral obligation to breach confidentiality, and it may be wrong to do so, particularly when the breach may produce other harms. However, 3 is still more difficult. For example, if there is only a low probability that the health problems of a nation's president will lead him or her to use nuclear weapons in utterly inappropriate circumstances, would this possibility be sufficient to justify blowing the whistle? The remote chance of substantial harm to millions of people, both now and in the future, could easily be sufficient to justify a breach of confidentiality.

We generally cannot have a high degree of confidence in our attempts to measure probability and magnitude of harm. Uncertainty may appear on several different levels, including diagnosis, prognosis, and likelihood of harmful outcomes. For example, in one case a psychiatrist used hypnotic techniques to help a pilot recall suppressed information about his responsibility for the crash of a commercial plane. The information obtained through hypnosis indicated that it would be risky for the pilot to fly again, at least for the immediate future, but the risks were not precisely measurable and the therapist was unable to convince the pilot that he should not fly until he could solve his problems. Confidentiality was strictly maintained. Six months after returning to the cockpit, the pilot made an error of judgment that led to the crash of a jet on a transatlantic flight, resulting in the loss of many lives.[62]

Suppose that a pilot of a commercial jet informs his physician that his forty-five-year-old mother was diagnosed as having Huntington's disease. The physician has to determine whether to disclose to the airline this pilot's fifty percent risk of having the disease, in the event the pilot fails to reveal it.[63] (The development of a test for a genetic marker for Huntington's disease now makes it possible to determine with ninety-five percent accuracy whether a person will develop the disease.) These cases involve difficult matters of judgment of determining the probability and magnitude of a harm (or benefit) that will justify the disclosure of confidential information. There is no formula for deciding such cases that escapes the need for the risk-benefit assessments discussed above and in Chapter 5.

When the Assembly of District Branches and the Board of Trustees of the American Psychiatric Association annotated the principles of medical ethics for psychiatry in 1973, they held, with special reference to court-ordered disclosures of confidences, that "When the psychiatrist is *in doubt*, the right of the patient to confidentiality and, by extension, to unimpaired treatment, should be given priority."[64] The standard of proof in this statement is not clear. It may mean either that psychiatrists should respect confidentiality if they have any doubts at all or that they should respect confidentiality if they are not convinced beyond a reasonable doubt. The standard of "any doubt" should, we suggest, be rejected, because it amounts to a ready excuse for no disclosure under any conditions.

Nonetheless, the health-care professional should seek alternative and more acceptable ways of realizing a benefit or preventing a harm before disclosing confidential information. Rarely is the breach of confidentiality justified if a morally and legally acceptable alternative exists. In one case, a physician had to determine whether to disclose a patient's homosexuality to his prospective wife, who was also the physician's patient. Although the physician chose to respect the rule of confidentiality, he was obligated, we believe, to try to persuade the young man to tell his prospective wife. A more radical approach would have been to discuss marriage and sexuality with the young woman, so that she might have pressed her prospective husband for more information. Because she was his patient, the physician had a stronger obligation to disclose information to her than he would have had if she had been a stranger, and this obligation makes his complete inaction less acceptable.[65] The formulation of this case antedates the AIDS crisis. Because a prospective husband's homosexual activities would today increase the risk of the transmission of the AIDS virus to his sexual partners, a physician's obligation to disclose such information to a prospective wife is correspondingly increased.

In recent years there has been widespread controversy about whether physicians and other health-care professionals should notify spouses and lovers that a patient has tested positive for exposure to HIV and thus can probably infect others through sexual intercourse or other exchanges of body fluids, particularly sharing needles in intravenous drug use. In Case 2, after several seeks of dry persistent coughing and more recently night sweats, a bisexual man visits his family physician, who arranges for a test to determine whether he has antibodies to HIV that indicate he has been infected with the virus. When the physician informs the patient that his test is positive, that his wife is at risk of infection, and that their children could lose both parents, the patient refuses to tell his wife and insists that the physician maintain absolute confidentiality. The physician reluctantly yields to this demand. Only in the last few weeks of his life does the patient allow his wife to be informed of the nature of his illness, and her test shows that she is also antibody-positive for HIV. When related symptoms appear a year later, she angrily accuses the physician of violating his moral responsibility to her and her children.[66]

Legal and moral rules of confidentiality are evolving in response to the AIDS crisis; this evolution is occurring in part by reflection on where this kind of case fits into the range of cases faced previously. For example, comparisons may be drawn with legal requirements to report sexually transmitted diseases to public health officials who then trace sexual contacts, and also with the therapist's obligation to warn potential victims of a client's violence, as articulated in the *Tarasoff* case.[67] In 1988, in the U.S. there is a legal requirement for health professionals to report cases of AIDS, but in most jurisdictions there is no legal obligation to report patients who have been infected with the AIDS virus, who may not have symptoms for several years.

There is a strong ethical argument based on beneficence and nonmaleficence for informing spouses and sexual partners that a particular person has tested positive for exposure to the AIDS virus and thus must be presumed to be infectious, even if the patient insists on maintaining confidentiality. The conditions identified earlier for justified breaches of confidentiality, as well as other prima facie principles and rules, are applicable here—a person is at risk of serious harm, the disclosure would probably prevent that harm (unless the spouse or lover is already infected, but even then he or she may be able to seek treatment and protect others from exposure), the breach is necessary to prevent that harm (after unsuccessful efforts to persuade the person who has HIV infection to disclose the information or to grant permission for the disclosure), and the breach of confidentiality is limited to the amount and kind of information that is necessary to protect others.

This last condition is important, because disclosure to people other than the spouse or lover that a person has HIV infection may have serious repercussions in view of widespread discrimination against people who have HIV infection. In addition, the disclosure to others, including to other family members who are not sexual partners, is generally unnecessary to protect them, because of solid evidence that the AIDS virus is not spread through casual contact or even through familial contact unless there is exposure to body fluids. In one case, a nurse in an emergency room told a woman that her elderly father had AIDS as a result of a blood transfusion years before; the disclosure was made because the daughter was functioning as the care-giver in the home and thus needed to take the kinds of precautions that care-givers routinely take in hospital settings. However, where there is no risk to others, there is no justification for disclosure without the patient's consent. Curiosity by others, whether family members or employers or friends, is not a sufficient reason.

The debate about rules of confidentiality in the AIDS epidemic is complicated because the risk of HIV infection is largely limited to intimate consensual contact, because there may be a long period of infectiousness before any symptoms appear, because AIDS appears to be universally fatal and virtually all HIV-infected persons will probably develop AIDS over time, and because there is no successful treatment. A fundamental question is which rule of confidentiality would save the most lives in the long run in these circumstances: One that permits or perhaps requires notification of spouses or lovers or one that guarantees strict confidentiality. Answers to this question hinge on disputed claims about the importance of voluntary testing in changing behavior and reducing risky conduct over time. One argument is that people who have been exposed to the AIDS virus but who do not yet have symptoms will be reluctant to seek testing unless confidentiality is protected; they will thus fail to obtain valuable information that could reduce risks to others. A counterargument is that the carefully limited breaches of confidentiality—namely disclosure only to sexual partners or needle-sharing partners who are at reasonable risk of harm—

would not deter people from seeking testing and medical attention. According to this counterargument people would still seek and accept testing if they were informed that confidentiality would be breached only under strictly limited conditions and then only to parties at reasonable risk of harm.[68]

In conclusion, we have argued that rules of medical confidentiality are not at present well delineated and would profit from a thorough restructuring. On the one hand, if we are to live up to the principle of respect for autonomy, patients often should be told more about practices of confidentiality, should consent to the inclusion of information in their records, and should have access to those records, as well as retaining some control over access to those records. On the other hand, sometimes the demands of respect for autonomy may have to yield to other moral demands such as the rights of others.

Rules of fidelity

The nature and place of fidelity

Paul Ramsey maintains that the fundamental ethical question in research, medicine, and health care is, "What is the meaning of the faithfulness of one human being to another?"[69] Ramsey interprets faithfulness along theological lines as covenant fidelity, but it is often expressed in philosophy in terms of fidelity or promise keeping and in law in terms of contracts, trust, or fiduciary relations. Ramsey appears to view fidelity as the fundamental ethical principle from which all other principles can be derived. Under this interpretation the principle becomes so broad that it serves as a summary term for morality, parallel to older uses of *righteousness*. Few theologians and philosophers would concur with Ramsey in making fidelity the fundamental moral principle, but many would accept it as one among several moral principles or rules.[70]

We believe the obligation of fidelity or promise keeping is best understood in terms of rules derived from the basic moral principles discussed in previous chapters: Rules of fidelity are rooted in respect for autonomy as well as utility.[71] These principles provide a strong warrant for an individual's obligation to keep promises as well as for an institution of promising. Upon making a promise, people create expectations on the part of others, who then rely on the promise and have a valid claim to its being kept.[72] As our framework implies, many moral obligations are independent of our voluntary agreements, commitments, or promises to perform them. Promising can account for only a portion (though a significant portion) of our obligations in research, medicine, and health care, and other moral principles and rules also limit obligations engendered by promises.

Most obligations of positive beneficence in health care rest on fidelity-generating contracts and role relations. In establishing a relationship with a patient the physician makes an implicit or explicit promise to seek the patient's welfare. This promise appears in the physician's pledge or oath upon entry into the profession or in the profession's code of ethics. A related promise is that the physician will not abandon the patient: "Once having undertaken a case, the physician should not neglect the patient, nor withdraw from the case without giving notice to the patient, the relatives, or responsible friends sufficiently long in advance of withdrawal to permit another medical attendant to be secured."[73] Abandonment would be a breach of faith, as well as a failure to discharge the obligation of beneficence.

The content of specific obligations of fidelity depends on the promises that were made, the expectations that were legitimately engendered, the nature of the special relationships, and the like. For example, in Case 25, discussed in Chapter 5, it might be argued that Shimp created legitimate expectations on the part of his cousin, McFall, when he agreed to undergo the tests for compatibility and to donate bone marrow to his dying cousin if they matched. Shimp's decision not to complete the tests after starting them could be viewed as a form of betrayal under the obligation of fidelity, although he had no obligation to undergo the tests or to donate bone marrow in the first place. Likewise, it might be argued that although the pregnant woman has a right to terminate her pregnancy by an abortion, her decision not to abort and to carry the pregnancy to term engenders certain moral (not necessarily legal) obligations of nonmaleficence and beneficence to the fetus. In such cases, by exercising their autonomy in certain ways, people change the structure of obligations and rights and in so doing limit their future autonomy from a moral (even if not from a legal) standpoint.

Similar conclusions can be reached about confidentiality, which also often depends on special relationships and explicit or implicit promises. For example, in an epidemiological study of what happens to people who are antibody-positive for HIV but do not yet have signs of AIDS or AIDS-related complex, some investigators indicated that they would use the information they received only for epidemiological purposes. However, a researcher noticed that an antibody-positive subject had not informed his lover and continued to practice unprotected sex with that person. In considering whether to warn the lover, this researcher had to weigh his specific promise of confidentiality against the obligation to prevent harm.[74]

Contracts and models

As a legal category, *contract* refers to voluntary agreements between parties that create or alter legal obligations. Contracts play a large role in human interactions, and their importance is indicated by legal sanctions. Contracts became progressively significant in law and ethics as contractual relations supplanted status relations in the modern era, especially when contracts became central in capitalistic markets. While everyone agrees that individuals have moral obligations to act in good faith in making and carrying out contracts and that contracts based on fraud or duress are not enforceable, what counts as a valid contract and whether biomedical ethics should make the language of contracts central are less clear.

Case 23, the case of Baby M, is an example of controversies about the legal enforcement of a contract for surrogate motherhood when the surrogate mother changes her mind and intends to keep the baby. Critics contend that such contracts should be voided because they are immoral and resemble unenforceable contracts for prostitution and the sale of children. Others, however, argue that surrogate-mother contracts should be recognized as valid and enforceable under carefully defined circumstances—perhaps including a prior psychological examination, counseling, and a waiting period. One way to limit issues of the validity of the contract is to approach disputes about the child of a surrogate arrangement as analogous to typical custody disputes and to resolve them in terms of the best interests of the child.[75]

Some proponents of the centrality of fidelity in biomedical ethics oppose the model of contract and propose instead a model of *covenant*. Part of this dispute centers on how to describe and how to structure health-care relationships, particularly between physicians and patients. On the one hand, defenders of the covenant model criticize contracts as individualistic (i.e., based exclusively on acts of individual autonomy), minimalistic (specifying only the moral minimum of the relationship), externalistic (emphasizing external actions rather than the spirit of the relationship and the character of the agents), and legalistic (focused on legal enforcement). These critics favor the language of loyalty and faithfulness as well as reliance on virtues rather than on principles and rules.[76] Defenders of a contract model reply that a covenant is only a special form of contract that emphasizes moral relationships such as fidelity and that medical ethics is best understood in terms of a broader nexus of contracts between society, the professions, and patients.[77]

However, there are many reasons not to reduce health-care relationships either to a literal, metaphorical, or hypothetical contract or to fidelity to the provisions of contracts. These relationships involve a range of moral considerations including the principles and rules we have already identified and the ideals and virtues discussed in Chapter 8. For better or worse, relations between health-care professionals and patients and between researchers and subjects usually have some contractual elements, which may be specific and may be legally enforceable. But to recognize such contractual elements is not to reduce obligations in those relations to contractual obligations.

From our standpoint, it is misleading to try to capture the relationships between health-care professionals and patients in any single metaphor or model such as contractors, partners, parents, friends, or technicians.[78] No single metaphor or model adequately expresses the complexity of health care or the moral principles and rules that should govern such relationships. For this reason we have refrained from analyzing these relationships through metaphors and models, referring to them only in passing.

Conflicts of fidelity in physicians' roles

THIRD-PARTY INTERESTS. Physicians, nurses, and hospital administrators sometimes find their role obligations in conflict with other obligations to patients. For example, they may have a therapeutic contract with a party other than the patient, and the contractor may not be the beneficiary. If someone promises John Doe to look after his children after his death, the promisor has an obligation to John Doe even though the children are the primary beneficiaries.[79] When parents bring a child to a physician for treatment, the physician's primary responsibility is to serve the child's interests, although the parents made the contract. Courts have often allowed adult Jehovah's Witnesses to reject blood transfusions for themselves, while rightly refusing to allow them to reject medically necessary blood transfusions for their children (see Case 12). In some cases, parents may be charged with child neglect if they fail to seek or permit highly desirable medical treatment, even if the treatment is not necessary to save the child's life.[80]

A physician has a fundamental responsibility to the patient, who may be incompetent, even if a third party establishes the initial contract. The physician (prima facie) ought to act in the patient's best interests, even if it is necessary to seek a court order to authorize surgery, a blood transfusion, or the like.[81] Other familial interests, such as avoiding the depletion of financial resources, should not be considered unless the threshold has been reached that significant interests of the patient would not be served by continued or new treatment.[82] Here the criterion is still that of the patient's interest rather than the family's interest. There may be major disagreements about what would be in the patient's interest, but in circumstances of conflict the physician has no basic responsibility to abide by a family's assessment, which may be controlled by the family's interest rather than the patient's interests. (See Chapter 4, pp. 179–80.)

INSTITUTIONAL INTERESTS. The above examples focus on the conflict between the interests of the patient, who is the beneficiary, and the interests of another party, such as a parent, who makes the contract with the health-care professional. In related types of conflict it may be less clear exactly what the health-care professional owes the "patient." Examples include a physician's contract to examine applicants for positions in a company or to determine whether applicants for insurance policies are good risks. In such cases, the health-care professional may rightly not think of the person examined as his or her patient. The professional has certain responsibilities of due care, but they may not be as comprehensive or as stringent as the responsibilities that apply in a typical physician-patient relationship. They would include care in examinations so as not to injure the individual, such as by exposure to excessive X-rays.

In some jurisdictions the health-care professional may not have a legal obligation to disclose the discovery of a disease to the examinee. For example, in one preemployment physical examination, X-rays indicated that a woman who subsequently was hired had tuberculosis, yet the physician and the employer did not disclose these findings to her. After three years, the employee became ill with tuberculosis and was hospitalized for a prolonged period. In this case, the court held that the woman's only recourse was workmen's compensation. It disallowed her suit against her employer and the physician who examined her, on grounds that there was no established patient-physician relationship and hence no legal obligation to disclose the information to her.[83] From a moral standpoint, however, both the employer and the physician had an obligation to disclose the information. The examinee had a legitimate expectation of disclosure in the absence of a specific disavowal of that responsibility. This obligation of disclosure stems from the principles of beneficence and respect for autonomy.

What obligation of disclosure exists in situations of conflict where institutional interests might be at stake? Suppose a company requires regular physical examinations of all employees by a physician. The physician's contract requires disclosure to the company about employees' health conditions that might affect their work. If the company uses materials such as kepone or benzene that might be hazardous to its employees and the physician discovers symptoms of a disease that might be directly related to working conditions, what obligation does the physician have to report these findings to the employees? Does he or she have the same obligation if the employer expressly forbids such disclosures to employees? At a minimum, we suggest, health-care professionals have a moral responsibility to oppose, avoid, and withdraw from contracts that would require them to withhold information of significant benefit to examinees.

In another type of situation, a health-care professional may be under contract or otherwise obligated to an institution to provide care for a group of individuals. In these cases, there can be no doubt that physicians, for example, owe "due care" to individuals who become their patients under a third-party contract. Examples include health-care professionals in industries, prisons, and the armed services. Care of the patient may come into conflict with institutional needs, but the patient's needs may or may not take precedence. Difficult cases for this rule emerge on the battlefield, where triage may be different from triage in the peacetime emergency room. In war the needs of the military may dictate

that certain patients be given priority—for example, because they can be returned to active duty—even when medical needs establish a different priority.

In addition to triage and other allocation decisions that are in part contingent
upon institutional needs, health-care professionals in military and other institutions sometimes are called on to make judgments about sickness and health
based on institutional values. In 1966, an Air Force newsletter reported that a
twenty-six-year-old staff sergeant gunner who had been on active duty in Vietnam for seven months and had flown more than one hundred missions developed a fear of flying because several of his acquaintances had been killed. The
diagnosis was gross stress reaction, "manifested by anxiety, tenseness, a fear
of death expressed in the form of rationalizations, and inability to function. His
problem was 'worked through' and insight . . . was gained to the extent that
he was returned to full flying duty in less than six weeks."[84] This case raises
significant questions about the point at which a health-care professional should
refuse to engage in military or other service on the grounds that he or she
cannot combine responsibility to patients with institutional needs in that setting.

Some actions grossly violate canons of medical ethics and thereby warrant
disobedience to orders rather than conformity to them. An example is an order
for a physician to help torture a prisoner in order to gain information.[85] There
are borderline cases, too, such as the one reported in the Air Force newsletter.
But in principle physicians and psychotherapists can function in the military
and can render valuable care to wounded soldiers, even in an unjust war, without violating moral principles. They render service to the soldier as a human
being rather than to the soldier as a soldier, and thus, according to the international laws of war, they are not legitimate targets for direct attack.[86]

CLINICAL TEACHING. Conflicts of fidelity often emerge in institutions that serve
multiple functions, such as institutions that educate health professionals through
the care of patients. The use of patients for teaching purposes need not violate
the prohibition against treating persons merely as means, because such patients
may choose to become participants in the training of professionals or the generation of scientific knowledge. If patients understand the divided loyalties of
teaching hospitals, are not subjected to undue risks, and are protected in other
ways (for example, by the rules of privacy and confidentiality), they can be
legitimate partners with teachers in the training of professionals. Indeed, some
studies indicate that many patients find bedside rounds (a declining practice) to
be "a positive experience that should be continued."[87] In addition to general
disclosure and consent upon entry, there should be specific disclosures. For
example, the patient should be told who will be on the surgical team and who
will be in charge.[88] The principle of justice also requires that any burdens of
participation, even if these burdens are only minor inconveniences, not be ine-

quitably assigned to poorer and less educated patients—a criterion also for the selection of subjects in research.[89]

Conflicts of fidelity in nursing

Perhaps in no area of health care are conflicts among obligations of fidelity more pervasive and morally troubling than in nursing. Although the same principles and rules apply to all health-care professionals, what they imply for the conduct of any particular person will depend on the structure of health care, its roles, its conventions, and its practices. For example, if a patient has a right to the truth about his or her condition, we still must ask who, among the various possible agents, has the obligation to make the disclosure. Answers to such questions often hinge on a more general understanding of moral responsibility in nursing.

Two coauthors describe the setting of nursing as follows: "Traditionally, nurses have been discouraged from developing and acting on their own ethical judgments. Although the institutions of nursing and medicine developed separately until the late eighteenth century, the increasing importance of the hospital in health care brought nursing under the dual command of physicians and hospital administrators."[90] Recent codes of nursing ethics reflect still other transitions. They define the moral responsibility of nurses in sharply different ways from the codes of even two decades earlier. For example, in 1950, the first code of the American Nurses' Association stressed the nurse's obligation to carry out the physician's orders, but the 1976 revision stressed the nurse's obligation to the client. Whereas the original code emphasized the nurse's obligation to protect the reputation of associates, the later code emphasized the obligation to safeguard the client and the public from "incompetent, unethical or illegal" practices of any person.

A similar dramatic shift appears in the codes of ethics of the International Council of Nursing. An earlier code stated that "the nurse is under an obligation to carry out the physician's orders intelligently and loyally and to refuse to participate in unethical procedures." It did not, however, define such procedures. The revised code of 1973 marks a definite shift. Instead of viewing the nurse as responsible primarily to the physician or to the institution, it holds that "the nurse's primary responsibility is to those people who require nursing care." Many nurses even conceive their role to be that of "patient advocate."[91]

Alterations in these codes reflect important changes in the profession of nursing, but their implications have not been fully clarified or implemented in institutions. Consequently, nurses may have to choose between discharging responsibilities to the physician and to the institution on the one hand and to the patient on the other.[92] Consider Case 15: Mrs. R., who is approximately forty-five years old, a divorcee, and the mother of teenage daughters who live with her, suffers from multiple sclerosis. She often comes to the emergency room of the local community hospital for treatment of acute episodes of asthma. The physician has ordered "no code" (no cardiopulmonary resuscitation) in case Mrs. R. suffered a cardiac arrest. The nurses believe that the physician made the decision without discussing it with Mrs. R. or the family, and they are not sure what Mrs. R. would want because she is often depressed when she comes to the emergency room and has not expressed her wishes.

What ought a nurse to do in these circumstances?[93] The nurse should first ascertain whether the patient's wishes have been determined and are being respected. If Mrs. R. competently and voluntarily requested or consented to the "no code" order, and if Mrs. R. and the physician are in agreement, the "no code" order should be followed. But if Mrs. R. enters the emergency room and suffers a cardiac arrest before this information can be obtained, the nurse and others may legitimately ignore the "no code" and provide the treatment ordinarily indicated in such cases. Should the nurse discover that the physician has ordered "no code" against the express wishes of Mrs. R., the nurse should refuse to follow the order. (We will return to conscientious refusals in the next chapter.) Because this case involves important moral principles, including respect for autonomy and beneficence, the nurse should not be satisfied with a refusal to carry out the "no code" order. The nurse has pledged, through nursing codes, to seek to have the physician's order countermanded in order to protect the patient's best interest and wishes. The nurse may also have a responsibility to goad the hospital to develop clearer and more satisfactory policies governing CPR.

Significant conflicts between health-care professionals can be expected as long as there are major differences in degrees of participation in decision making and in degrees of closeness and distance in the delivery of care. There will probably be political if not moral problems as long as some professionals make the decisions and order their implementation by other professionals who have not participated in the decision making. The several cases in which nurses have blown the whistle on parents and physicians who have decided not to treat seriously handicapped newborns and have required others to implement their decisions are unfortunate and, we think, largely avoidable conflicts.

There are no second-order rules to enable professionals to resolve all the dilemmas created by conflicts between rules of fidelity and other principles and rules. However, it is often possible for professionals to clarify the nature and weight of their obligation of fidelity—for example, whether there is an implicit or explicit contract—and also to take special care to avoid some contracts or roles linked with expectations that would necessitate major compromises with other principles and rules. If substantive resolutions are not possible, there may nonetheless be procedural solutions for many forms of conflict between obligations of fidelity and other obligations.

Conflicts of fidelity in clinical research

The Declaration of Geneva of the World Medical Association affirms that "the health of my patient will be my first consideration." But can this principle be affirmed under all conditions in the context of research involving patients (or other human subjects)? The dual roles of research scientist and clinical practitioner may conflict and present a range of problems similar to those discussed above. As an investigator, the physician acts to generate scientific knowledge that will ultimately benefit individual patients. As a clinical practitioner, he or she may have specific contracts and responsibilities for care and in general must act in the patient's best interests. Both roles may benefit the sick; but the scientific role primarily aims to benefit future patients, whereas the clinical role seeks to benefit particular patients now. Responsibility to future generations may conflict with "due care" for particular patients.

Research involving human subjects must satisfy several conditions, including the pursuit of important knowledge, a reasonable prospect that the research will generate the knowledge that is sought, the necessity of using human subjects (e.g., the Nuremberg code holds that "the experiment should be such as to yield fruitful results for the good of society, unprocurable by other methods or means of study"), favorable balance of benefits to the subject and the society over risks to the subject, and fair selection of subjects.[94] Only after these conditions have been met, as attested by researchers and by an institutional review board, is it appropriate to ask subjects to participate. Consent is necessary for the research to be with human subjects, rather than merely on them,[95] but it is not sufficient by itself to justify the research.

Limiting contracts between potential subjects and investigators to research that passes the above tests has been criticized as paternalistic.[96] However, because society encourages extensive research and because investigators and subjects are unequal in knowledge and vulnerability—especially if sick patients are involved—it is morally appropriate to prevent potentially exploitative contracts, to protect privacy and confidentiality, and to provide compensation for injuries incurred in research.[97]

RANDOMIZED CLINICAL TRIALS. The above observations apply to nontherapeutic research, which offers no prospect of medical benefit to the subject, and also to therapeutic research, which offers some prospect of medical benefit to the patient-subject. Among the forms of therapeutic research, controlled clinical trials are sometimes necessary in order to confirm that an observed effect, such as reduced mortality from a particular disease, is the result of a particular treatment rather than some unknown variable in the patient population. A control group receives either a standard therapy or a placebo—a procedure or substance, such as a sugar pill, that the investigator believes is pharmacologically or biomedically inert for the patient's condition—in order to allow investigators to determine whether an experimental therapy is more effective and safer than a standard therapy or a placebo.

Among the controlled trials to determine the effectiveness and safety of treatment, the randomized clinical trial (RCT) is widely used. Instead of trying to match patients for variables so that some of the matched patients can receive A and some B, the RCT randomly assigns patients to different therapies or placebos. Randomization is designed to keep variables other than the particular treatments under examination from distorting the study. RCTs are often preferred to observational or retrospective studies on grounds that their results have a higher degree of validity by eliminating bias in assignment and reducing the effects of extraneous variables.

RCTs may be single-blind (the subject does not know whether he or she is in the control group or the experimental group), double-blind (neither the subject nor the investigator knows), or unblinded (all parties know). Double-blind studies are designed specifically to reduce bias in observations and reports by subjects and physicians. Blinding the physician-investigator, according to some interpretations, also serves an ethical function, because it obviates the conflict of interest present in both providing therapy and performing research.

Even though RCTs are generally sound ways to generate knowledge, they are not free of moral questions. In Chapter 3, we discussed whether informed consent could and should be given by subjects in these trials. But there are other questions as well. For example, are RCTs as essential as their proponents say? Can they be used without compromising acknowledged responsibilities to patients?[98] The increased certainty of the results is only a matter of degree, and there might be moral reasons for preferring a less conclusive method if it would more adequately fulfill obligations to current patients. It seems inconsistent with serving the patient's best interests to select a treatment randomly for the patient. Such random allocation is just what the patient does not expect his or her physician to do or to permit to be done by others. No two patients are alike, and it is essential that a physician be able to modify the individual course of therapy, as required by the patient's best interests. But is this axiom of medical ethics consistent with controlled trials? Are the current patient's interests sacrificed to those of future patients? Can statistically significant results be achieved if physicians are allowed to act on this principle of the patient's best interests? Finally, to return to the problems of Chapter 3, is the entire structure of RCTs consistent with the obligation to obtain informed consent?[99]

Proponents of RCTs often argue that RCTs do not violate moral obligations to patients because they are only used in circumstances in which there is genuine doubt about the merits of existing, standard, or new therapies. No patient, they note, will receive a treatment known to be less effective or more dangerous than another available alternative. Because current patients, in effect, are not asked to make any sacrifices, who could object to this use of RCTs, especially when they promise benefit to future patients?

Prior to initiating an RCT, there is usually some evidence about a treatment's safety or efficacy, even relative to other treatments, and one of the major questions is, "What will count as knowledge and what will be sufficient to convince others?" The standard of statistical significance that is widely used—probability of at least 0.05, which means that there is less than a one-in-twenty chance that there is no difference in effects and that the difference results from a variable other than the treatments—is reasonable and well established, but the convention involves a normative choice about which cutoff establishes significance.[100] The convention has also been criticized as arbitrary, despite its well-entrenched position.

Two vivid recent examples indicate some controversies about the use of RCTs. According to one report (see Case 27), a controlled double-blind experiment on a new drug, adenine arabinoside (ara-A), indicated that it is an effective treatment for herpes simplex encephalitis, a disease fatal to approximately seventy percent of those who contract it. Of the ten people given the placebo, seven died, one suffered severe damage, and two recovered to lead reasonably normal lives. Of the eighteen who received ara-A, five died, six had serious brain or nerve damage, and seven recovered to lead reasonably normal lives. The ten who received the placebo were given standard treatment, which mainly consists of palliative care because no treatment prior to ara-A had been found to be effective.

Critics charge that it was not necessary to have a placebo group instead of historical controls. Because ara-A had already been shown to be effective and nontoxic in some localized herpes simplex hominis infections, and because no other treatment prevented mortality and serious brain and nerve damage, moral questions have been raised about giving anyone the placebo. Defenders of the research respond that the mortality rate of herpes simplex encephalitis was not known prior to the research because the disease is so difficult to diagnose apart from brain biopsies and that it was not known whether ara-A would be toxic when administered with large amounts of fluid to such patients. The research was stopped when the above statistics emerged, but several scientists contend that it was stopped prematurely, before statistically significant evidence had emerged about effectiveness and toxicity. They note that because of the small groups involved, it is misleading to say that 20 percent of the recipients of the placebo and 38.8 percent of the recipients of ara-A had reasonable recovery. If only one person, the next placebo recipient, had had reasonably normal recovery, the figures would have been much closer.[101]

A similar conflict erupted over placebo-controlled trials of AZT (azidothymidine) in the treatment of AIDS, as Case 28 reports. After it had earlier proved to be ineffective in the treatment of cancer, AZT was shelved for several years by its manufacturer, Burroughs Wellcome, only to be removed in the massive search for some effective agent in the treatment of AIDS. Promising laboratory tests were followed by a trial (phase I) to determine the safety of AZT among AIDS patients. Several patients showed clinical improvement during the trial. Because AIDS is believed to be universally fatal, many people argued that compassion should dictate making it immediately available to all AIDS patients and perhaps to patients with ARC (aids-related complex) or those who are antibody-positive to the AIDS virus. Not only did the company have an inadequate supply of the drug for all AIDS patients, but it followed a placebo-controlled trial of AZT to determine its effectiveness for certain groups of AIDS patients (as federal regulations require). A computer randomly assigned some AIDS patients to AZT and others to a placebo, in this case a sugar pill. For several months, no major differences emerged in effectiveness, but then patients receiving the placebo began to die at a significantly higher rate. Of the 137 patients on the placebo, 16 died; of the 145 patients on AZT, only 1 died. In view of these results, the trial was terminated on the advice of a data and safety monitoring board. Subjects who had received the placebo in the trial were, as promised, the first to receive the drug.

Future research will have to compare other drugs with AZT as the standard drug, and placebo-controlled trials will probably be considered unethical, at least for certain groups of patients. However, it is not known how effective AZT will be over time (it does not cure the underlying disease) or how toxic it will prove to be. Beginning in early 1987, the drug was distributed according to strict criteria because the supply was inadequate for all AIDS patients, there was inadequate evidence about its effectiveness for some groups of patients, and there was uncertainty about whether the risks of the drug (e.g., its toxicity) would outweigh its benefits to patients with ARC. Proponents of compassion for present patients have raised questions about starting such a placebo-controlled trial when the disease appears to be universally fatal and there is no promising alternative to the new treatment. They also raise questions about when to stop a trial and how broadly to distribute a new treatment.[102]

Even if there are neither scientific nor ethical grounds for opposing a particular randomized clinical trial of two treatments that are roughly equal in safety and efficacy, patients may have strong preferences for one treatment or the other. Suppose two surgical procedures for treating the same disease appear to have the same survival rate (say, an average of fifteen years), and suppose we test their effectiveness by an RCT. The patient might have a preference if treatment A has little risk of death during the operation but a high rate of death after ten years, while treatment B has a high risk of death during the operation or postoperative recovery but a low rate of death after recovery (say, for thirty years). A patient's age, family responsibilities, and other circumstances might lead to a preference for one over the other.[103] If there is no known difference in the rates of survival after two procedures, patients may have a strong preference for the less invasive or less disfiguring procedure, as they did in trials of treatments for breast cancer that are discussed below. Some research institutions can legitimately accept only patients willing to participate in research projects related to their diseases, but patients should generally be able to choose between treatments if both treatments are available.

Because patients commonly assume that decisions about their treatments are made in their best interests, and not in the interests of a research design, the physician-researcher should disclose all significant alternatives to patient-subjects so that they can make an informed judgment about participation. One relevant item of information is the method used to determine who receives a particular treatment. Some contend that disclosure of the allocation system would cause distress to the patient or would lead some patients to refuse to participate in the research. They also argue that disclosure of such matters is not necessary because patients do not need to know how the allocation is made between two treatments that appear to be equally effective and equally risky. However, because the physician-researcher has dual responsibilities, he or she has a fiduciary obligation to inform patient-subjects of every item directly relevant to their decisions, including conditions that might involve the physician-researcher in a conflict of interest.[104]

This obligation of disclosure is not always met. In Denmark, a randomized clinical trial (Case 29) was conducted to assess the value of intestinal bypass in the treatment of gross obesity. One hundred thirty patients received surgery and were compared with sixty-six patients who received medical treatment. The subjects—at least the ones receiving medical treatment—did not give informed consent, because the researchers withheld relevant information and used deception. As the researchers reported, "We did not ask for informed consent for randomization. Patients allocated to medical treatment were told that surgery had to be postponed for an undetermined period primarily because liver-biopsy findings showed fatty infiltration" (even though this statement was untrue).[105]

THE USE OF PRERANDOMIZATION. One controversial development in RCTs has been the use of prerandomization. In conventional RCTs, the patient is screened for eligibility and then informed about the study, the different arms of treatment or placebo (if one is used), the risks and benefits, and the method of assignment to the different arms. If the patient consents to participate, he or she is randomized to one arm of the study. In prerandomization there is a shift in the time of randomization, so that it occurs prior to the patient's consent to participate.

The National Surgical Adjuvant Project for Breast and Bowel Cancers designed an important study of treatments of breast cancer to determine whether survival rates differed among patients randomly assigned to simple mastectomy versus lumpectomy with or without radiation. However, this RCT had such a low rate of patient participation that researchers thought it might have to be discontinued because an inadequate number of subjects threatened the canons of statistical significance. Two statisticians associated with the project describe the problem:

A major problem with the protocol appeared to be the lack of acceptability of the randomization. Physicians were reluctant to approach patients at the time of the operation about chance assignment to surgical therapies that involved either removal or cosmetic preservation of the breast. Patients also had difficulty dealing with randomization. In many cases, patients were not even certain whether or not they had a breast cancer and yet they were being asked to consider quite dissimilar surgical procedures if cancer was found at the time of the surgery. Further, even when the patient knew the diagnosis, it was disquieting not to know which surgery would be performed, i.e., whether she would wake up with or without a breast.[106]

For this RCT to be ethically justified, it had to be reasonable to assume that neither treatment was superior to the other in survival rates; but under these conditions, considerations of quality of life become central in decisions to participate, and women's preferences for the less invasive and disfiguring surgery would be reasonable. A survey of physicians who decided not to enter all of their patients in this nationwide RCT identified several moral and nonmoral difficulties:

(1) concern that the doctor-patient relationship would be affected by a randomized clinical trial (73 percent), (2) difficulty with informed consent (38 percent), (3) dislike of open discussions involving uncertainty [including uncertainty about the superior treatment and about which treatment patients would receive through randomization] (22 percent), (4) perceived conflicts between the roles of scientist and clinician (18 percent), (5) practical difficulties in following procedures (9 percent), and (6) feelings of personal responsibility if the treatments were found to be unequal (8 percent).[107]

However after prerandomization was adopted, the accrual rate increased sixfold and the trial was salvaged, producing sound evidence that the survival rates are as good with the less disfiguring surgery for early breast cancer.[108]

Although the outcome of this RCT was scientifically decisive and significant, critics have raised moral questions about the method of prerandomization. The major question for many critics is how the simple shift in time from randomization to prerandomization could result in increased patient accrual without some distortion in the information patients received, particularly in view of the physicians' stated reasons for their reluctance to enroll all of their eligible patients. It is possible that although they had no preference for one treatment over the other, some patients refused conventional randomization because of its uncertainty—that is, because of their lack of knowledge about which treatment they would receive. But there seems to be no evidence to support this hypothesis.[109] It would be odd if rational behavior under randomization could shift so dramatically under prerandomization.[110] Many suspect that disclosure of information becomes distorted, perhaps unconsciously, when the physician knows the assigned treatment in advance.[111] At the very least, the process of obtaining informed consent under conditions of prerandomization merits unusually careful scrutiny in order to ensure adequate disclosure.

There is more general and justified opposition to another version of prerandomization that only solicits consent from patients who receive the experimental treatment, not the standard treatment, although those receiving the standard treatment are followed through chart review. In addition to problems of scientific validity—for example, the groups are different in that one group knows something the other group does not—ethical problems are evident in one description of the values of this approach: "The proposed new design has the desirable feature that the physician need only approach the patient to discuss a single therapy. The physician need not leave himself open, in the eyes of the patient, to not knowing what he is doing and 'tossing a coin' to decide the treatment."[112] But if it is a genuine and ethical RCT, it will involve something like tossing a coin, and the physician-researcher should not hide that relevant fact.

EARLY TERMINATION OF CLINICAL TRIALS. Physician-researchers may also face difficult questions about whether to stop an experiment before its completion, and even before they have sufficient data to support the preliminary conclusions. If a physician determines that a patient's condition is deteriorating and that the patient's interests dictate withdrawal from the research, the physician should be free to act on behalf of the patient, assuming that he or she does not act in opposition to the express wishes of the patient. Some research designs take advantage of emerging evidence to alter the protocol; and some play the winner by utilizing what appear to be the best therapies until they fail.[113] But in an RCT it may be difficult to determine whether the experiment as a whole should be stopped even if some physician-researchers insist that they are satisfied by the evidence. As we noted earlier, some researchers contend that the trial of ara-A was stopped before the evidence became statistically convincing. They maintain that, as a result, there exists no definitive determination that ara-A is superior to standard, palliative care.

One procedural proposal to handle the ethical conflict involves a differentiation of roles. It recommends an advisory committee to determine whether to continue or stop a trial. Such a committee "must consider the impact of its decision on the treatment of future patients. Although an individual physician may only be responsible for treating his current patients, the advisory committee must act as if the care of future patients rests in their hands, because their recommendations are likely to influence therapy for the many patients to follow.''[114]

This differentiation of roles by using an advisory committee—particularly in a double-blind RCT—may be procedurally sound, but it relocates rather than resolves central ethical questions. The advisory committee must then determine when, if ever, it is legitimate to impose some risks on current patients in order to benefit future ones by increasing confidence that one treatment is superior to another or to a placebo in terms of safety or effectiveness or both.

Patient-subjects may also face questions about whether to withdraw from an RCT prior to its termination or completion of their scheduled participation. Consent forms typically indicate that subjects may withdraw at any time, without detriment to their care.[115] However, several questions, particularly about the disclosure of information, are relevant to a patient-subject's decision to withdraw from an RCT. Of special importance is the question of the disclosure of interim data and early trends. Trends are often misleading and are later shown to be temporary aberrations, but they might be relevant to a patient-subject's decision to continue to participate. They represent the kind of evidence that might be decisive for patients (and their physicians), although the evidence would not satisfy statisticians on the subject.

Some hold that the research physician's commitment to the welfare of his or her patients offers the best protection, even if a research protocol has been authorized by an institutional review board. Others, however, contend that we should differentiate roles so that physicians do not use their patients in research. The point is not that a person cannot be both an investigator and a clinician but that a person should not assume both roles for the same patient-subject.[116] A similar argument from conflict of interest concludes that the physician who is to transplant a heart from A to B should not be allowed to determine when A is dead.

Proposals for these procedures will depend in part on conceptions of human nature and convictions about the importance of reducing conflicts of interest. In many cases role differentiation may obviate some of the moral conflicts. Nevertheless, answers to procedural questions will not be satisfactory unless we also have answers to more substantive questions. At stake is not merely who can and should protect patients' interests but how much weight should be given to the interests of current patients and how much to interests of future patients.

Our view is that medical knowledge and scientific progress are vital goals, but particular protocols are often optional. Our obligations to future patients are strong enough that we should permit, encourage, and support research that can generate knowledge without violating the rights and interests of current patients. But the obligation of beneficence to future generations of patients is generally less stringent than the obligation to benefit the sick, who already have a special relationship with health-care professionals. It is important to avoid making RCTs a ritual or a necessary canon of acceptable research. RCTs are often important but not always indispensable and could be replaced by historical controls in some trials.

Conclusion

In this chapter, we have applied the four principles of respect for autonomy, nonmaleficence, beneficence, and justice to relationships in research and health care. We have concentrated on rules derived from these principles—the rules of veracity, fidelity, confidentiality, and privacy—and their conflicts. In each instance, we have explored the basis, meaning, limits, and stringency of these rules in the context of professional and patient or subject relationships. These rules, like the principles on which they depend, are prima facie binding, and our analysis has indicated some conditions under which each can be overridden.

Morality includes more than these principles and rules. When conflicts occur between prima facie obligations, we often recognize that the character traits of a person who must make a judgment are no less important than obligations derived from principles and rules. Several times in this chapter we have appealed to the importance of virtues such as truthfulness and trustworthiness. Any adequate ethical theory must also attend to these virtues, to integrity, which is often expressed in terms of conscience, and to moral ideals. We turn to these topics in the final chapter.

Notes

1. Some of these derivative moral rules might be appropriately described as derivative moral principles, but for simplicity of analysis we use the term *rules*. We believe these rules are best understood as derivative from one or more of the four basic moral principles. We refer to them as rules rather than as a rule because they generally involve several distinct and specific requirements.
2. Henry Sidgwick, *The Methods of Ethics*, 7th ed. (London: Macmillan, 1907), pp. 315–16.
3. G. J. Warnock, *The Object of Morality* (London: Methuen, 1971), pp. 85–86.
4. See Alan Donagan, *The Theory of Morality* (Chicago: University of Chicago Press, 1977), p. 88; and Charles Fried, *Right and Wrong* (Cambridge, Mass.: Harvard University Press, 1978), chap. 3.
5. See W. D. Ross, *The Right and the Good* (Oxford: Clarendon Press, 1930), chap. 2.
6. Sissela Bok stresses the harm of lies to the one lied to, to the liar, and to social trust. See *Lying: Moral Choice in Public and Private Life* (New York: Pantheon

Books, 1978), pp. 188 et passim. For discussions of utilitarianism and veracity, see David Lewis, "Utilitarianism and Truthfulness," *Australasian Journal of Philosophy* 50 (May 1972): 17–19; and Peter Singer, "Is Act-Utilitarianism Self-Defeating?" *Philosophical Review* 81 (1972): 94–104. See also Arnold Isenberg, "Deontology and the Ethics of Lying," *Philosophy and Phenomenological Research* 24 (1964): 465–80; and Roderick M. Chisholm and Thomas D. Feehan, "The Intent to Deceive," *Journal of Philosophy* 74 (March 1977): 143–59.

7. *Truman* v. *Thomas,* 611 P.2d 902 (Cal. 1980), at 906, quoting *Cobbs* v. *Grant,* 502 P.2d at 10.

8. This case is discussed in Bettina Schöne-Seifert and James F. Childress, "How Much Should the Cancer Patient Know and Decide?" *CA-A Cancer Journal* 36 (March–April 1986): 85–94.

9. See Donald Oken, "What to Tell Cancer Patients: A Study of Medical Attitudes," *Journal of the American Medical Association* 175 (1961): 1120–28; William D. Kelly and Stanley R. Freisen, "Do Cancer Patients Want to Be Told?" *Surgery* 27 (1950): 822–26; Dennis H. Novack et al., "Changes in Physicians' Attitudes toward Telling the Cancer Patient," *Journal of the American Medical Association* 241 (1979): 897–900. For a valuable survey and analysis of various studies, see Robert M. Veatch and Ernest Tai, "Talking about Death: Patterns of Lay and Professional Change," *Annals of the American Academy of Political and Social Science* 447 (January 1980): 29–45.

10. For several reasons for the change, see Veatch and Tai, "Talking about Death," and Novack et al., "Changes in Physicians' Attitudes."

11. Novack et al., "Changes in Physicians' Attitudes."

12. See Bok's discussion of similar arguments in *Lying,* chap. 15. For her discussion of the obligation of veracity as presented in various codes, see Sissela Bok, "Truthtelling," *The Encyclopedia of Bioethics,* ed. Warren T. Reich (New York: Free Press, 1978), Vol. IV.

13. James Boswell, *Life of Johnson,* Vol. IV, p. 306, as quoted in Donagan, *The Theory of Morality,* p. 89.

14. See Bok, *Lying,* chap. 1, for a discussion of the distinction between truth and truthfulness.

15. See "Huntington's Disease: Some Prefer Not to Know," *Medical World News* 15 (April 5, 1974).

16. See, for example, several studies in the *American Journal of Medical Genetics* 26 (1987), esp. C. Mastromauro, R. H. Myers, and B. Berkman, "Attitudes toward Presymptomatic Testing in Huntington's Disease," pp. 271–82.

17. Kimberly A. Quaid et al., "The Decision to Be Tested for Huntington's Disease," *Journal of the American Medical Association* 257 (1987): 3362.

18. See Robert Veatch, *Death, Dying and the Biological Revolution* (New Haven: Yale University Press, 1976), chap. 6.

19. Margery W. Shaw, "Testing for the Huntington Gene: A Right to Know, a Right Not to Know, or a Duty to Know?" *American Journal of Medical Genetics* 26 (1987): 243–46.

20. Ronald Bayer, Carol Levine, and Susan M. Wolf, "HIV Antibody Screening: An Ethical Framework for Evaluating Proposed Programs," *Journal of the American Medical Association* 256 (1986): 1768–74.

21. Perry L. Bartelt and Marjorie A. Bowman, letter to editor, *Journal of the American Medical Association* 258 (1987): 1604.

22. See Robert Veatch, *Case Studies in Medical Ethics* (Cambridge, Mass: Harvard University Press, 1977), pp. 137–39.

23. Charles L. Bosk, *Forgive and Remember: Managing Medical Failure* (Chicago: University of Chicago Press, 1979).

24. Joan Vogel and Richard Delgado, "To Tell the Truth: Physician's Duty to Disclose Medical Mistakes," *UCLA Law Review* 28 (1980): 55.

25. Ibid., pp. 52–94. "Aside from their need for information to evaluate treatment, patients may simply want to know what has happened to them. The Golden Rule supports a duty to disclose; if we were malpractice victims we would presumably wish to be notified rather than kept in ignorance of the damage that has been done to our bodies" (p. 61, n. 55).

26. See Jonathan Alter with Peter McKillop, "AIDS and the Right to Know: A Question of Privacy," *Newsweek*, August 18, 1986, pp. 46–47.

27. James Fitzjames Stephen, *Liberty, Equality and Fraternity* (New York: Henry Holt, 1873); Samuel Warren and Louis Brandeis, "The Right to Privacy," *Harvard Law Review* 4 (1890): 193–220. The latter is reprinted in Ferdinand D. Schoeman, ed. *Philosophical Dimensions of Privacy: An Anthology* (New York: Cambridge University Press, 1984). Schoeman's anthology contains a helpful bibliography. See also David O'Brien, *The Right to Privacy: Its Constitutional and Social Dimensions: A Comprehensive Bibliography* (Austin: University of Texas Law School, 1980). Our analysis of privacy has benefited from an unpublished paper by Michael Duffy and from discussion with him. We were unable to take account of another important book in this chapter, Anita Allen, *Uneasy Access: Privacy for Women in a Free Society* (Totowa, N.J.: Rowman and Allanheld, 1987).

28. *Pierce v. Society of Sisters*, 268 U.S. 510 (1925); *Meyer v. Nebraska*, 262 U.S. 390 (1923).

29. For example, see *Wisconsin v. Yoder*, 406 U.S. 205 (1972); *Stanley v. Georgia*, 394 U.S. 557 (1969); *Loving v. Virginia*, 388 U.S. 1 (1967); *Skinner v. Oklahoma*, 316 U.S. 535 (1942).

30. *Griswold v. Connecticut*, 381 U.S. 479 (1965) [on contraception]; *Roe v. Wade*, 410 U.S. 113 (1973) [on abortion]. In *Griswold*, Justice William O. Douglas, writing the majority opinion for the Court, rested his decision on privacy, but four separate opinions by members of the majority cited different grounds to justify their concurrence in the result. Not all were based on a right to privacy.

Historically, the earliest expression of the privacy right was derived from two common-law doctrines, libel and copyright law, and not from the Constitution. At that time, the right was limited to protecting individuals from those who would pry into, observe, or publicize personal matters. In an influential 1960 article that preceded *Griswold*, William Prosser argued that the common law of privacy protects not one but four different privacy interests: (1) an interest in freedom from intrusion into solitude and personal affairs, (2) an interest in freedom from disclosure of potentially embarrassing facts about one's person, (3) an interest in freedom from publicity that falsely represents one's views or conduct, and (4) an interest in freedom from appropriation of one's name or likeness for the advantage of another. The constitutional right developed from these inherently subjective privacy interests. See William L. Prosser, "Privacy," *California Law Review* 48 (1960): 383–423. For a critique of the latter, see Edward J. Bloustein, "Privacy as an Aspect of Human Dignity: An Answer to Dean Prosser," *New York University Law Review* 39 (1964): 962–1007.

31. See, for example, Tom Geret, "Redefining Privacy," *Harvard Civil Rights–Civil Liberties Law Review* 12 (1977): 233; Jeffrey Reiman, "Privacy, Intimacy and Personhood," *Philosophy and Public Affairs* 6 (1976): 26; Comment, "A Taxonomy of Privacy," *California Law Review* 64 (1976): 1447. See also Laurence Tribe, *American Constitutional Law* (Mineola, N.Y.: Foundation Press, 1978), pp. 886–96.

32. Ferdinand D. Schoeman, "Privacy: Philosophical Dimensions of the Literature," in Schoeman, ed., *Philosophical Dimensions of Privacy*, p. 3.

33. Ruth Gavison, "Privacy and the Limits of Law," *Yale Law Journal* 89 (January 1980): 428; reprinted in Schoeman, ed. *Philosophical Dimensions of Privacy*, pp. 346–402.

34. Richard Wasserstrom, "Privacy: Some Arguments and Assumptions," *Philosophical Law,* ed. Richard Bronaugh (Westport, Conn.: Greenwood Press, 1978); reprinted in Schoeman, ed., *Philosophical Dimensions of Privacy*, pp. 317–332.

35. Charles Fried, "Privacy: A Rational Context," *Yale Law Journal* 77 (1968): 475–93; reprinted in Schoeman, ed., *Philosophical Dimensions of Privacy*, pp. 203–22.

36. Warren and Brandeis, "The Right to Privacy."

37. Thomson, "The Right to Privacy," *Philosopy and Public Affairs* 4 (Summer 1975): 295–314, reprinted in Schoeman, ed., *Privacy*, pp. 272–89. For criticisms of Thomson's important essay, see Thomas Scanlon, "Thomson on Privacy," and James Rachels, "Why Privacy is Important," *Philosophy and Public Affairs* 4 (Summer 1975): 315–333. (Rachels' essay is reprinted in Schoeman, ed., *Privacy*, pp. 290–99.)

38. Fried, "Privacy: A Rational Context."

39. Joel Feinberg, "Autonomy, Sovereignty, and Privacy: Moral Ideas in the Constitution?" *Notre Dame Law Review* 58 (February 1983): 445–92.

40. W. A. Parent, "Recent Work on the Concept of Privacy," *American Philosophical Quarterly* 20 (October 1983): 343.

41. H. J. McCloskey, "Privacy and the Right to Privacy," *Philosophy* 55 (January 1980): 36.

42. See Bok, *Lying,* chap. 14 et passim.

43. *Head* v. *Colloton,* 331 NW 2d 870 (Iowa 1983). See also Paul Lansing, "The Conflict of Patient Privacy and the Freedom of Information Act," and Robert A. Burt, "Coercion and Communal Morality," both in *Journal of Health Politics, Policy and Law* 9 (Summer 1984): 315–22, 323–24; and Arthur Caplan et al., "Mrs. X and the Bone Marrow Transplant," *Hastings Center Report* 13 (June 1983): 18–19.

44. David Zimmerman, commentary on "Mrs. X and the Bone Marrow Transplant," *Hastings Center Report* 13 (June 1983): 18.

45. The literature on HIV infection and AIDS must be constantly updated. For some helpful reports as of 1988, see Institute of Medicine and National Academy of Sciences, *Confronting AIDS* (Washington, D.C.: National Academy Press, 1986); and several articles in *Science* 239 (1988), esp. LeRoy Walters, "Ethical Issues in the Prevention and Treatment of HIV Infection and AIDS," pp. 597–603.

46. See Health and Public Policy Committee, American College of Physicians; and the Infectious Diseases Society of America, "Acquired Immunodeficiency Syndrome," *Annals of Internal Medicine* 104 (1986): 578. See also the references in notes 45 and 48. Some parts of the argument in this section appeared in James F. Childress,

"An Ethical Framework for Assessing Policies to Screen for Antibodies to HIV," *AIDS and Public Policy Journal* 2 (Winter 1987): 28–31.

47. Michael Mills, Constance B. Wofsy, and John Mills, "The Acquired Immunodeficiency Syndrome: Infection Control and Public Health Law," *New England Journal of Medicine* 314 (1986): 932.

48. For a strong argument that, at least in 1988, "mandatory premarital screening in a population with a low prevalence of infection is a relatively ineffective and inefficient use of resources," see Paul D. Cleary et al., "Compulsory Premarital Screening for the Human Immunodeficiency Virus: Technical and Public Health Considerations," *Journal of the American Medical Association* 258 (1987): 1757–62.

49. Gene W. Matthews and Verla S. Neslund, "The Initial Impact of AIDS on Public Health Law in the United States—1986," *Journal of the American Medical Association* 257 (1987): 345; Walters, "Ethical Issues," p. 598; Mark A. R. Kleiman, "Prostitution Isn't 'Victimless' with AIDS Here," *Wall Street Journal*, June 1, 1987, p. 22.

50. For statements about confidentiality in other codes (for example, in nursing) and in other societies, see *The Encyclopedia of Bioethics*, ed. Warren T. Reich (New York: Free Press, 1978), Vol. IV, Appendix, "Codes and Statements Related to Medical Ethics."

51. Mark Siegler, "Confidentiality in Medicine—A Decrepit Concept," *New England Journal of Medicine* 307 (1982): 1518–21.

52. Barry D. Weiss, "Confidentiality Expectations of Patients, Physicians, and Medical Students," *Journal of the American Medical Association* 247 (1982): 2695–97.

53. Sissela Bok, *Secrets: On the Ethics of Concealment and Revelation* (New York: Random House, Vintage Books, 1984), p. 119.

54. *Bratt* v. *IBM*, 467 N.E. 2d 126 (1984).

55. William Winslade, "Confidentiality," *Encyclopedia of Bioethics*, ed. Reich, Vol. I, 194–200.

56. *Tarasoff* v. *Regents of the University of California*, California Supreme Court, 17 California Reports, 3rd Series, 425, decided July 1, 1976.

57. Ibid.

58. D. Schmid et al., "Confidentiality in Psychiatry: A Study of the Patient's View," *Hospital and Community Psychiatry* 34 (1983): 353–55.

59. Paul S. Appelbaum et al., "Confidentiality: An Empirical Test of the Utilitarian Perspective," *Bulletin of the American Academy of Psychiatry and the Law* 12 (1984): 109–16.

60. See James F. Childress, *Civil Disobedience and Political Obligation* (New Haven: Yale University Press, 1971); and John Rawls, *A Theory of Justice* (Cambridge, Mass.: Harvard University Press, 1971), chap. 6.

61. See Schöne-Seifert and Childress, "How Much Should the Cancer Patient Know and Decide?"

62. Bernard B. Raginsky, "Hypnotic Recall of Aircrash Cause," *International Journal of Clinical and Experimental Hypnosis* 17 (1969): 1–19.

63. Aubrey Milunsky, *The Prevention of Genetic Disease and Mental Retardation* (Philadelphia: W. B. Saunders, 1975), p. 75.

64. "The Principles of Medical Ethics with Annotations Especially Applicable to Psychiatry," *American Journal of Psychiatry* 130 (September 1974): 1063.

65. Harvey Kuschner, Daniel Callahan, Eric J. Cassell, and Robert M. Veatch, "The Homosexual Husband and Physician Confidentiality," *Hastings Center Report* 7

(April 1977): 15–17. See also Robert Veatch, *A Theory of Medical Ethics* (New York: Basic Books, 1981), chap. 7.

66. For a discussion, see Grant Gillett, "AIDS and Confidentiality," *Journal of Applied Philosophy* 4 (1987): 15–20, from which this case study has been adapted.

67. On the legal situation in the United States, see Harlon L. Dalton, Scott Burris, and the Yale AIDS Law Project, *AIDS and the Law* (New Haven: Yale University Press, 1987).

68. For this debate, see Gillett, "AIDS and Confidentiality," and Case Studies, "AIDS and a Duty to Protect," *Hastings Center Report* 17 (February 1987): 22–23, with commentaries by Morton Winston and Sheldon H. Landesman.

69. Paul Ramsey, *The Patient as Person* (New Haven: Yale University Press, 1970), p. xii.

70. An example is W. D. Ross, who viewed fidelity as one of the prima facie principles that should govern human conduct; as we saw earlier, he even derived the obligation of veracity from this principle. Ross, *The Right and the Good*, p. 21.

71. Charles Fried has grounded the obligation of promise keeping in respect for autonomy. See Charles Fried, *Contract as Promise: A Theory of Contractual Obligation* (Cambridge, Mass.: Harvard University Press, 1981), p. 16. In addition, Rawls has plausibly contended that the principle of fidelity is only a special case of the principle of fairness applied to social practices of promising. Rawls, *A Theory of Justice*, p. 344.

72. Henry Sidgwick correctly observed that "the essential element of the Duty of Good Faith seems to be not conformity to my own statement [i.e., veracity], but to expectations that I have intentionally raised in others." Sidgwick, *Methods of Ethics*, p. 304. Contrast G. J. Warnock, *The Object of Morality*, chap. 7.

73. American Medical Association Council on Ethical and Judicial Affairs, *Current Opinions—1986* (Chicago: American Medical Association, 1986), 8.10.

74. This case was prepared by John Fletcher.

75. See *Matter of Baby M*, 537 A.2d. 1227 (N.J. 1988).

76. See, for example, Ramsey, *The Patient as Person;* William May, *The Physician's Covenant* (Philadelphia: Westminster Press, 1984); Leon Kass, *Toward a More Natural Science: Biology and Human Affairs* (New York: Free Press, 1985). In general, we favor *fidelity* in discussing specific obligations and *faithfulness* in discussing traits of character, but we sometimes use *loyalty* for both, especially for the latter.

77. See Veatch, *A Theory of Medical Ethics*.

78. See James F. Childress, *Who Should Decide? Paternalism in Health Care* (New York: Oxford University Press, 1982), chap. 1.

79. See H. L. A. Hart's discussion in "Are There Any Natural Rights?" *Philosophical Review* 64 (1955): 175–91.

80. See summary of In re *Sampson*, 317 NYS 2d (1970), in Angela Holder, *Medical Malpractice Law* (New York: John Wiley, 1975), p. 17.

81. See, for example, Anthony Shaw, "Dilemmas of 'Informed Consent' in Children," *New England Journal of Medicine* 289 (1973): 885–94. See also Anthony Shaw, Judson C. Randolph, and Barbara Manard, "Ethical Issues in Pediatric Surgery: A National Survey of Pediatricians and Pediatric Surgeons," *Pediatrics* 60 (October 1977): 588–99.

82. Even more complicated problems may emerge in the treatment of a pregnant woman and an unborn fetus, particularly if the fetus is viewed as a patient, because of

technological developments including intrauterine surgery and if the pregnant woman's interests and the fetus's interests conflict. See Case 22. See also Watson A. Bowes and Brad Selgestad, "Fetal versus Maternal Rights: Medical and Legal Perspectives," *Obstetrics and Gynecology* 58 (August 1981): 209–14; John C. Fletcher, "The Fetus as Patient: Ethical Issues," *Journal of the American Medical Association* 246 (1981): 722–23; and William R. Barclay et al., "The Ethics of In Utero Surgery," *Journal of the American Medical Association* 246 (1981): 1550–55.

83. Holder, *Medical Malpractice Law*, p. 19. A summary of *Lotspeich v. Chance Vought Aircraft Corporation*, 369 SW 2d Tex (1963). For a recent argument that "the ethical and legal principles derived from other aspects of providing medical care can be similarly applied in responding to dilemmas posed by caring for working patients," with the legal (but not ethical) exception for the preemployment examination, see Linda Rosenstock and Amy Hagopian, "Ethical Dilemmas in Providing Health Care to Workers," *Annals of Internal Medicine* 107 (1987): 580.

84. *PACAF Surgeon's Newsletter* 7 (December 1966): 5; reprinted in *Hastings Center Report* 6 (February 1976): 20 (with commentary). See also Veatch, *Case Studies in Medical Ethics*, pp. 245–58. For further discussion of the physician in the military, see Robert M. Goldwyn and Victor W. Sidel, "The Physician and War," *Ethical Issues in Medicine: The Role of the Physician in Today's Society*, ed. E. Fuller Torrey (Boston: Little, Brown, 1968), pp. 325–46.

85. See L. Sagan and A. Jonsen, "Medical Ethics and Torture," *New England Journal of Medicine* 294 (1976): 1428.

86. See Ingrid Detter De Lupis, *The Law of War* (Cambridge: Cambridge University Press, 1987), chap. 9.

87. Eugene W. Linfors and Francis A. Neelson, "The Case for Bedside Rounds," *New England Journal of Medicine* 303 (1980): 1231.

88. According to the AMA, there are rules against substituting a surgeon without the patient's knowledge or consent: "it is the operating surgeon to whom the patient grants consent to perform the operation." Even though this surgeon may use the assistance of residents and others, it is not appropriate for the resident or another physician to become the operating surgeon without the patient's knowledge or consent. AMA Council on Ethical and Judicial Affairs, *Current Opinions—1986*, 8.13.

89. See Bradford H. Gray, *Human Subjects in Medical Experimentation* (New York: Wiley-Interscience, 1975); and National Commission for the Protection of Human Subjects of Biomedical and Behavioral Research, *The Belmont Report* (Washington, D.C.: DHEW, 1978).

90. Martin Benjamin and Joy Curtis, "Ethical Autonomy in Nursing," in *Health Care Ethics*, ed. Donald VanDeVeer and Tom Regan (Philadelphia: Temple University Press, 1987), p. 394. See Andrew Jameton, "When Roles and Rules Conflict," *Hastings Center Report* 7 (1977): 22–23; and Arlene B. Dallery, "Professional Loyalties," *Holistic Nursing Practice* 1 (1986): 64–72.

91. See Gerald Winslow, "From Loyalty to Advocacy: A New Metaphor for Nursing," *Hastings Center Report* 14 (June 1984): 32–40; and Natalie Abrams, "A Contrary View of the Nurse as Patient Advocate," *Nursing Forum* 17 (1978): 258–67.

92. For helpful discussions of these conflicts, see Benjamin and Curtis, "Ethical Autonomy in Nursing," and *Ethics in Nursing*, 2d ed. (New York: Oxford University Press, 1986). See Anne J. Davis and Mila A. Aroskar, *Ethical Dilemmas and Nursing Practice*, 2d ed. (Norwalk, Conn.: Appleton-Century-Crofts, 1983), p.

49. See also Leah Curtin and Josephine Flaherty, *Nursing Ethics: Theories and Pragmatics* (Bowie, Md.: Robert J. Brady, 1982); Andrew Jameton, *Nursing Practice: The Ethical Issues* (Englewood Cliffs, N.J.: Prentice-Hall, 1984); Catherine P. Murphy and Howard Hunter, eds., *Ethical Problems in the Nurse-Patient Relationship* (Boston: Allyn and Bacon, 1983); James L. Muyskens, *Moral Problems in Nursing: A Philosophical Investigation* (Totowa, N.J.: Rowman and Littlefield, 1982); Stuart F. Spicker and Sally Gadow, eds., *Nursing: Images and Ideals* (New York: Springer, 1980).

93. See Mila Aroskar, Josephine M. Flaherty, and James M. Smith, "The Nurse and Orders Not to Resuscitate," *Hastings Center Report* 7 (August 1977): 27–28; and R. R. Yarling and B. J. McElmurry, "Rethinking the Nurse's Role in 'Do Not Resuscitate Orders,' " *Advances in Nursing Science* 5 (1983): 1–12.

94. See the Nuremberg code and *The Belmont Report* of the National Commission for the Protection of Human Subjects. See also James F. Childress, *Priorities in Biomedical Ethics* (Philadelphia: Westminster Press, 1981), chap. 3; LeRoy Walters, "Some Ethical Issues in Research Involving Human Subjects," *Perspectives in Biology and Medicine* (Winter 1977): 193–211; and Robert M. Veatch, *The Patient as Partner: A Theory of Human Experimentation Ethics* (Bloomington: Indiana University Press, 1987).

95. John C. Fletcher, "The Evolution of the Ethics of Informed Consent," in *Research Ethics,* ed. Kare Berg and Knut Erik Tranoy (New York: Alan R. Liss, 1983).

96. E. L. Pattullo, "Institutional Review Boards and the Freedom to Take Risks," *New England Journal of Medicine* 307 (1982): 1156–59.

97. See James F. Childress, "Compensating Injured Research Subjects: I. The Moral Argument," *Hastings Center Report* 6 (December 1976): 21–27.

98. For recent valuable assessments of RCTs, see the essays in *Journal of Medicine and Philosophy* 11 (November 1986) devoted to "Ethical Issues in the Use of Clinical Controls"; Bruce Miller, "Experimentation on Human Subjects: The Ethics of Random Clinical Trials," in *Health Care Ethics,* ed. Donald VanDeVeer and Tom Regan (Philadelphia: Temple University Press, 1987); and Robert J. Levine, *Ethics and the Regulation of Clinical Research,* 2d ed. (Baltimore: Urban and Schwarzenberg, 1986). A thorough, critical study of RCTs appears in Charles Fried, *Medical Experimentation: Personal Integrity and Social Policy* (New York: American Elsevier, 1974). For other criticisms, see Milton C. Weinstein, "Allocation of Subjects in Medical Experiments," *New England Journal of Medicine* 291 (1974): 1278–85. For defenses of RCTs, see David P. Byar et al., "Randomized Clinical Trials: Perspectives on Some Recent Ideas," *New England Journal of Medicine* 295 (1976): 74–80; and several writings by Thomas Chalmers, including Thomas C. Chalmers et al., "Controlled Studies in Clinical Cancer Research," *New England Journal of Medicine* 287 (1972): 75–78; L. W. Shaw and T. C. Chalmers, "Ethics in Cooperative Clinical Trials," *Annals of the New York Academy of Science* 169 (1970): 487–95; and Thomas Chalmers, "The Clinical Trial," *Milbank Memorial Fund Quarterly/Health and Society* 59 (Summer 1981): 324–39.

99. R. Burkhardt and G. Kienle, "Controlled Clinical Trials and Medical Ethics," *Lancet* 2 (1978): 1356–59. See Miller, "Experimentation on Human Subjects," p. 151.

100. See Loretta Kopelman, "Consent and Randomized Clinical Trials: Are There Moral or Design Problems?" *Journal of Medicine and Philosophy* 11 (November 1986): 322.

101. For some of the controversy and references, see Case 27.

102. See the references in Case 28 for the sources for this case presentation.

103. See Weinstein, "Allocation of Subjects in Medical Experiments," p. 1280.

104. See Fried, *Medical Experimentation*, p. 71.

105. See the Danish Obesity Project, "Randomised Trial of Jejunoileal Bypass versus Medical Treatment in Morbid Obesity," *Lancet* (1979): 1255.

106. C. Redmond and M. Bauer, "Statisticians' Report on Prerandomization," *NSABP Progress Report* (Pittsburgh: National Surgical Adjuvant Project for Breast and Bowel Cancers, 1979), as quoted in Kenneth F. Schaffner, "Ethical Problems in Clinical Trials," *Journal of Medicine and Philosophy* 11 (November 1986): 306.

107. K. Taylor, R. Margolese, and C. L. Soskolne, "Physicians' Reasons for Not Entering Eligible Patients in a Randomized Clinical Trials of Surgery for Breast Cancer," *New England Journal of Medicine* 310 (1984): 1363.

108. B. Fischer et al., "Five-Year Results of a Randomized Clinical Trial Comparing Total Mastectomy and Segmental Mastectomy With or Without Radiation in the Treatment of Breast Cancer," *New England Journal of Medicine* 312 (1985): 665–73.

109. Don Marquis, "Prerandomized Clinical Trials Are Unethical," *Journal of Medicine and Philosophy* 11 (November 1986): 380.

110. Marcia Angell, "Patient Preferences in Randomized Clinical Trials," *New England Journal of Medicine* 310 (1984): 1385–87.

111. See S. S. Ellenberg, "Randomized Designs in Comparative Clinical Trials," *New England Journal of Medicine* 310 (1984): 1404–8; Marquis, "Prerandomized Clinical Trials Are Unethical," p. 377. Contrast Kopelman, "Consent and Randomized Clinical Trials," pp. 334–36. It should also be noted that Marquis has serious reservations about "the conduct of many conventionally randomized clinical trials" as well (p. 382).

112. M. Zelen, "A New Design for Randomized Trials," *New England Journal of Medicine* 300 (1979): 1243.

113. Schaffner writes, "Suffice it to say that the [adaptive] designs did not live up to their promise and to the best of my knowledge have never been used in actual clinical trials." "Ethical Problems in Clinical Trials," p. 305. Joseph B. Kadane has proposed another version of adaptive designs, by using new Bayesian technology for eliciting the opinions of medical experts, which are conditioned on specific predictor variables and held in a computer for updating according to information generated in the trial. He argues that such a method, currently being used in a trial at Johns Hopkins, would give patients a fairer shake in clinical trials. "Progress Towards a More Ethical Method for Clinical Trials," *Journal of Medicine and Philosophy* 11 (November 1986): 385–404.

114. Byar et al., "Randomized Clinical Trials," p. 78, commenting on a proposal by Chalmers et al., "Controlled Studies in Clinical Cancer Research," pp. 75–78.

115. There are experiments in which a subject agrees not to withdraw after a certain time. For example, in a bone marrow transplant experiment, total body irradiation is used to prepare the recipient to receive the bone marrow. At that point the recipient would die if the subject-donor were permitted to withdraw.

116. See Fried, *Medical Experimentation*, pp. 160–61.

8

Ideals, Virtues, and Conscientiousness

Throughout this book we have concentrated on the justification of acts and policies. Principles and rules have been employed to support claims about obligations and rights. In this final chapter we examine other aspects of morality—in particular, moral ideals, virtues, and conscientiousness. These categories are consistent with our earlier categories. Whereas principles and rules determine morally required actions, moral ideals identify a dimension beyond the required, and virtues point to moral character. This chapter, then, is about a dimension of morality that complements and augments the discussion in the first seven chapters.

Moral ideals

Actions that are extraordinary and praiseworthy

Two levels of moral standards need to be distinguished in order to discuss moral ideals: ordinary moral standards and extraordinary moral standards. The first level is limited to moral standards that bind everyone. On the second level, which is a morality of aspiration, agents adopt ideals that do not bind everyone. These optional ideals are chosen autonomously and transcend ordinary morality. Those who realize these ideals can be praised and admired, whereas those who fall short cannot be rightly blamed, condemned, or coerced by others.

With the addition of ideals, we have at least four categories of moral action: (1) actions that are right and obligatory (such as truth telling); (2) actions that are wrong and prohibited (such as murder); (3) actions that are permissible, neither wrong nor obligatory but morally neutral; and (4) actions that are optional but also meritorious and praiseworthy. We have concentrated in earlier chapters on (1) and (2), mentioning (3) only in passing. In this section we are concerned with (4), and in later sections we will turn to the virtues, which do not constitute a category of moral action.

We begin with supererogatory actions, which represent a special type of ideal.[1] The etymological root of *supererogation* means paying or performing more than is required. As a general concept in moral theory, it has several features. First, a supererogatory act is neither required nor forbidden by the standards of common morality. Second, supererogatory acts are undertaken for the welfare of others beyond what obligation requires. Thus, these acts are optional, although agents may not themselves consider their actions morally optional. Many heroes and saints, for example, describe their actions in the language of *ought, duty,* and even *necessity:* "I had to do it." "I had no choice." "It was my duty." The point of this language is to express a personal sense of obligation that does not apply to others. Some accounts deny the literal appropriateness of this language, interpreting it as a form of moral modesty designed to deflect merit or praise that might be showered on the person.[2] Certainly one's personal belief that an action is obligatory does not make it obligatory rather than supererogatory.[3] The individual is free to regard the action as personally required and also free to view failure as grounds for guilt; but no one is free to view a supererogatory ideal as a general moral requirement.

Not all supererogatory acts are extraordinarily demanding, costly, or risky. Examples include generosity, gift-giving, and complying with requests made by other persons. For example, acts of volunteering to participate in nontherapeutic research that is not demanding, costly, or risky may be neither obligatory nor extraordinary; yet the acts are still supererogatory because they involve the personal and discretionary. The case is similar with low-risk organ and tissue donations; but many different actions fall under donation, and such gifts may sometimes be obligatory because of the principle of beneficence (see Chapter 5). Some special relationships between the parties—for example, debts of gratitude—might create an even stronger moral obligation to donate. However, as we argue below, the problem of distinguishing the obligatory from the nonobligatory is severe in these cases, and we can perhaps best conceive these acts as virtuous rather than obligatory.

Saints and heroes

Among the several different types of supererogatory actions, some heroic and saintly actions merit attention, because they provide developed models of supererogation. At the end of Albert Camus's *The Plague,* Dr. Rieux decides to make a record of those who fought the pestilence. It is to be a record of "what had to be done . . . despite their personal afflictions, by all who, while unable to be *saints* but refusing to bow down to pestilences, strive their utmost to be *healers*."[4] Although unable to be saints, these healers are heroes, because they accept major risks and thus go beyond the obligations ordinarily associated with the role of healer.

J. O. Urmson has helpfully distinguished between minor and major saints and heroes.[5] Minor saints and heroes live up to their obligations where others generally would not; major saints and heroes go beyond their obligations where others generally would not. Examples of major saints include St. Francis, Mother Teresa, Albert Schweitzer, and Martin Luther King, Jr. Examples of major heroes include those soldiers, political prisoners, and ambassadors who take substantial risks to save endangered persons by acts such as falling on hand grenades or resisting political tyrants. Scientists and physicians who experiment on themselves in order to generate knowledge that can benefit others can also be major heroes. Daniel Carrion injected into his arm blood from a patient with verruga peruana (an unusual disease marked by many vascular eruptions of the skin and mucous membranes as well as fever and severe rheumatic pains), only to discover that it had given him a fatal disease (Oroya fever). Werner Forssman performed the first heart catheterization on himself, walking to the radiological room with the catheter sticking into his heart.[6] More recently, a French researcher, Dr. Daniel Zagury, injected himself with an experimental AIDS vaccine, holding that this was "the only ethical line of conduct."[7]

This distinction between heroes and saints, here conceived through moral rather than religious criteria, is not rigidly fixed. In general, as Urmson suggests, the hero acts when others would succumb to fear of dangers to self-preservation, including health and survival, whereas the saint acts when others would yield to desires for such goods as pleasure. But other characteristics are also important. Saintliness requires consistent fulfillment or transcendence of obligation over time. A final judgment about a person's saintliness thus cannot be made until his or her record is substantially complete. By contrast, regardless of past conduct, a person may become a hero instantly, through a single action, such as taking a major risk while trying to save someone's life.

A physician or nurse who works long days at low pay for several years in a poverty-stricken area might easily be a saint. Even if his or her actions appear to be required by a role, such as a position in a clinic in the slums, acceptance of that role with its responsibilities is beyond the demands of obligation. We probably would not view such a person as a moral saint if we thought he or she lacked important traits of character and had not discharged other obligations. However, the physician or nurse may become a hero by actions on a single occasion, such as by overcoming fear of death in order to serve briefly in a plague-stricken city.

Some health professionals who have cared for AIDS patients after the mid-1980s have insisted that heroism is not involved because the risks are minimal. Yet in the early 1980s, before there was solid evidence about the transmission of the disease, those who cared for AIDS patients often were moral heroes, and some types of care of HIV-infected patients may still qualify as heroic. The spread of AIDS has raised questions about how much risk health professionals are obligated to assume in order to care for patients, and thus about the threshold between ordinary role obligations and extraordinary self-imposed standards. This debate is not about whether there are limits to role obligations but about what those limits are.

Moral saintliness or sainthood has always been recognized as a difficult, if not impossible, ethical ideal because of the demands it places on human beings throughout their lives. A major moral saint is as close to morally good and worthy as circumstances permit.[8] Such a person's life is dominated by a commitment to benefit others, even at significant inconvenience, and can be a form of perfectionism. But a perfectionist ideal and commitment in one dimension of life may also lead the agent to neglect other dimensions of human life. One might even challenge the assumption that "it is always better to be morally better."[9] We can ask whether saints have fallen short in some dimension of life such as education, exercise, or family life by sacrificing too many non-moral interests. Similar points may hold for moral heroes who act at substantial sacrifice. The best human life may include some moral relaxation or even moral holidays, not by violating moral principles and rules but by not always seeking moral excellence at the expense of other valuable concerns.

That some heroic acts are morally praiseworthy does not entail that all heroic acts are, on balance, praiseworthy. Many factors, especially motives, can affect the overall evaluation of heroic acts and agents. If, for example, we believe a physician went to a plague-stricken city motivated primarily by a desire to gain public recognition or to have experiences that could serve as the basis of a profitable book, we are not likely to praise his or her acts.

Furthermore, people who take risks in accord with higher, but optional, ideals sometimes do not merit our moral praise, because they neglect or violate moral obligations in the process. Ill-advised and unduly risky acts of beneficence might be criticized for their heroic quality. Imagine, for example, that a physician volunteers to take the grave risk of serving in a plague-stricken city that has attracted the world's sympathy, and imagine that there are no other physicians or medical services in the small town he leaves unprotected in his absence. It is possible that his heroic action should be condemned rather than praised.

Related issues emerge when physicians, courts, guardians, and society at large have to decide how to respond to offers of supererogatory and sometimes heroic actions that go beyond ordinary obligations. These issues may be especially poignant when deciding whether to accept a living donor's offer of a kidney or bone marrow for transplantation. Several questions arise of the sort explored in Chapter 3. Does the prospective donor adequately understand the risks and benefits? What information, if any, is relevant to a decision if the person understands little about the risks and benefits? Are the risks unreasonable? These questions can be especially difficult in the instance of supererogatory gifts that are based more on family love, indebtedness, and loyalty than on informed consent.

We have so far excluded cases of natural affection that involve assumptions of risk or sacrifices for relatives or friends (e.g., a mother entering a burning house to rescue her child), but they now merit notice. Suppose a mother offers to donate a kidney to her child. If there is a good match and the mother has no physical or psychological conditions that would make her donation too risky, her offer should probably be accepted. If questioned, she may indicate that she did not calculate probable benefits and risks but rather decided to be a donor before hearing information about risks and benefits. She may argue that she had no other choice, which does not mean that she did not make an informed choice. Even if a donor decides immediately upon learning that a family member needs a transplant, he or she may be acting autonomously from a sense of either moral obligation or aspiration and may have all the morally relevant information.[10]

However, we might rightly refuse to allow individuals to undertake some heroic actions even when their decision is informed and voluntary. Should we, for example, be willing to remove a woman's only kidney for transplantation to her son if she requested the procedure? Any decision must carefully weigh the factual circumstances—for example, whether the mother is doomed to die shortly because of some other illness or whether she could do well on dialysis. Under some circumstances it would be justifiable to accept the kidney. If, however, we consider a mother's informed and voluntary decision to give her heart to her son, we have a strong reason for refusing to accept her offer. In this case, we face not the risk but the certainty of a heroic death in which we become a direct causal link. The mother may want to make a moral sacrifice for her son, but her request may be resisted in these circumstances. We are not obligated to help her be faithful to her conception of what she ought to do. A refusal to assist is valid not only on grounds of the professional's autonomy rights (see Chapter 7) but also because the action would violate the (prima facie) rule against killing in medicine (see Chapter 4).

Consider also heroic actions by strangers. The medical profession is generally suspicious of living unrelated donors of kidneys, especially if they want to donate a kidney to a stranger. By the late 1960s, there had been approximately sixty living unrelated donors who were not also spouses of the recipients or who had not undergone a nephrectomy for other reasons. Since that time there have been few transplants of kidneys from living unrelated donors.[11] Nonetheless, research on attitudes indicates a broad consensus that the gift of a kidney to a stranger is reasonable and proper—a clear challenge to the medical profession's reluctance to use living unrelated donors.[12]

This issue turns in part on defensible conceptions of reasonable risk. The donation of a kidney to a stranger does not involve so much risk to the donor that questions should automatically be raised about his or her competence to decide. Some opponents of a policy of accepting donations to strangers argue that volunteers are emotionally unstable; proponents of a more permissive policy argue that giving a kidney enhances the donor's self-esteem and, in this light, is neither irrational nor unreasonable. In some circumstances—for example, the donor has a medical condition that would make the donation extremely dangerous—medical practitioners might violate their obligation to do no harm by removing an organ for transplantation. Again, if the donor's act would increase the risks for others, we might also have grounds for refusing the gift—for example, if a widow with three small children wants to donate a kidney to a stranger. But these refusals should be tempered by an appreciation that the reasonableness of a risk is generally extremely difficult to assess.

The continuum from obligation to supererogation

There is a tendency in contemporary ethical theory to classify anything in the domain of morality either as a matter of obligation or as beyond obligation, thus omitting what might be situated between the two. However, as we saw in Chapters 2 and 5, we often distinguish between strong and weak demands of the moral life, and between forms of beneficence that are strictly obligatory, other forms of beneficence that are borderline, and still others that are not obligatory. (See pp. 197–203.) These distinctions suggest that a continuum runs from strong obligation through weaker forms of obligation and on to the domain of the morally unrequired, including lower-level supererogation (e.g., assisting a person lost on the city streets), and ending with higher-level supererogation (e.g., heroic and saintly acts). This continuum, then, moves from the strictest obligation to the most arduous personal ideal.

Obligation		Beyond Obligation (Supererogation)	
Strong Obligation	Weak Obligation	Ideals Beyond the Obligatory	Saintly and Heroic Ideals

The continuum runs from the strictly required to the nonrequired in the moral life, with rough rather than sharp breaks in between. Just as in Chapter 5 we could not with precision distinguish obligatory and nonobligatory beneficence, so we can only make broad distinctions across the whole of the moral life. For example, an absence of charitableness and a failure of generosity are defects in the moral life, even if they are not failures of obligation. The category of obligation (or duty) does not even exhaust what we ought to do, as various interpretations of the general form ''X ought to do it'' indicate. *Ought* in this sentence might mean (among other things) ''is required by duty,'' ''should do it because it is the most honorable or decent thing to do,'' or ''should do it because it is the best thing to do.'' Terms such as *ought,* then, operate across the boundary between obligation and that which exceeds obligation.

What role the concepts of a weak obligation and supererogation should play in different moral theories is an open question. Some moral theories have been criticized because of their failure to accommodate some part of this moral terrain. It has been argued, for example, that act utilitarians cannot account for the category of supererogation because if an act would produce more good than any alternative act for all affected parties, including the agent, then it is obligatory; if it would not maximize good outcomes, then it is wrong.[13] However, rule utilitarians can recognize supererogation, along lines proposed by David Heyd. Some acts are supererogatory ''just because the adoption of a rule making them obligatory would not have good consequences, even though individual voluntary performance of these acts is of great value.''[14] This point holds especially for negative in contrast to positive utilitarianism. Because negative utilitarianism focuses on the reduction of pain and suffering, the actual promotion of happiness could be viewed as optional but praiseworthy.

There is also debate about whether a deontologist such as Kant, with his central category of duty, can find a place for supererogation. But even if a strict Kantian ethic leaves it no room, it can be incorporated into other deontological perspectives. Just as deontologists can consider consequences, so they can recognize some features of acts as morally significant without construing them as obligations or duties.

Although important, the obligation/nonobligation distinction may have been overplayed in contemporary moral theory. The distinction is not as sharp as some theories suggest and does not exhaust the relevant alternatives. The distinction has also been mistakenly interpreted as a way of distinguishing between moral obligation and that which is not even advised, recommended, urged, or encouraged by morality. This approach obscures the richness and variety of the moral life.

Other ideals

Before we conclude this section, ideals other than supererogation deserve mention. First, there is the ideal of autonomous persons. In Western individualism, the autonomous person—the one who chooses his or her life plans and acts independently of both external authority and the manipulative or coercive actions of others—has often been praised. The failure to distinguish this ideal of autonomy from the principle of respect for autonomy has led to many confusions in biomedical ethics, especially to the confusion that the principle neglects community and tradition. The principle imposes a prima facie requirement that we not control the choices and actions of others. An ideal of the autonomous person is neither a presupposition nor an implication of this principle. Recognition of this ideal and praise for the autonomous person require additional premises not required for a defense of the principle. We have serious doubts whether this ideal of autonomy is defensible apart from major qualifications, and we also question whether it has anything to do with morality.[15] That is, we doubt the propriety of even classifying the ideal of being an autonomous person as a moral ideal.

Second, ideals may be social or communal rather than individualistic. Ideals of community and threats to those ideals have often been invoked in debates about biomedical ethics. For example, the practice of buying and selling blood has been criticized not only because of its ineffectiveness, inefficiency, and danger but also because of what it symbolizes and expresses about a community and its values.[16] Similar arguments have been offered against buying and selling organs such as kidneys and against various forms of human experimentation that carry risk of injury, pain, or mutilation. In assessing policies to increase the supply of organs for transplantation, one might argue for the ethical preferability of donation over presumed consent on grounds that a policy of express donation symbolizes and sustains a community of altruism, even if a policy of presumed consent is ethically acceptable.[17] Such arguments sometimes focus on what these practices produce—such as the hardening of public sensibilities—and they sometimes focus on the values these practices symbolize and express.

A striking example of an appeal to the ideal of community appears in Robert Burt's criticism of public policies that permit decisions to allow impaired newborns to die.[18] Even if the decisions are based on the newborns' best interests, he argues, such policies fail to express and ultimately undermine American communal ideals. Social legitimation of withholding life-sustaining treatment from impaired newborns "could lead to the repudiation of the inclusive communal ideal," could create a society of "fearful strangers," and "will press parents beyond the right to withhold lifesaving treatment toward the belief that they have a 'duty' to withhold this treatment because our society has clearly signalled both its unwillingness to extend a communal relationship to these children and a consequent inhospitality—an intolerance, perhaps—for their very existence." Furthermore, he believes that the social recognition of the parental right implies not only that "parents alone have the right to decide but that they are alone in making this decision." Hence, unless they are heroic, parents may decide to let the infant die because of inadequate communal support. The loss of this social ideal of community, Burt fears, will have negative implications and consequences for the retarded, elderly, and gravely ill, no less than for impaired newborns.

Finally, some ideals concern how we act and not merely what we do. They direct attention to the mode of performing actions.[19] Consider kindness. A health professional could discharge all the obligations imposed by the principles and rules in this book without doing so in a kindly fashion. For example, a physician might respect a patient's autonomy and disclose all related and needed information in a gruff, blunt manner, while standing by the doorway as if in a hurry to depart. Recognition of appropriate and ideal modes of acting, even in discharging obligations, implies that there are many different ways to go beyond or to exceed one's obligation without being heroic or saintly.

Health professionals who are morally good are usually inclined—without the prod of obligation—to do what is right and to realize personal and communal ideals. Their goodness is not limited to their conformity to "the moral law" or to action in accordance with a sense of obligation. Such persons exhibit a virtuous moral character, a subject that deserves examination in its own right.

Virtue and character

In addition to judgments about right acts and moral ideals, we make judgments about the moral goodness and badness of persons and about the praise and blame they merit. We judge their traits of character, including their virtues and vices. We thus evaluate the moral worth of agents no less than their actions. Without these additional themes, our view of the moral life would be truncated.

In recent years several philosophers and theologians have argued that ethics should abandon its preoccupation with principles, rules, and dilemmatic situations. Following the classical tradition shaped by Plato and Aristotle, they have urged that we return to the fundamental question, "Who should I be?" In this revival of virtue ethics, morality is viewed principally as the expression of a person's virtuous character, rather than as action in accordance with principles and rules.[20]

From the perspective of a theory like Kant's, moral worth is derived from a good will directed at the fulfillment of moral requirements. However, we generally have less admiration for a person who acts beneficently from a sense of obligation than for a person who acts in the same way from well-formed virtues, without needing motivation by rules, obligations, or external sanctions. As Philippa Foot has observed, "The man who acts charitably out of a sense of duty is not to be undervalued, but it is the other who most shows virtue and therefore to the other that most worth is attributed."[21] For Foot and many recent neoclassical writers, Aristotle's theory of the virtues is more acceptable than Kant's theory of duty in evaluating moral worth.

The concept of virtue

We will understand the term *virtue* in general to refer to a trait of character that is valued as a human quality. A moral virtue is a trait of character that is morally valued. Virtues, then, can be nonmoral and even contramoral or immoral. Admirable traits such as calmness and competitiveness are virtues but not moral virtues; they may be character traits of a person who consistently performs immoral actions.[22] Even some traits close to moral virtue, such as devotion and patience, are virtues but not specifically moral virtues.

Some have defined moral virtue as a disposition to act or a habit of acting in accordance with moral obligations and ideals.[23] On this simple definition, the moral virtue of nonmalevolence, for example, is nothing but the trait a person has of abstaining from causing harm to others when it would be wrong to harm them. However, this approach fails to account for all that needs to be covered by the concept of moral virtue. No less vital, from the perspective of virtue ethics, is the agent's motivational structure in abstaining from harm. A nonmalevolent person not only has a disposition to act nonmalevolently but has a morally appropriate desire to do so. The person has a moral reservation about acting in a harmful way. Having only the motive to act in accordance with a rule of obligation is thus not morally sufficient for virtue (even if it is morally sufficient for a theory of moral obligation).

Imagine that a person performs his or her obligation because it is an obligation but regrets and intensely dislikes being placed in a position in which the interests of others must override his or her own. Such a person, let us imagine, does not love, feel friendly toward, or cherish others and respects others only because obligation requires it. Such a person can nonetheless, on a theory of moral obligation, perform a morally right action, have a disposition to perform that action (because the person has a disposition to follow rules and perform duty), and act commendably because the right action is performed. In short, the act is right and the actor is not blameworthy, but neither the person nor the act is virtuous. To be virtuous is not only be disposed to bring about a good state of affairs but also to desire what is good. It is possible to be disposed to do what is right, to intend to do it, and to do it, while also desiring to be able to avoid doing it.

In one case, a man is willing to donate his kidney to his cousin, not as an act of altruism or love but because they have mutually agreed to a financial payment for the kidney. A psychiatrist questions whether this is an acceptable motive for donation. This action would be morally praiseworthy under the right motivation but is not morally praiseworthy under this motive. Generalizing from this case, we can ask whether persons who routinely perform morally right actions from nonmoral motives, such as motives of self-interest, can be morally praiseworthy. The answer is that an act can be judged the morally right act when done from an inferior motive, but knowledge of the motive makes a difference in our assessment of the morality of the agent who performs the action. Persons who exhibit traits of acting on inferior motives would be judged deficient in virtue, even if they consistently performed actions that are right actions from the moral point of view.

Traits alone are virtues in this analysis; single motives are virtues only in an extended sense. However, motives can be virtuous, and single motives can provide evidence of virtue. A distinction should thus be drawn between a virtue, a virtuous act, and a virtuous motive. *Virtuous act* refers to an action that conforms to a moral standard of virtue. For example, a kindly act conforms to the standard of kindness that represents the virtue of kindness. *Virtuous motive* similarly refers to a motive that conforms to a moral standard of virtue.

Finally, another important distinction is between a virtuous trait of a person and a virtuous person. The latter refers to a person who has many virtues and thus is a person of high moral character. *High* indicates that there are degrees of being a virtuous person, in accordance with the number and degree of virtues possessed.

The special place of the virtues

The special place of the virtues has been stressed in contemporary biomedical ethics by writers who focus on discernment and on the importance of desiring to acting morally.

The first emphasis on discernment, which is closely associated with practical wisdom (or classical prudence), is illustrated by two claims in the literature. It has been maintained that the attempt in obligation-oriented theories to replace the judgments of health-care professionals with rules, codes, or procedures will not result in better decisions. The argument is that discernment has a special role that action-guides cannot play.[24] It has also been argued that rather than using rules and government regulations to protect subjects in research, the more reliable protection is the presence of an "informed conscientious, compassionate, responsible researcher."[25] These are claims that character development is more important than conformity to rules and that virtues should be inculcated and cultivated over time, through educational interactions, role models, and so on.

The second argument for the special place of the virtues concentrates on having the desire to do what is good and right. Gregory Pence contends:

The ultimate argument why moral issues in medical experimentation [and other areas of medicine and health care] should be discussed in the framework of virtues, is that almost any experimenter can get around any informed consent document [or any such system of rules generally] if he really so desires. . . . [We should create] a climate in which experimenters desire not to abuse their subjects—a point harking back to our definition of the good person as one who has the right kind of desires.[26]

This argument provides a significant reason for incorporating the virtues into biomedical ethics and in medical education, but the argument needs expansion along the following lines.

A morally good person with the right kind of desires or motivational structure is more likely than a bad person to understand what should be done, more likely to be motivated to perform the acts that are required, and even more likely to form and act on moral ideals. A person we trust to do what is morally right is one who has an ingrained motivation and desire to perform right actions—the person who from his or her character cares about a morally appropriate response. The person who simply follows rules of obligation, and otherwise exhibits no special moral character, may not be trustworthy. Not the rule follower, then, but the person disposed by character to be generous, caring, compassionate, sympathetic, fair, and so on, is the one we will recommend, admire, praise, and hold up as a moral model. To discharge obligations with great reluctance, without caring about the outcome, and even wishing that the obligation could be avoided altogether, is only to satisfy an external standard of conduct, perhaps from a fear of sanctions, while the inner motivation lacks moral worth.

The person who is virtuous or has high moral character is more likely to have morally good intentions and motives, and such a person is correspondingly more likely to perform right and good actions. This is the most vital link between good persons and right actions, and it has important implications for assessments of praise and blame. If a virtuous person makes a mistake in judgment or suffers a moral lapse in conduct, thereby performing a morally wrong act, he or she will be less blameworthy than a scoundrel who performed the same act. The person's character, which provides a link with good intentions, forms part of the background of our judgments of praise and blame and shapes our use of these categories as we interpret an agent's actions.

In his chronicle of life under the Nazi SS in the Jewish ghetto in Cracow, Poland, Thomas Keneally describes a physician faced with a grave dilemma: either inject cyanide into four immobile patients or abandon them to the *SonderKomando*, who were at that moment emptying the ghetto and had already proved that they would brutally kill all captives and patients. This physician, Keneally reports, "suffered painfully from a set of ethics as intimate to him as the organs of his own body."[27] Here is a person of the highest moral character and virtue, motivated to act rightly and even heroically, yet who had no idea what to do. Ultimately, with uncertainty and reluctance, the physician elected nonvoluntary active euthanasia for the four doomed patients (using forty drops of hydrocyanic acid)—an act almost universally denounced by the canons of professional medical ethics. Even if one thinks that the physician's act was wrong and blameworthy, a judgment we would reject, no one could reasonably make a judgment of blame or demerit directed at the physician's character. Having already risked death by choosing to remain at the patients' beds in the hospital rather than take a prepared escape route, the physician is a moral hero.

Judgments of an agent's merit and praiseworthiness or demerit and blameworthiness are always tied to the person's motives, not merely to the person's actions, in the sense that the reason why the person acted is central in our determination of merit or demerit. To speak of a good and praiseworthy action is elliptical for our evaluation of the motive underlying action. That is, a praiseworthy action is a sign of a praiseworthy motive and derives its merit from that motive. Indeed, a virtuous action is a sign of and derives its merit from a virtuous motive,[28] a motive that conforms to the evaluative standard for a particular virtue or set of virtues. Naturally, a virtuous person exhibits a wide range of virtuous motives. We can speak of a continuum of quality in a person's motivation, running from (in the ideal) a person of character who has the full complement of virtuous traits to those who lack more and more of those traits.[29]

An instructive study of the role of our assessments of virtue and character, as well as their place in our judgments of praise and blame, appears in Charles L. Bosk's *Forgive and Remember: Managing Medical Failure*, an ethnographic study of the way two different surgical services in "Pacific Hospital" handle medical failure, especially on the part of surgical residents.[30] Bosk found that these surgical services distinguish, at least implicitly, between different sorts of error or mistaken action. The first is technical: The professional discharges role responsibilities conscientiously, but his or her technical skills or information fall short of what the task requires; every surgeon can be expected to make this sort of mistake occasionally. The second sort of error is judgmental: A conscientious professional develops and follows an incorrect strategy; these errors can also be expected. Attending surgeons forgive momentary technical and judgmental errors but remember them in case a pattern develops indicating that a person lacks the technical and judgmental skills to be a competent surgeon. The third sort of error is normative: This error violates standards of conduct, particularly by a failure to discharge obligations conscientiously. At this point a moral judgment about the person enters. Bosk contends that technical and judgmental errors are subordinated in importance to normative errors, because every conscientious person can be expected to make "honest errors" or "good faith errors." Normative errors are especially serious because a pattern indicates a defect of moral character, where moral character is understood in terms of good faith or conscientiousness.

Bosk's study as well as other examples in biomedicine help us understand how persons of high moral character acquire a reservoir of good will when it comes to our assessment of the praiseworthiness or blameworthiness of their actions. The conscientious surgeon can make a mistake and not be blamed in the same way a person defective in conscientiousness would be blamed—even if the mistake made by the two persons is identical. Fraud in medical research provides an instructive example. A single act of padding or tampering with data, although undoubtedly a morally serious matter, might nonetheless be pardonable if performed by a person of integrity who succumbed to temptation and broke the rules in a weak moment. A similar violation by a person of lower moral character may not be pardonable. Fraud in medical research is not merely a matter of breaking rules—although that violation is important—but of the character of the person involved. In part, we want to know whether the person is generally trustworthy.

In November 1986, the president of Harvard University's Dana-Farber Cancer Institute announced that a research investigator had tampered with data reported in an article published in *Science*. In an interview with a reporter, the researcher offered his "reasons": "There was a lot of pressure in the lab, and I didn't have the courage to tell them" that earlier results could not be replicated. Whether this error should be deemed pardonable is not a matter to be decided merely by this single case of failed courage. Until more is known about this man's character, we rightly would withhold our full and final assessment of blame.[31] Most of us, after all, have a moral character that varies over time in its strength and predictability, and often when variation occurs (e.g., from occasional moral weakness) we retain our view of typical moral behavior. A person's character may be virtuous in some respects (e.g., he or she may be conscientious and compassionate) but suffer from deficiencies in other respects (e.g., he or she may lack patience and tolerance). Thus, in evaluating persons, we need to take account of the full range of their traits of character.

The compatibility of virtues and principles

The special role of the virtues in ethical theory should not be construed as evidence for a primary role, as if a virtue-based theory were more important than or could replace obligation-based theories. The two kinds of theory have different emphases, but they are compatible and mutually reinforcing. As the case of the Cracow physician shows, persons of good moral character sometimes have trouble discerning what is right and may be the first to recognize that they need to determine right or good acts by recourse to principles, rules, consequences, and ideals. Hence, a discussion of the morality of acts remains indispensable in establishing what morally good people should do.

A plausible thesis in moral theory is that for every moral principle or rule there is a corresponding moral virtue, that is, a corresponding trait or disposition to act. This correspondence can be depicted in schematic form:[32]

Action-Guides [correspond to] Virtue Standards

Ordinary Principles	Fundamental Obligations	Primary Virtues
	Derivative Obligations	Secondary Virtues
Exceptional Principles	Ideals of Action	Ideals of Virtue

In this schema, action guides that are exceptional standards are the moral ideals discussed in the previous section. Here principles are extended to a new level beyond the demands of common morality, as moral ideals, and the category of obligation (as well as duty) fades away.

The point of the above schema is not that virtue standards are equivalent to standards of obligation. The point is that both types of standards are general and complementary in the moral life. The following list, which is not intended to be a complete catalogue, illustrates the correspondence or correlation between both fundamental and derivative action-guides and virtues, as well as ideals.

Fundamental Obligations
  Respect for autonomy
  Nonmaleficence
  Beneficence
  Justice

Derivative Obligations
  Veracity
  Confidentiality
  Privacy
  Fidelity

Ideals of Action
  Forgiveness
  Generosity
  Compassion
  Kindness

Primary Virtues
  Respectfulness
  Nonmalevolence
  Benevolence
  Justice or Fairness

Secondary Virtues
  Truthfulness
  Confidentialness
  Respect for Privacy
  Faithfulness

Ideals of Virtue
  Forgiveness
  Generosity
  Compassion
  Kindness

This list could be expanded to include many other obligations, ideals, and virtues. For example, gratitude in response to generous actions might be considered either a derivative obligation or an ideal action (or both), and gratefulness would be a corresponding virtue.

Nevertheless, this programmatic approach does not easily accommodate all the important virtues, because some do not straightforwardly correlate to action-guides.[33] Consider, for example, some virtues that are indispensable to morality as a whole. These may be called general or "second-order" virtues, in contrast to specific or first-order virtues that more directly correspond to action-guides.[34] Three virtues of this description are prudence (already discussed as discernment or practical wisdom), courage, and self-control (often called temperance), which along with justice have been traditionally known as the cardinal virtues.[35] Another virtue, conscientiousness, will be discussed in the last section of this chapter. Other virtues might be similarly cited, although there is debate about whether many of these virtues—such as hopefulness, meekness, and long-sufferingness—are moral virtues. Beyond this problem it must be acknowledged that for numerous moral virtues our language is at best untidy for making connections between virtues and obligations. One virtue may encompass many obligations and ideals, and one obligation or ideal may correspond to many virtues.

More important still is that virtue standards provide no clear distinction between ideal virtues that surpass common morality and virtues that everyone is expected to manifest, whereas an ethics of action-guides, by contrast, readily acknowledges a division into obligatory actions and nonobligatory actions. An obligation theory by its nature requires that a principle specify what is obligatory and what exceeds obligation. But a virtue-based theory has a less pressing need for this distinction, because the virtues do not inherently require actions. This difference does not show that obligation-based and virtue-based theories are incompatible; it merely indicates that one adds a perspective on the moral life that the other does not inherently contain. This analysis makes it possible to take a more comprehensive view of the moral life. Although the relations between the various pieces of the moral life are not always tidy, no theory should seek tidiness at the expense of comprehensiveness.

The role of virtues in professional ethics

Some virtues are correlated with professional obligations and ideals, as professional codes often indicate. Insisting that the medical profession's "prime objective" is to render service to humanity (reward or financial gain being a "subordinate consideration"), an AMA code in effect from 1957 to 1980 urged the physician to be "an upright man," "pure in character and . . . diligent and conscientious in caring for the sick." It also endorsed the virtues that Hippocrates commended: modesty, sobriety, patience, promptness, and piety. However, in contrast to its first code in 1847, the AMA over the years has deemphasized virtues. The references that remained in the 1957 version were perfunctory and marginal; and the 1980 version eliminated almost all traces of the virtues, except for the admonition to "expose those physicians deficient in character or competence."

Different conceptions of the health-care professions suggest different virtues. For example, if medicine is conceived in paternalistic terms, the physician's virtues will differ from those drawn from a conception of medicine as a contract. In the paternalistic model, virtues of benevolence, care, and compassion are dominant; in other models, especially an autonomy model, virtues of respectfulness (for autonomy) and fairness are more prominent. For example, in one paternalistic conception of the physician's role, arrogance is seen as a virtue and as preferable to humility,[36] whereas arrogance is not likely to even make the list of virtues in an autonomy model.

A classic example of this struggle over the proper set of virtues and their priority is found in Thomas Percival, who wrote the most influential treatise on medical ethics in the last two centuries—a work that formed the substantive basis of the first AMA code. Percival argued from the premise that the patient's best medical interest is the proper goal of medicine to conclusions about the physician's proper traits of character. Recognizing the dependence of patients, he counseled physicians that authority should direct the profession's understanding of its virtues, which, for Percival, are invariably aimed at beneficence. In an overt attempt to balance truthfulness against benevolence, he upheld benevolent deception by arguing that

To a patient, therefore, perhaps the father of a numerous family, or one whose life is of the highest importance to the community, who makes inquiries which, if faithfully answered, might prove fatal to him, it would be a gross and unfeeling wrong to reveal the truth. His right to it is suspended, and even annihilated; because, its beneficial nature being reversed, it would be deeply injurious to himself, to his family, and to the public. And he has the strongest claim, from the trust reposed in his physician, as well as from the common principles of humanity, to be guarded against whatever would be detrimental to him. The only point at issue is, whether the practitioner shall sacrifice that delicate sense of veracity, which is so ornamental to, and indeed forms a characteristic excellence of the virtuous man, to this claim of professional justice and social duty.[37]

Virtues of nurses also hinge on conceptions of the nursing profession and its role responsibilities. In the traditional model of nursing, the nurse, as "handmaiden" of the physician, is expected to cultivate the passive virtues of obedience and submission. In contemporary models, active virtues are more prominent. For example, if the nurse's role is perceived as patient advocacy, nurses will emphasize other virtues such as respect for persons, justice, persistence, and courage.[38] Even if the same virtue—conscientiousness, for example—appears in different models, its content may be specified differently. Obedience to rules is demanded in the traditional model, but constant attention to patients' rights is emphasized in contemporary autonomy models, especially those that call on the nurse to be a patient's advocate.

One difficulty in determining the content of the virtues for professionals can be seen in the language of *detached concern* or *compassionate detachment*, terms sometimes used to identify a primary characteristic of a good physician or a good nurse. Compassion is an "attitude toward another, characteristically involving imaginative dwelling on the condition of the other person, an active regard for his good, a view of him as a fellow human being, and emotional responses of a certain degree of intensity" and duration.[39] Compassion presup-

poses sympathy, has affinities with mercy, and is expressed in acts of beneficence. A physician who lacked compassion would generally be viewed as deficient; yet compassion also may cloud judgment and preclude rational and
effective responses. Constant contact with suffering can overwhelm and even
paralyze a compassionate physician. Hence medical education is designed to
inculcate detachment as well as compassion. In the final analysis, a judgment
about the importance and proper balance of these attitudes of compassion and
detachment will depend in part on the kinds of acts they produce, and thus our
moral judgments will again require principles, rules, and ideals.

The relation between character and the general virtue of trustworthiness is
also pertinent. The recent decline of trust in medicine is evidenced by the dramatic rise in medical malpractice suits and adversarial relations between health-
care professionals and the public. Among the contributing causes of the erosion
of trust are pluralism of values, the loss of intimate contact between physicians
and patients, the increased use of specialists, and the growth of large, impersonal, and bureaucratic medical institutions. These factors have undermined the
kind of interaction that over time would permit knowledge of the professional's
or the patient's character and would provide an adequate basis for trust. Our
willingness to trust health-care professionals depends essentially on our assessment of their character and professional competence. To trust others is to have
confidence in and to rely on them to act in certain ways.[40] Insofar as trust is
viewed as central in the doctor-patient relationship, virtues and character are
likely to be emphasized, and action-guides—especially institutional or government rules—are likely to be seen as intrusions. However, when strangers interact in health care, character will generally play a less significant role than
principles and rules that are backed by sanctions.[41]

Whether rules or character traits serve us best, morally speaking, may vary
from one context to the next. Thus, the character assessments that work well
for surgeons making judgments about other surgeons (e.g., in the hospital studied by Bosk) may not work well for patients who encounter physicians as
strangers. Here the person's conformity to rules, principles, and even explicit
contracts backed by sanctions may be essential to proper moral relationships.
Many physicians believe that they cannot trust many of their patients, especially if something goes wrong and litigation looms as a possibility. As a consequence, many physicians welcome mutually agreed-upon rules, require signed
documentation of mutual decisions, and practice defensive medicine.

The need for rules encourages the establishment of public boundaries and
sanctions. Public rules remind us of the moral minimum expected of everyone,
and sanctions may both deter morally good (but imperfect) persons from suc-
cumbing to temptations to cut moral corners and prevent morally untrustworthy
persons from immoral conduct. These external sanctions include criminal pros-
ecutions and civil suits, loss of professional standing or position, and blockage

of access to professional practice. Other sanctions have also been proposed, such as enforceable rules for how editors of journals should handle submitted scientific papers based on unethical research. According to the Declaration of Helsinki of the World Medical Association (1964, revised in 1975), "reports of experimentation not in accordance with the principles laid down in this Declaration should not be accepted for publication." The assumption is that researchers will refrain from unethical research if they know they will not be able to publish their results.[42]

A reliance on principles and rules, accompanied by sanctions, does not entail a general presumption of distrust of researchers, physicians, and other health-care professionals. A presumption of trust can be combined with a recognition that people who are generally trustworthy may sometimes fail to perceive what they ought to do and may sometimes lack sufficient motivation to do it. What Robert Dahl holds about government applies also to rules and sanctions in biomedical ethics: "It seems wiser to design a government on the assumption that people will not always be virtuous and at times surely will be tempted to do evil, yet where they will not lack for the incentive and the opportunities to act according to their highest potential."[43]

Research involving human subjects provides an example of the balance required. On the one hand, government regulations in the United States for institutions receiving federal funds now require that research involving human subjects be conducted according to certain ethical standards—for example, the research must have an acceptable ratio of benefits to risks for subjects, and investigators must obtain the subject's (or proxy's) informed consent. These regulations also require that a local institutional review board (IRB), including public representatives, evaluate research proposals according to those standards; the IRB may approve or disapprove the research or require the researcher to modify the protocol or consent form. On the other hand, IRBs generally do not know whether the researchers actually follow their guidelines. These IRBs presume that researchers will follow their approved protocols without needing a police force to monitor conduct. Reports of infractions appear sporadically from various sources. When IRBs investigate these reports, they often determine that the researchers were not sufficiently conscientious in a particular case but that they generally conduct their research in an ethical manner. However, a pattern of misconduct suggests that a researcher is indifferent or unconscientious. In that event, a specific presumption of distrust may be warranted, and careful monitoring or even suspension of research may be appropriate.

If IRBs operated with a general presumption of distrust, apart from specific evidence of abuse, this approach would require detailed and inflexible regulations, the expenditure of vast amounts of time and energy in documentation, and the need for advocates, auditors, and monitors.[44] These procedures could have a serious impact on the community of researchers and on progress in medical research. Determining whether such a set of procedures should be adopted depends on the defensibility of a general presumption of the trustworthiness of researchers, a presumption that their traits of character will enable them to judge what ethical standards require in the context of research and dispose them to follow those requirements.

Virtues in moral deliberation

We have argued that there is an important and complementary role for the virtues in the moral life and also in ethical theory. In conclusion, it may be asked what explicit role, if any, virtues and character may play in deliberation about and justification of moral judgments. A major criticism is that they can make little if any contribution to deliberations about what we should do, but this point can easily be overstated. Virtue theorists rightly point out that a virtuous person can often more readily discern what is right than can a mere rule follower. Virtues and character may therefore play a significant role in deliberation about a course of action.

After reflecting on a situation, an agent may conclude that no specific action is required but may still wonder what he or she should do. The agent may even ask, "What would a good person do?" or "What would a good health-care professional do?" (*Good* in these questions refers not to technical or judgmental skills but to moral goodness.) Consider this example (and compare Case 11). Mr. X suffers from Huntington's chorea and believes that he would be better off dead. He carefully considers suicide in light of his obligations to others and concludes that his suicide would not violate any obligations. Nevertheless, he wonders whether a good or virtuous person would commit suicide; in particular, he worries that his contemplated act is cowardly rather than courageous. Dr. Y, who is Mr. X's physician, also considers his responsibility in terms of moral principles and rules, concluding that Mr. X has the right to commit suicide and that it would not be wrong for Mr. X to exercise that right in his circumstances. Nevertheless, Dr. Y wonders what a good or virtuous physician would do. Would trying to persuade Mr. X not to commit suicide be meddlesome or kindly?[45]

This example indicates some of the limits of moral principles and rules. Rights and obligations simply do not always suffice to determine appropriate conduct. In particular, they do not determine all forms of good, ideal, and virtuous ways of life, many of which are shaped by religious and civic communities and personal commitments.[46]

Conscientious persons and actions

As we saw earlier in examining Bosk's study of "Pacific Hospital," we often evaluate ourselves and others in terms of the general virtue of conscientiousness, a critical virtue for establishing an agent's trustworthiness. This virtue has both motivational and procedural components. The conscientious person is motivated to perform right actions and follows procedures to discern those actions. An action is thus conscientious if the agent has tried to determine what is right, intends to do what is right, and has the motive of doing what is right because it is right.

The virtue of conscientiousness is sometimes associated with deontological theories, but conscientiousness is also recognized in many utilitarian theories. A utilitarian may view conscientiousness as a settled commitment to follow the principle of utility and to follow a procedure to determine which action would maximize utility. The rule utilitarian and the rule deontologist may hold similar or even identical views of the procedure to determine what is right. We have defended one such procedure throughout this book. For us, conscientiousness as a procedural virtue involves carefully considering prima facie principles and rules relevant to a situation, determining when one outweighs or overrules another if they conflict, seeking alternatives to infringing any principles or rules, and minimizing that infringement.

The nature of conscience

We will first concentrate on the nature of conscientiousness, noting in particular what it means to act out of conscience. In viewing conscientiousness as a procedural and motivational virtue, we may seem to be neglecting what many people have in mind when they view conscience as a faculty or authority in moral decision making. We are all familiar with such slogans as "Let your conscience be your guide" and "Just follow your conscience." For some who invoke these maxims, conscience appears to be the final authority in moral justification. However, we believe another account more adequately explains conscientiousness.

Consider the following two cases. First, Lael Tucker Wertenbaker describes the last months of her husband's life in *Death of a Man* and writes at one point about her husband's physician: "He would have done anything for us that was not against his own deepest conscience."[47] Second, in Case 38, George, who is unemployed, believes that he cannot accept a particular job because of his moral scruples about research on chemical and biological warfare. Yet he needs the position to restore family stability and to meet his children's needs. Furthermore, the other candidate for the position would pursue the research uncritically if he received the position. George has an opportunity to help his family and perhaps to prevent a destructive fanatic from obtaining the position, but his conscience stands in the way.

What precisely is conscience in these cases? In our analysis, conscience is not a special moral or psychological faculty but rather is a form of self-reflection on one's acts and their rightness or wrongness, goodness or badness. Under this description conscience often comes into play in critical reflection and judgment on past acts. It also appears as a bad conscience, in the form of feelings of guilt, shame, and disunity or disharmony, as the agent recognizes his or her acts as wrong. The experience of a bad conscience does not, however, signify bad moral character. Only people who affirm moral standards and strive to live up to them will be troubled by their failures to do so; only they will experience a bad conscience.[48] A good conscience, by contrast, is associated with such nouns as *integrity, wholeness,* and *peace* and with such adjectives as *quiet, clear,* and *easy.*[49]

Conscience is personal by virtue of an agent's consciousness of and reflection on his or her acts in relation to his or her own standards. An agent may or may not also apply these standards to the conduct of others. Perhaps George would have raised moral questions about anyone's participation in research on chemical and biological welfare, and perhaps a Roman Catholic gynecologist would hold that it is universally wrong to perform an abortion. But they also may hold only themselves to such standards. Even if they view their standards as universalizable, it would be odd, even absurd, for one of them to say, "My conscience indicates that you should not do that." In judging others or advising them about their conduct, we may consult our consciences by imagining what we would think or feel if we were to act in a certain way. We may then say that someone else ought not to engage in that conduct, and we may present a justification of our claim; but we cannot justify this admonition by saying, "I would have a guilty conscience if he did that." Perhaps we would have guilty consciences if we failed to advise him or attempt to stop him, but any reasons we offer for his abstention from that conduct must involve general principles or rules.

When people claim that their actions are conscientious, they usually indicate that they are doing what they believe to be right and that they have followed the appropriate procedure to determine what is right. They may make stronger claims if they feel compelled to resist the demands of others to act in ways that they believe to be wrong. In the face of such demands they may claim that if they were to perform the act in question—for example, perform an abortion or torture a prisoner—they would violate their consciences. For example, in one case, M, a nurse changes her mind about assisting with abortions and "refuses in conscience" to assist, although she has no problem giving care to or being supportive of patients who come to the unit for abortions. She is aware that her "moral conflict" generates another moral conflict within the nursing staff that she wishes could be avoided, but her conscience is uncompromising.

A violation of conscience can result in unpleasant feelings of guilt or shame and also in a loss of integrity, wholeness, peace, and harmony. Conscientious agents who feel these consequences acutely sometimes make predictive appeals to their consciences that involve dramatic language: "I couldn't live with myself if I did that." "I would hate myself." "I could not look at myself in the mirror." As kidney donors have been known to exclaim, "I had to do it. I couldn't have backed out, not that I had the feeling of being trapped, because the doctors offered to get me out. I just had to do it."[50] Such poignant statements indicate that for the agents in question some ethical standards are so important and fundamental that their violation would diminish their integrity and result in severe guilt or shame. These claims thus focus on conscience as a personal sanction.[51]

Agents who make such statements also believe that they will not be able to forget the deed, which will shadow and disrupt their lives over time, and that they cannot deny that the deed is theirs or shift the responsibility for it to someone else. Interesting examples include military physicians who believe they have to answer first to their consciences and may be unable to plead "superior orders" when commanded by a superior officer to commit what they believe to be a moral wrong. When Capt. Howard B. Levy, a military physician, refused in 1966 to obey his commander's order to establish and operate a program in dermatology for Special Forces Aid Men, he argued that to obey the order would implicate him in war crimes committed by Special Forces in Vietnam and would—for him, as a physician—be a violation of medical ethics.[52] Any person who makes such claims might be a victim of self-deception, might later be able to forget the act or change his views, or might later find a legitimate reason to shift the responsibility to someone else. But for this physician, at this time, his conscience would not allow him to perform the act.

The role of conscience in moral justification

When agents appeal to their consciences to explain or justify their refusal to perform acts, they have made a judgment that must be justified by appeals to general principles and rules. Conscience is personal but not self-certifying from the moral point of view. But if conscience is not a substantive ground of moral judgments, we face some puzzles. What is it to consult conscience and to have a conflict of conscience? When people consult their consciences, they examine their moral convictions to determine what they really think and feel; they consider their principles and rules to determine their relevance to the situation at hand. Conscience unaided will give agents only one answer: Do what you believe you ought to do, or else. Consulting conscience is thus only one step in the examination of one's moral convictions and is not morally sufficient. Despite a long tradition to the contrary,[53] conscience is formal and empty if left exclusively to its own workings.

A conflict of conscience occurs when a person faces two conflicting moral demands, neither of which can be met without a partial rejection of the other.

The dilemma may be particularly painful because both courses of action seem firmly required from the perspective of conscience. Sometimes a person even confronts "dirty hands," because all available courses of action involve a serious wrong. In Case 38, George's conscience may direct him both to refuse the position because it involves immoral research on chemical and biological warfare and to accept the position because it will prevent the research from being pursued by fanatics and will also benefit his family. It might be argued that George has misconstrued his situation and that his apparent conflict of conscience is merely an instance of a doubtful conscience, one that is ambivalent or unsure about the relevant standards and their weights in the situation. Perhaps, however, George believes with sound reason that he faces a genuine moral tragedy, a belief that lies at the heart of his conflict of conscience.

Those who proclaim "Let your conscience be your guide" or "Just follow your conscience" need not hold that conscience is either a sufficient or an infallible guide. They can and usually do recognize the possibility of an erroneous conscience. Many theologians across the centuries have held that it is blameworthy to act against conscience even if it is erroneous. These theologians not only hold an individual blameless for a wrongful action done out of conscience; they hold that an action done against conscience is necessarily culpable. That is, agents are culpable if they fail to follow their conscience. The reason is that in acting against conscience, agents must intend the violation of moral standards. These intentions are morally blameworthy even if the agents fail to do anything materially wrong.[54] The point is simple but important: People should do everything possible to ensure that their consciences are properly informed by relevant moral principles and rules, but finally they must act autonomously, in accord with their best judgment. To act against that judgment would be to intend to do what they believe morally wrong.

This point does not imply that we should acquiesce to the demands of conscience whatever their content. Conscientious judgments may be seriously mistaken, and claims of conscience may be rationalizations for immoral acts. As we have seen, conscientiousness requires the critical examination of personal convictions by general moral standards and thorough evidence about the facts of the situation. Nothing less will stand the test of justification.

Conscientious objection

A person's conscience may lead to resistance to the demands of others in the form of conscientious objection or conscientious refusal. Suppose a nurse believes that a doctor's order to turn off a respirator for a patient is unethical. The nurse may judge the doctor's order so unethical that he or she should report it to the proper authority as well as refuse to implement it. Alternatively, the nurse may think that cooperation in the doctor's order would involve complicity in a moral wrong, although he or she is not convinced that others would act wrongly in disconnecting the machine. In this second circumstance, the nurse may not feel compelled to expose the matter to others. In effect, the nurse says to the physician, "I see that the arguments you give are sufficient for you to judge that you are doing the right thing by switching off the machine. I do not doubt that you *are* acting according to your conscience, but *my* conscience tells me differently."[55] Similarly, a gynecologist may be conscientiously opposed to abortions without calling into question the conscientious convictions of others. He or she may not even oppose a liberal abortion law but may draw a personal line at material cooperation in abortion procedures.

In situations of interpersonal conflict, agents have to determine not only how they will act in light of their consciences but also how they will respond to the claims of conscience made by others, including their colleagues and patients. The general guidelines for an appropriate response derive from our discussion of respect for autonomy in Chapter 3. The right to have one's autonomy respected—or the right of self-determination—entails the right of conscientious action. The rules for justified interferences with autonomous actions are equally applicable to conscientious actions. It is therefore possible to justify overriding a person's conscientious action if that action imposes serious risks on others, invades the autonomy of others, or treats others unjustly. But individuals and the society bear a heavy burden of proof in arguing that coercion of conscience is necessary to protect others from harm, to respect others' autonomy, or to preserve fairness.

In some cases, the society may be able to respect an individual's conscientious objection by pursuing its goal in other ways. It may fairly require other forms of service by the objector, such as hospital service in lieu of military service. Occasionally the society may be able to protect the individual's conscience by performing the act for the person, who only objects to performing it himself or herself. For example, some Jehovah's Witnesses hold that the prohibition against taking blood forbids them to consent to blood transfusions but that court-ordered transfusions would not be their responsibility. In one case (Case 13), Judge J. Skelly Wright granted a hospital the right to give blood transfusions to a woman without her consent or her husband's consent. The transfusions were deemed medically necessary because she had lost two-thirds of her body's blood supply from a ruptured ulcer. Wright determined that neither the woman nor her husband wanted her death but that they could not conscientiously consent to the blood transfusions. By granting a court order, he thought he could adequately protect their consciences while saving her life.[56]

However, removal of responsibility by medical practitioners or by the state is not a strategy that will work for all conscientious refusers of medical treatments. For example, some Jehovah's Witnesses hold that blood transfusions contaminate the recipients even if responsibility belongs exclusively to physicians and the state. On grounds of respect for autonomy, we agree with the court decision in Case 12 to allow a woman with such convictions to refuse a blood transfusion while ordering a transfusion for her infant. However, because infants cannot be situated under the categories of either autonomy or conscientiousness, we still need to consider the responsibilities the hospital and the state have to care for such infants, who as a result of transfusions may be considered by their families to be contaminated.

In medicine and health care, conflicts of conscience—within persons and between persons—sometimes emerge because people believe that a particular role obligation or some order that descends from a hierarchical structure of authority is unethical. Such conflicts are especially acute when A orders B to perform an action that B believes to be wrong, as in the case of the nurse who believed it was wrong to follow an order to turn off a respirator. In one study of the perceptions of ethical problems by nurses and doctors, the members of both groups acknowledged ethical conflicts within the health-care team. However, most nurses perceived the differences of ethical opinion to be between the nurse and the physician, whereas almost all of the physicians saw the differences to be between physicians, not between nurses and physicians. A partial explanation may be found in the working relationship: "Doctors write orders; nurses carry them out. Potential conflicts are exacerbated because nurses' close contact with patients leads them to see the results of medical intervention far more intensely than do physicians. Also, physicians see themselves as accountable to other physicians, and to patients and their families, but not to nurses."[57]

We saw above that a person may conscientiously refuse to perform an action without judging others by his or her standards. In many such conscientious refusals, the agent does not try to stop others from performing the act but only says, "Not through me."[58] One difficult issue concerns the extent to which physicians are obligated to manage the patient as the patient elects, especially if the patient refuses a procedure in a context the physician views as medically unconscionable or requests a procedure the physician finds morally objectionable, such as abortion, amniocentesis for sex selection, or laetrile for cancer therapy.

In one case, a young unmarried intern requested a sterilization procedure because she did not like available contraceptives and did not want children. Her gynecologist could not in good conscience perform the procedure because she thought it was not in the young woman's best interests to preclude the possibility of having children later.[59] However, the gynecologist did not try to prevent the woman from getting someone else to perform the operation. In such cases the physician usually has a moral obligation to refer or to transfer the patient to another physician. Such an obligation appears in many recent natural death acts, which do not require unwilling physicians to carry out a patient's so-called living will but do require them to make a reasonable effort to transfer the patient to another physician.

If it is morally permissible for the physician to withdraw from the case, and he or she plans to do so, then this plan, too, should be disclosed to the patient, because it may reasonably affect the patient's decision. If the physician wishes to withdraw from the case because the patient's requests or refusals seem morally or professionally repugnant, the physician's conscientious convictions should be respected, and he or she should be free to withdraw—assuming, however, that the requested actions are not among the responsibilities one generally accepts in agreeing to be someone's physician. This appeal to the autonomy rights of the physician rests on the premise that the physician's basic values and beliefs would be violated by carrying out the patient's request. The patient's autonomy should not be purchased at the price of the physician's parallel right.

In addition to situations in which health-care professionals refuse on grounds of conscience to carry out a patient's wishes or institutional orders, there are situations in which professionals wonder about the degree of participation and complicity in what they take to be a moral wrong. Traditional moral theology has distinguished several different degrees of cooperation with evil actions by others. In formal cooperation, the agent consents to and actively participates in the morally wrong actions of others, whereas in material cooperation the agent does not consent even though his or her actions are to some extent involved in the wrongdoing. Material cooperation in wrongdoing can be justified only if the agent's own actions are not morally wrong and if there are compelling reasons for participation. For example, Catholic moral theology has allowed an assistant to a surgeon performing an "evil operation" of abortion or sterilization to cooperate by sterilizing instruments, preparing the patient, and administering the anesthesia.[60]

Despite its shortcomings, this traditional doctrine attempted to deal with the reality that agents in complex circumstances may be unable to detach themselves totally from what they believe to be moral evil. Where total disassociation is impossible, conscientious agents have to decide how far they can cooperate without violating their consciences. For example, they may have to make such decisions while in military service in what they believe to be an unjust war, in a bureaucratic health-care institution that has adopted unjust policies, or in research they consider unjustified (see Case 38).

In a striking example, some physicians and hospitals have tried to disassociate themselves from evil by refusing to participate in medical preparedness programs that may be part of plans for nuclear war or increase the likelihood of nuclear war. In October 1981, sixty physicians at Contra Costa Hospital in San Francisco refused a Defense Department request to pledge at least fifty civilian beds for the care of military casualties who would be airlifted from overseas in the event of a large-scale war. A year earlier the Defense Department had established the Civilian-Military Contingency Hospital System (CMCHS), a voluntary contingency planning program, to obtain fifty thousand beds in civilian hospitals for military casualties in the event of "a future large-scale conflict overseas [that] could begin very rapidly and produce casualties at a higher rate than any other war in history." Although this plan was supported by the American Medical Association and the American Hospital Association, it was opposed by Physicians for Social Responsibility, who agreed with the medical staff at Contra Costa—and several other hospitals—that participation "would offer tacit approval for the planning of a nuclear war." The Defense Department insisted that CMCHS was limited to conventional warfare overseas, but critics stressed the serious risk of escalation even in a conventional war.

Supporters of the plan insisted that "the medical ethical issue at hand is that of care for sick and injured young servicemen and women—not the morality of nuclear war." They believed that advance planning and coordination could improve care in the event of war. One critic, physician Jack Geiger, argued that it is "precisely the professional commitment to the protection and preservation of human life that would make it unethical for any physician to participate in either civilian or military 'disaster' plans specifically designed to attempt to cope with the consequences of nuclear war." In contrast to ordinary medical disaster plans, he argued, nuclear war disaster plans may increase the likelihood of the disaster occurring because they provide false assurance that medical care can enable the society to survive and even win a nuclear war. Steven Goodman, a physician, describes the dilemma: "On the one side there is the perception of unnecessarily lost lives if we do not adopt the CMCHS, and on the other a possible increased risk of nuclear war if we do. . . . If there is even a grain of truth in either of the two sides, a physician pledged to 'do no harm' is faced with a profoundly difficult moral choice."[61]

Conscientious refusal, withdrawal, or disassociation may not be sufficient moral responses if the agent believes that others are violating fundamental and universal obligations, such as nonmaleficence and justice. For instance, nurses and others might have believed that such obligations were violated in Case 7, in which a physician refused to inform a patient that she had cancer, and Case 15, in which an order not to resuscitate had been written apparently without the patient's informed consent. In such cases, agents may believe that it is necessary to try to ensure or prevent certain actions. After unsuccessful appeals to appropriate officials in the hierarchy, they may decide that it is warranted and necessary to blow the whistle in order to direct public attention to the actions in question. Examples include nurses, social workers, and others blowing the whistle to secure treatment for handicapped newborns whose physicians and families have ordered no treatment.[62]

When we encounter serious moral disagreements or conflicts of conscience, we may legitimately rely on procedures and on such second-order virtues as conscientiousness. As John Rawls notes, "In times of social doubt and loss of faith in long established values, there is a tendency to fall back on the virtues of integrity: truthfulness and sincerity, lucidity and commitment, or, as some say, authenticity." [63] The maintenance of mutual trust in situations of serious moral conflict often depends on the willingness of the parties involved to preserve the second-order virtues and to abide by procedures. Even when the conflicts are too serious or too profound to permit mutual trust, conscientiousness in taking further steps should still involve a willingness to consider and reconsider one's position.

Conclusion

In this chapter, we have moved beyond the obligations and rights created by the four basic moral principles and by derivative moral rules. Ideals, virtues, and convictions of conscience support and enrich the moral framework of principles developed in the previous five chapters. Ideals transcend obligations and rights, and some virtues enable individuals to perceive the implications of and dispose them to act in accord with principles and rules as well as ideals. Our examination of moral ideals, virtues, and conscience has also returned us to the discussion in Chapters 1 and 2 of the limits of moral principles and rules.

Throughout this book, we have attempted to present a moral point of view on the activities of researchers, physicians, nurses, and other health professionals who daily make important moral decisions. But the answers provided by a treatise in biomedical ethics are limited. Ethical theory does not create the morality that guides professionals' decisions and actions. It can only cast light on and supplement that morality, in part by analyzing and appraising moral justifications, their presuppositions, and their implications. The obligations, virtues, and ideals analyzed in this book are basic and indispensable threads in the moral life, but the moral life is a still richer fabric with other threads in its weave.

Notes

1. We are indebted to David Heyd, *Supererogation: Its Status in Ethical Theory* (Cambridge: Cambridge University Press, 1982); and to J. O. Urmson, "Saints and Heroes," *Essays in Moral Philosophy*, ed. A. I. Melden (Seattle: University of Washington Press, 1958), pp. 198–216. Other valuable analyses include Joel Feinberg, "Supererogation and Rules," *Ethics* 71 (1961): 276–88; Roderick M. Chisholm, "Supererogation and Offense: A Conceptual Scheme for Ethics," *Ratio* 5 (1963): 1–14; and Millard Schumaker, *Supererogation: An Analysis and Bibliography* (Edmonton: St. Stephen's College, 1977). Historically, supererogation has been invoked in religious debates between Roman Catholics and Protestants about whether human acts and motives can generate religious merit before God.

2. Heyd, *Supererogation*, pp. 138–39.

3. Ibid.

4. Albert Camus, *The Plague*, trans. Stuart Gilbert (New York: Random House, Vintage Books, 1972), p. 286 (italics added).

5. Urmson, "Saints and Heroes."

6. Jay Katz, ed., *Experimentation with Human Beings* (New York: Russell Sage Foundation, 1972), pp. 136–40.

7. Philip J. Hilts, "French Doctor Testing AIDS Vaccine on Self," *Washington Post*, March 10, 1987, p. A7. For a thorough discussion of self-experimentation in medicine, see Lawrence K. Altman, *Who Goes First?: The Story of Self-Experimentation* (New York: Random House, 1987).

8. Susan Wolf, "Moral Saints," *Journal of Philosophy* 79 (August 1982): 419–39.

9. Ibid. For a critical response to Wolf's argument, see Robert Merrihew Adams, "Saints," *Journal of Philosophy* 81 (May 1984): 392–401.

10. See Carl H. Fellner and John R. Marshall, "Kidney Donors—The Myth of Informed Consent," *American Journal of Psychiatry* 126 (March 1970): 1245–51. On p. 1250, they write: "all relevant data are immediately available to him" (i.e., the renal donor). See also Robert M. Eisendrath et al., "Psychological Considerations in the Selection of Kidney Transplant Donors," *Surgery, Gynecology and Obstetrics* 129 (August 1969): 243–48.

11. Carl H. Fellner, "Organ Donation: For Whose Sake?" *Annals of Internal Medicine* 79 (October 1973): 590. For arguments against using living donors of kidneys, see Thomas Starzl, "Will Live Organ Donations No Longer Be Justified?" *Hastings Center Report* 15 (April 1985): 5. Contrast Andrew Levey, Susan Hou, and Harry L. Bush, Jr., "Kidney Transplantation from Unrelated Living Donors," *New England Journal of Medicine* 314 (April 1986): 914–16.

12. See Carl H. Fellner and Shalom H. Schwartz, "Altruism in Disrepute," *New England Journal of Medicine* 284 (March 1971): 582–85.

13. Alan Donagan, "Is There a Credible Form of Utilitarianism?" in *Contemporary Utilitarianism*, ed. Michael D. Bayles (New York: Doubleday Anchor Books, 1968), pp. 187–202.

14. Heyd, *Supererogation*, p. 88.

15. See John Benson, "Who Is the Autonomous Man?" *Philosophy* 58 (1983): 5–17. For serious reservations about these ideals as ideals of moral autonomy or of nonmoral autonomy, see Gerald Dworkin, "Moral Autonomy," in *Morals, Science and Sociality*, Vol. III of The Foundations of Ethics and Its Relationship to Science, ed. H. Tristram Engelhardt, Jr., and Daniel Callahan (Hastings-on-Hudson, N.Y.: Hastings Center, 1978); and Ruth R. Faden and Tom L. Beauchamp, *A History and Theory of Informed Consent* (New York: Oxford, 1986), chap. 7, esp. pp. 235–41.

16. Richard Titmuss, *The Gift Relationship* (New York: Pantheon, 1971).

17. This position is defended by Paul Ramsey, *The Patient as Person* (New Haven: Yale University Press, 1970).

18. Robert Burt, "The Ideal of Community in the Work of the President's Commission," *Cardozo Law Review* 6 (1984): 267–84.

19. See Peter A. French, *The Scope of Morality* (Minneapolis: University of Minnesota Press, 1979), esp. chap. 7. For other discussions of ideals, see R. M. Hare, *Freedom and Reason* (Oxford: Clarendon Press, 1963), chap. 8; P. F. Strawson, "Social Morality and Individual Ideal," in *Christian Ethics and Contemporary Philos-*

ophy, ed. Ian T. Ramsey (New York: Macmillan, 1966), pp. 280–98; and A. S. Cua, *Dimensions of Moral Creativity: Paradigms, Principles, and Ideals* (University Park: Pennsylvania State University Press, 1978).

20. For an influential defense of the Aristotelian perspective, see Alasdair MacIntyre, *After Virtue* (Notre Dame: University of Notre Dame Press, 1981). For a statement of the primacy of character in Christian ethics, see Stanley Hauerwas's various writings, including *A Community of Character: Toward a Constructive Christian Social Ethic* (Notre Dame: University of Notre Dame Press, 1981). For an assessment of the virtues in biomedical ethics, see Earl E. Shelp, ed., *Virtue and Medicine* (Dordrecht: D. Reidel, 1985); William F. May, "The Virtues in a Professional Setting," *Soundings* 68 (Fall 1984): 245–66; and Gregory Pence, *Ethical Options in Medicine* (Oradell, N.J.: Medical Economics, 1980). Other relevant works include Philippa Foot, *Virtues and Vices* (Oxford: Basil Blackwell, 1978); James Wallace, *Virtues and Vices* (Ithaca: Cornell University Press, 1978); Lawrence C. Becker, "The Neglect of Virtue," *Ethics* 85 (January 1975): 110–22; and, for a guide to recent literature, Gregory E. Pence, "Recent Work on Virtue," *American Philosophical Quarterly* 21 (October 1984): 281–96.

21. Foot, *Virtues and Vices*, pp. 12–14.

22. See Michael Slote, *Goods and Virtues* (Oxford: Clarendon Press, 1983), chap. 4.

23. This form of definition has been defended by Alan Gewirth, "Rights and Virtues," *Review of Metaphysics* 38 (1985): 751, and earlier by William Frankena. Edmund Pincoffs presents a definition of virtue in terms of desirable dispositional qualities of persons. See *Quandaries and Virtues: Against Reductivism in Ethics* (Lawrence: University Press of Kansas, 1986), pp. 9, 73–100. We acknowledge that we accepted a definition similar to these definitions in the first two editions of this book.

24. Leon R. Kass, "Ethical Dilemmas in the Care of the Ill," *Journal of the American Medical Association* 244 (October 1980): 1811.

25. H. K. Beecher, "Ethics and Clinical Research," *New England Journal of Medicine* 274 (1966): 1354–60.

26. Pence, *Ethical Options in Medicine*, p. 177.

27. Thomas Keneally, *Schindler's List* (New York: Penguin Books, 1983), pp. 176–80.

28. This formulation is indebted to John Mackie, *Hume's Moral Theory* (London: Routledge and Kegan Paul, 1980), p. 79.

29. See Gregory W. Trianosky, "Supererogation, Wrongdoing, and Vice: On the Autonomy of the Ethics of Virtue," *Journal of Philosophy* 83 (January 1986): esp. 36.

30. Charles L. Bosk, *Forgive and Remember: Managing Medical Failure* (Chicago: University of Chicago Press, 1979). Bosk also recognizes a fourth type of error: "quasi-normative errors" based on the attending's protocols.

31. See Boyce Rensberger, "Harvard Researchers Retract Published Medical 'Discovery,'" *Washington Post*, November 23, 1986, pp. A1, A8.

32. This schema has been adapted, with significant modifications, from Tom L. Beauchamp, *Philosophical Ethics* (New York: McGraw-Hill, 1982), chap. 5.

33. For a critique of the approach we have taken, see several writings by Gregory Trianosky, including "Supererogation, Wrongdoing, and Vice: On the Autonomy of the Ethics of Virtue"; "Virtue, Action, and the Good Life: A Theory of the Virtues," *Pacific Philosophical Quarterly*, forthcoming; and "Rightly Ordered Ap-

petites: How to Live Morally and Live Well," *American Philosophical Quarterly*, 25 (1988): 1–12.

34. See William Frankena, *Ethics*, 2d ed. (Englewood Cliffs, N.J.: Prentice-Hall), p. 64.

35. These cardinal virtues were drawn from Plato rather than Aristotle. See Josef Pieper, *The Four Cardinal Virtues* (Notre Dame: University of Notre Dame Press, 1965).

36. See Franz J. Ingelfinger, "Arrogance," *New England Journal of Medicine* 303 (December 1980): 1507–11. For an assessment of various models of the relations between physicians and patients, including paternalism, see Tom L. Beauchamp and Laurence McCullough, *Medical Ethics* (Englewood Cliffs, N.J.: Prentice-Hall, 1984), esp. chap. 2; Edmund D. Pellegrino and David C. Thomasma, *For the Patient's Good* (New York: Oxford University Press, 1988), esp. part I; and James F. Childress, *Who Should Decide? Paternalism in Health Care* (New York: Oxford University Press, 1982). These models of professional roles, responsibilities, and virtues also imply roles and virtues for patients.

37. Thomas Percival, *Medical Ethics; or a Code of Institutes and Precepts, Adapted to the Professional Conduct of Physicians and Surgeons* (Manchester: S. Russell, 1803), pp. 165–66.

38. For an analysis of models of nursing, see Dan W. Brock, "The Nurse-Patient Relation: Some Rights and Duties," in *Nursing: Images and Ideals*, ed. Stuart F. Spicker and Sally Gadow (New York: Spring Publishing, 1980), pp. 102–24. See also Gerald Winslow, "From Loyalty to Advocacy: A New Metaphor for Nursing," *Hastings Center Report* 14 (June 1984): 32–40.

39. Lawrence Blum, "Compassion," in *Explaining Emotions*, ed. A. O. Rorty (Berkeley: University of California Press, 1980).

40. See H. J. N. Horsburgh, "Trust and Social Objectives," *Ethics* 72 (1961): 28, and "The Ethics of Trust," *Philosophical Quarterly* 10 (October 1960): 343–54. See also Annette Baier, "Trust and Antitrust," *Ethics* 96 (1986): 231–60; and Bernard Barber, *The Logic and Limits of Trust* (New Brunswick, N.J.: Rutgers University Press, 1983).

41. See Robert M. Veatch, "Against Virtue: A Deontological Critique of Virtue Theory in Medical Ethics," in *Virtue and Medicine*, ed. Shelp, pp. 329–45.

42. A sanction other than refusal of publication has also been proposed, in order to procure the benefits of scientifically valid (though unethical) research as well as to deter unethical research. The editor of the journal could publish the article but with an editorial on the ethical reservations about the conduct of the research, perhaps accompanied by the researcher's response. See Robert J. Levine, *Ethics and Regulation of Clinical Research*, 2d ed. (Baltimore: Urban and Schwarzenberg, 1986), pp. 28–31. A similar approach was taken by the editor of *Lancet* in publishing the results of a study of intestinal bypass surgery in which the control patients were deceived. The editor defended this decision as a contribution to the ethical debate as well as to science. "Bypassing Obesity," *Lancet* (December 1979): 1275. See Case 29 for more details.

43. Robert A. Dahl, *After the Revolution? Authority in a Good Society* (New Haven: Yale University Press, 1970), p. 137.

44. Levine, *Ethics and Regulation of Clinical Research*, p. 349. Levine's analysis has influenced this paragraph and the previous one.

45. These examples are influenced by James Bogen, "Suicide and Virtue," in *Suicide:*

The Philosophical Issues, ed. M. Pabst Battin and David Mayo (New York: St. Martin's Press, 1980), pp. 286–92.

46. Although we have not discussed the "theological virtues," such as faith, hope, and love, religious communities frequently require their adherents to follow what the broader society might consider as ideals. Furthermore, such communities frequently claim additional resources, such as grace, to enable individuals to live up to those requirements. Nevertheless, some of these communities also recognize different levels of moral activity; an example is the traditional Roman Catholic distinction between the precepts of natural law that bind all people and the counsels of perfection for those who aspire to excellence.

47. Lael Tucker Wertenbaker, *Death of a Man* (Boston: Beacon Press, 1974).

48. Hannah Arendt, *Crises of the Republic* (New York: Harcourt, Brace, Jovanovich, 1972), p. 62.

49. For a discussion of these themes, especially integrity, see Peter Winch, *Moral Integrity* (Oxford: Basil Blackwell, 1968); Bernard Williams, "A Critique of Utilitarianism," in J. J. C. Smart and Bernard Williams, *Utilitarianism: For and Against* (Cambridge: Cambridge University Press, 1973), esp. pp. 108–18; and Bernard Williams, *Moral Luck: Philosophical Papers 1973–1980* (Cambridge: Cambridge University Press, 1981), esp. pp. 40–53. Because he is concerned to defend integrity against charges of moral self-indulgence, Williams insists that integrity is not a virtue, not a disposition that yields motivations; rather, "one who displays integrity acts from those dispositions and motives which are most deeply his." Nevertheless, it makes sense to refer to claims of conscience as motive statements that invoke integrity, and it is possible to do so without falling into objectionable moral self-indulgence. See James F. Childress, "Appeals to Conscience," *Ethics* 89 (July 1979): 315–35, from which several of the following points are drawn.

50. Carl H. Fellner, "Organ Donation: For Whose Sake?" *Annals of Internal Medicine* 79 (October 1973): 591.

51. See Childress, "Appeals to Conscience." See also Larry May, "On Conscience," *American Philosophical Quarterly* 20 (January 1983): 57–67. It is difficult, if not impossible, to determine whether conscience as a motive in relation to other motives, such as fear, is necessary and sufficient, necessary but not sufficient, sufficient but not necessary, or neither necessary nor sufficient, to lead to the action. Determining the role of conscience in a person's action requires considering what the person would have done without conscience as a motive. See C. D. Broad, "Conscience and Conscientious Action," in *Moral Concepts,* ed. Joel Feinberg (Oxford: Oxford University Press, 1969), pp. 74–79.

52. See Robert M. Veatch's discussion of this case, *Case Studies in Medical Ethics* (Cambridge, Mass.: Harvard University Press, 1977), pp. 61–64.

53. In one of the most celebrated analyses of conscience, Joseph Butler argued in the eighteenth century that insofar as the supreme moral faculty of conscience governs, one lives in accordance with the dictates of human nature; if any other principle prevails, one has failed to do so. Obligation is erected on the law of nature in this theory: "Your obligation to obey this law, is its being the law of your nature. . . . Conscience does not only offer itself to show us the way we should walk in, but it likewise carries its own authority with it." *Sermons,* in *The Works of Joseph Butler, D.C.L.,* ed. W. E. Gladstone (Oxford: Clarendon Press, 1896), Vol. II, p. 71.

54. Alan Donagan, *The Theory of Morality* (Chicago: University of Chicago Press, 1977), pp. 131–38.

55. Alastair V. Campbell, *Moral Dilemmas in Medicine*, 2d ed. (Edinburgh: Churchill Livingstone, 1975), p. 25 (italics added).

56. *Application of President and Directors of Georgetown College*, 331F. 2d 1000 (D.C. Cir.), certiorari denied, 377 U.S. 978 (1964).

57. Gregory P. Gramelspacher, Joel D. Howell, and Mark J. Young, "Perceptions of Ethical Problems by Nurses and Doctors," *Archives of Internal Medicine* 146 (March 1986): 577–78.

58. See Williams, *Moral Luck*, esp. p. 50.

59. See Marc D. Basson, ed., *Rights and Responsibilities in Modern Medicine* (New York: Alan R. Liss, 1981), pp. 135–36, with discussions by Tom L. Beauchamp and Eric J. Cassell.

60. Daniel C. Maguire, "Cooperation with Evil," *Dictionary of Christian Ethics*, 2d ed., ed. James F. Childress and John Macquarrie (Philadelphia: Westminster Press, 1986), p. 129.

61. *CMCHS: In Combat, In the Community, Saving Lives . . . Together*, available from the Office of the Assistant Secretary of Defense (Health Affairs) at the Pentagon; John F. Beary, Jay C. Bisgard, and Philip C. Armstrong, "The Civilian Military Contingency Hospital System," *New England Journal of Medicine* 306 (1982): 738–40; Physicians for Social Responsibility Executive Committee, "Medical Care in Modern Warfare: A Look at the Pentagon Plan for the Civilian Sector," *New England Journal of Medicine* 306 (1982): 741–42; letters to the editor, *New England Journal of Medicine* 307 (1982): 751–53; Steven Goodman, letter to the editor, *New England Journal of Medicine* 307 (1982): 1578; Jay C. Bisgard, "The Obligation to Care for Casualties"; H. Jack Geiger, "Why Survival Plans Are Meaningless"; and James T. Johnson, "The Moral Bases of Contingency Planning," *Hastings Center Report* 12 (April 1982): 15–21. CMCHS was replaced by the National Disaster Medical System (NDMS), which emphasizes civilian emergencies as well as overseas conventional military conflicts. The moral debate has continued. See Jan Kirsch, "NDMS: Enlisting MDs in Nuclear War," and Jane M. Owen, "NDMS: A Plan That Can Save Lives," *Medical Ethics for the Physician* 1 (October 1986): 6–7, 10.

62. For a good analysis of professional noncompliance, especially in nursing, see Natalie Abrams, "Moral Responsibility in Nursing," in *Nursing*, ed. Spicker and Gadow, pp. 148–59.

63. John Rawls, *A Theory of Justice* (Cambridge, Mass.: Harvard University Press, 1971), p. 519.

Appendix

Case Studies

Case 1

Facts in the case

On October 27, 1969, Prosenjit Poddar killed Tatiana Tarasoff. Plaintiffs, Tatiana's parents, allege that two months earlier Poddar confided his intention to kill Tatiana to Dr. Lawrence Moore, a psychologist employed by the Cowell Memorial Hospital at the University of California at Berkeley. They allege that on Moore's request, the campus police briefly detained Poddar, but released him when he appeared rational. They further claim that Dr. Harvey Powelson, Moore's superior, then directed that no further action be taken to detain Poddar. No one warned plaintiffs of Tatiana's peril.

Plaintiffs, Tatiana's mother and father, . . . [allege] that on August 20, 1969, Poddar was a voluntary outpatient receiving therapy at Cowell Memorial Hospital. Poddar informed Moore, his therapist, that he was going to kill an unnamed girl, readily identifiable as Tatiana, when she returned home from spending the summer in Brazil. Moore, with the concurrence of Dr. Gold, who had initially examined Poddar, and Dr. Yandell, assistant to the director of the department of psychiatry, decided that Poddar should be committed for observation in a mental hospital. Moore orally notified Officers Atkinson and Teel of the campus police that he would request commitment. He then sent a letter to Police Chief William Beall requesting the assistance of the police department in securing Poddar's confinement.

Officers Atkinson, Brownrigg, and Halleran took Poddar into custody, but, satisfied that Poddar was rational, released him on his promise to stay away from Tatiana. Powelson, director of the department of psychiatry at Cowell Memorial Hospital, then asked the police to return Moore's letter, directed that all copies of the letter and notes that Moore had taken as therapist be destroyed, and "ordered no action to place Prosenjit Poddar in a 72-hour treatment and evaluation facility."

Plaintiff's second cause of action, entitled "Failure to Warn of a Dangerous Patient," . . . adds the assertion that defendants negligently permitted Poddar to be released from police custody without "notifying the parents of Tatiana Tarasoff that their daughter was in grave danger from Prosenjit Poddar." Poddar persuaded Tatiana's brother to share an apartment with him near Tatiana's residence; shortly after her return from Brazil, Poddar went to her residence and killed her.

Majority opinion in the case   TOBRINER, Justice

We shall explain that defendant therapists cannot escape liability merely because Tatiana herself was not their patient. When a therapist determines, or pursuant to the standards of his profession should determine, that his patient presents a serious danger of violence to another, he incurs an obligation to use reasonable care to protect the intended victim against such danger. The discharge of this duty may require the therapist to take one or more of various steps, depending upon the nature of the case. Thus it may call for him to warn the intended victim or others likely to apprise the victim of the danger, to notify the police, or to take whatever other steps are reasonably necessary under the circumstances. . . .

In each instance the adequacy of the therapist's conduct must be measured against the traditional negligence standard of the rendition of reasonable care under the circumstances. . . . In sum, the therapist owes a legal duty not only to his patient, but also to his patient's would-be victim and is subject in both respects to scrutiny by judge and jury. . . . Some of the alternatives open to the therapist, such as warning the victim, will not result in the drastic consequences of depriving the patient of his liberty. Weighing the uncertain and conjectural character of the alleged damage done the patient by such a warning against the peril to the victim's life, we conclude that professional inaccuracy in predicting violence cannot negate the therapist's duty to protect the threatened victim. . . .

We recognize the public interest in supporting effective treatment of mental illness and in protecting the rights of patients to privacy . . . and the consequent public importance of safeguarding the confidential character of psychotherapeutic communication. Against this interest, however, we must weigh the public interest in safety from violent assault.

The revelation of a communication under the above circumstances is not a breach of trust or a violation of professional ethics; as stated in the Principles of Medical Ethics of the American Medical Association (1957), section 9: "A physician may not reveal the confidence entrusted to him in the course of medical attendance . . . unless he is required to do so by law or unless it becomes necessary in order to protect the welfare of the individual or of the community." We conclude that the public policy favoring protection of the confidential character of patient-psychotherapist communications must yield to the extent to which disclosure is essential to avert danger to others. The protective privilege ends where the public peril begins. . . .

Minority opinion in the case   CLARK, Justice (dissenting)

Until today's majority opinion, both legal and medical authorities have agreed that confidentiality is essential to effectively treat the mentally ill, and that imposing a duty on doctors to disclose patient threats to potential victims would greatly impair treatment. . . .

Policy generally determines duty. Principal policy considerations include foreseeability of harm, certainty of the plaintiff's injury, proximity of the defendant's conduct to the plaintiff's injury, moral blame attributable to defendant's conduct, prevention of future harm, burden on the defendant, and consequences to the community.

Overwhelming policy considerations weigh against imposing a duty on psychotherapists to warn a potential victim against harm. While offering virtually no benefit to society, such a duty will frustrate psychiatric treatment, invade fundamental patient rights and increase violence.

The importance of psychiatric treatment and its need for confidentiality have been recognized by this court. "It is clearly recognized that the very practice of psychiatry vitally depends upon the reputation in the community that the psychiatrist will not tell. . . ."

Assurance of confidentiality is important for three reasons.

DETERRENCE FROM TREATMENT First, without substantial assurance of confidentiality, those requiring treatment will be deterred from seeking assistance. It remains an unfortunate fact in our society that people seeking psychiatric guidance tend to become stigmatized. Apprehension of such stigma—apparently increased by the propensity of people considering treatment to see themselves in the worst possible light—creates a well-recognized reluctance to seek aid. This reluctance is alleviated by the psychiatrist's assurance of confidentiality.

FULL DISCLOSURE Second, the guarantee of confidentiality is essential in eliciting the full disclosure necessary for effective treatment. The psychiatric patient approaches treatment with conscious and unconscious inhibitions against revealing his innermost thoughts. . . .

SUCCESSFUL TREATMENT Third, even if the patient fully discloses his thoughts, assurance that the confidential relationship will not be breached is necessary to maintain his trust in his psychiatrist—the very means by which treatment is effected. . . .

Given the importance of confidentiality to the practice of psychiatry, it becomes clear the duty to warn imposed by the majority will cripple the use and effectiveness of psychiatry. Many people, potentially violent—yet susceptible to treatment—will be deterred from seeking it; those seeking it will be inhibited from making revelations necessary to effective treatment; and, forcing the psychiatrist to violate the patient's trust will destroy the interpersonal relationship by which treatment is effected.

VIOLENCE AND CIVIL COMMITMENT By imposing a duty to warn, the majority contributes to the danger to society of violence by the mentally ill and greatly increases the risk of civil commitment—the total deprivation of liberty—of those who should not be confined. The impairment of treatment and risk of improper commitment resulting from the new duty to warn will not be limited to a few patients but will extend to a large number of the mentally ill. Although under existing psychiatric procedures only a relatively few receiving treatment will ever present a risk of violence, the number making threats is huge, and it is the latter group—not just the former—whose treatment will be impaired and whose risk of commitment will be increased.

This case is adapted from *Tarasoff* v. *Regents of the University of California,* California Supreme Court, 17 California Reports, 3d series, 425, decided July 1, 1976. The language is that of the court. The facts and majority opinion are written by Justice Tobriner. The dissenting opinion is written by Justice Clark. The comments are brief excerpts from each opinion.

Case 2

After experiencing dry, persistent coughing for several weeks and night sweats for ten days, a bisexual male visits his family physician. When the patient describes his symptoms and admits that he is bisexual, the physician orders a test to determine if the patient has antibodies to the human immunodeficiency virus (HIV), the virus that causes AIDS. The test results are positive and indicate that the patient has been infected with the virus, will probably develop full-blown AIDS over time, will probably die from the disease, and is probably capable of infecting others through sexual contact. In a long counseling session, the physician explains all this to the patient and discusses the risk of unprotected sexual intercourse to his wife, as well as the possibility that their children, now one and three years old, would be left without parents if his wife contracts the disease too. The patient refuses to allow the physician to disclose his condition to his wife. The physician finally and reluctantly accedes to this demand for absolute confidentiality. After surviving two episodes of opportunistic infection, the patient dies eighteen months later. Only during the last few weeks of his life does he allow his wife to be informed that he has AIDS. She is then tested and is found to be antibody positive, but she does not yet have any symptoms. However, a year later she goes to the doctor with dry cough, fever, and loss of appetite. She angrily accuses the physician of violating his moral responsibility to her and her children; she insists that she might have been able to take steps to reduce the risk to herself if she had only known the truth.

This case has been adapted from Grant Gillett, "AIDS and Confidentiality," *Journal of Applied Philosophy* 4 (1987): 15.

Case 3

A five-year-old girl had been a patient in a medical center for three years because of progressive renal failure secondary to glomerulonephritis. She had been on chronic renal dialysis, and the possibility of a renal transplantation was considered. The effectiveness of this procedure in her case was questionable. On the other hand, it was the feeling of the professional staff that there was a clear possibility that a transplanted kidney would not undergo the same disease process. After discussion with the parents, it was decided to proceed with plans for transplantation. Tissue typing was performed on the patient; it was noted that she would be difficult to match. Two siblings, age two and four, were thought to be too young to serve as donors. The girl's mother turned out not to be histocompatible. The father, however, was found to be quite compatible with his daughter. He underwent an arteriogram, and it was discovered that he had anatomically favorable circulation for transplantation. The nephrologist met alone with the father, and gave him these results. He informed the father that the prognosis for his daughter was quite uncertain. After some thought, the girl's father decided that he did not wish to donate a kidney to his daughter. He admitted that he did not have the courage, and that, particularly in view of the uncertain prognosis, the very slight possibility of a cadaver kidney, and the degree of suffering his daughter had already sustained, he would prefer not to donate. The father asked the physician to tell everyone else in the family that he was not histocompatible. He was afraid that if they knew the truth, they would accuse him of allowing his daughter to die. He felt that this would "wreck the family." The physician felt very uncomfortable about this request. However, he agreed to tell the man's wife that "for medical reasons" the father should not donate a kidney.

This case is reprinted by permission from Melvin D. Levine, Lee Scott, and William J. Curran, "Ethics Rounds in a Children's Medical Center: Evaluation of a Hospital-Based Program for Continuing Education in Medical Ethics," *Pediatrics* 60 (August 1977): 205.

Case 4

Mr. X, a fifty-four-year-old patient with a long history of nodular goiter, presented with recent growth of a thyroid mass and hoarseness. Surgery was performed following a biopsy diagnosis of anaplastic thyroid carcinoma. Only partial removal of the tumor was possible, however, and pulmonary metastases were also suspected. Three weeks after the operation, the patient complained of dyspnea, which proved to be caused by a local recurrence. Further tests revealed lung and bone metastases. Despite irradiation and chemotherapy, as well as palliative treatment, the patient died about three months after the initial diagnosis.

The patient, a hard-driving entrepreneur who dominated both his family and his business, was first told that there was a probability of "malignant cell transformation" in his thyroid gland. He immediately consented to the recommended surgery and was told afterward that the diagnosis had been confirmed and that the tumor had been successfully removed. The likelihood of lung metastases was not mentioned.

During a two-hour conversation, the physician then informed the patient's wife, son, and daughter-in-law of the patient's clinical status and his extremely bleak prognosis. The physician encouraged them to ask everything they wanted to know and answered every question with patience and empathy. The family decided to conceal the diagnosis and prognosis from the patient, and the treating physician accepted their decision. Mr. X was told only that he needed "preventive" treatment. After being informed of possible side effects, he enthusiastically consented to irradiation and chemotherapy. When he later developed dyspnea, it was explained as "postoperative swelling" that would subside with treatment. The true nature of his subsequent back pain was never discussed with him, and he never expressed any concern about its seriousness.

The family inquired daily about the patient's condition, either by phone or in person, and was treated very kindly by the staff. The patient himself complained that his recovery was too slow. During intermittent discharges from the hospital, he continued to work in his business—against medical advice—until he exhausted himself. In the hospital, the patient's complaints and harsh criticism of the nurses generated hostility, causing them to avoid him whenever possible. Mr. X was never offered a chance to talk about his impending death, since until the very end, everyone pretended that he would soon recover.

Bettina Schoene-Seifert and James F. Childress, "How Much Should Cancer Patients Know and Decide?" *CA—A Cancer Journal for Clinicians* 36, no. 2 (March–April 1986).

Case 5

A sixty-five-year-old retired army officer had several abdominal operations for gallstones, postoperative adhesions, and bowel obstructions. Because of chronic abdominal pain, loss of weight, and social withdrawal, he voluntarily entered a psychiatric ward. Although he had had a very productive military, teaching, and research career, he was now somewhat depressed and unkempt and had poor hygiene. Furthermore, he and his wife had curtailed their social activities because he could not control his pain without assuming awkward and embarrassing postures. He relied on six self-administered injections each day of Talwin (Pentazocine), which he believed to be essential to control his pain. He quoted the early literature to support his claim that Talwin is nonaddictive; later studies, however, indicated that it is addictive. Having used this medication for more than two years, he had so much tissue and muscle damage that he had difficulty finding injection sites. His goal for therapy was to "get more out of life in spite of my pain."

This psychiatric ward included individual behavior therapy programs, daily group therapy, ward government, and social activities, and the staff ignored pain behaviors in order to avoid reinforcing them. Their positive procedures included relaxation techniques, covert imagery, and cognitive relabeling. Although the patient had voluntarily admitted himself to this ward, where adjustment in medication was a clear expectation, he refused to allow direct modification of his Talwin dosage levels on the grounds that his experience showed that the level of medication was indispensable to controlling his pain. After considerable discussion with colleagues, the therapists decided to withdraw the Talwin over time without the patient's knowledge by diluting it with increasing proportions of normal saline. Although the patient experienced nausea, diarrhea, and cramps, he thought that these withdrawal symptoms were actually the result of Elavil (Amitriptyline), which the therapists had introduced to relieve the withdrawal symptoms. While the therapists did not use Elavil to deceive the patient, it served that purpose, for he blamed it for his discomfort. The staff had informed the patient that his medication regime would be modified but had not given him the details.

After three weeks of saline injections, the therapists explained what had been done. At first, the patient was incredulous and angry, but he asked that the saline be discontinued and the self-control techniques continued. When he was discharged three weeks later, he reported that he experienced some abdominal pain but that he could control it more effectively with the self-control techniques than previously with the Talwin. A follow-up six months later showed that he was still using the relaxation techniques and had resumed social activities and part-time teaching.

The therapists justified this deceptive use of a placebo on grounds of its effectiveness: "We felt ethically obliged to use a treatment that had a high probability of success. To withhold the procedure may have protected some standard of openness but may not have been in his [the patient's] best interests. We saw no option without ethical problems. Although it is precarious to justify the means by the end, we felt most obliged to use a procedure designed to help the patient achieve a personally and medically desirable goal."

Based on the description of an actual case provided by Philip Levendusky and Loren Pankratz, "Self-Control Techniques as an Alternative to Pain Medication," *Journal of Abnormal Psychology* 84, no. 2 (1975): 165–68. Several articles in this issue comment on this case report.

Case 6

A sixty-nine-year-old male, estranged from his children and with no other living relatives, underwent a routine physical examination in preparation for a brief and much anticipated trip to Australia. The physician suspected a serious problem and ordered more extensive testing, including further blood analysis (detailing an acid phosphatase), a bone scan, and a prostate biopsy. The results were quite conclusive: The man had an inoperable, incurable carcinoma—a small prostate nodule commonly referred to as cancer of the prostate. The carcinoma was not yet advanced and was relatively slow growing. Later, after the disease had progressed, it would be possible to provide good palliative treatment. Blood tests and X rays showed the patient's renal function to be normal. (The physician consulted with the urologist who had performed the prostate biopsy in order to confirm the diagnosis.)

The physician had treated this patient for many years and knew that he was fragile in several respects. The man was quite neurotic and had an established history of psychiatric disease—although he functioned well in society and was clearly capable of rational thought and decision making. He had recently suffered a severe depressive reaction, during which he had behaved irrationally and attempted suicide. This episode immediately followed the death of his wife, who had died after a difficult and protracted battle with cancer. It was clear that he had not been equipped to deal with his wife's death, and he had been hospitalized for a short period before the suicide attempt. Just as he was getting back on his feet, the opportunity to go to Australia materialized, and it was the first excitement he had experienced in several years.

This patient also had a history of suffering prolonged and serious depression whenever informed of serious health problems. He worried excessively and often could not exercise rational control over his deliberations and decisions. His physician therefore thought that disclosure of the carcinoma under his present fragile state would almost certainly cause further irrational behavior and render the patient incapable of thinking clearly about his medical situation.

When the testing had been completed and the results were known, the patient returned to his physician. He asked nervously, "Am I OK?" Without waiting for a response, he asked, "I don't have cancer, do I?" Believing his patient would not suffer from or even be aware of his problem while in Australia, the physician answered, "You're as good as you were ten years ago." He was worried about telling such a bald lie but firmly believed that it was justified.

This case was prepared especially for this volume. David Bloom, M.D., was a contributing consultant.

Case 7

Mrs. X, forty-five years of age, was diagnosed as having cancer of the colon with metastases to the lymph nodes. Miss N., a young but experienced nurse in the oncology unit, developed a good rapport with Mrs. X during the three days before the scheduled operation. Miss N. was off duty the day after surgery. When she returned, she could not locate the physician to ascertain what he had told the patient about her condition, and the associate nurse indicated that the patient had not requested or received any information from her. In talking to Mrs. X, Miss N. discovered that she did not know that the tumor was cancerous, that it had metastasized, or that her condition was serious. Mrs. X, however, was concerned about the sharp pain in her abdomen and specifically inquired about the results of the tests. She also wondered when she might be able to return to work. The nurses avoided direct answers to these questions, and Mrs. X's two daughters tried to divert the conversation. When Mrs. X asked, "Is everything all right?" no one answered.

Later, Mrs. X's daughters, who knew the truth, asked the nurse to reassure Mrs. X about her condition. They were worried about the possible impact of the truth, especially since Mrs. X had recently undergone very difficult divorce proceedings. They thought that she would not be able to bear this additional burden. Although the nurse made no promises, she did try to keep the conversation with Mrs. X as light as possible until she could talk to the attending physician—a procedure recommended by the head nurse. When the attending physician arrived in the patient's room, Mrs. X indicated that she felt "pretty good" but asked no questions. He left after a brief examination.

Later, when the nurse was finally able to talk to the physician, he indicated that no one had told Mrs. X about her cancer because such information would only cause her unnecessary anxiety and suffering. Furthermore, he ordered Miss N. not to disclose this information, warning her that he would consider such an act a violation of the patient's best interests and a breach of professional responsibility.

After talking again to the head nurse, who recognized the dilemma but advised her to follow the doctor's orders, Miss N. decided not to disclose the information to the patient, despite her uneasy conscience.

This case has been adapted from Rod R. Yarling, "Ethical Analysis of a Nursing Problem: The Scope of Nursing Practice in Disclosing the Truth to Terminal Patients," parts I and II, *Superior Nurse* (May 1978 and June 1978).

Case 8

Ralph Cobbs was admitted to a hospital for treatment of a duodenal ulcer. He was given a series of tests and was administered medication to ease his discomfort. He still continued to complain of lower abdominal pain and nausea. His family physician, Dr. Jerome Sands, concluded that surgery was indicated. He discussed prospective surgery with Mr. Cobbs and advised him in general terms of the risks of undergoing a general anesthetic.

Dr. Sands then called in Dr. F. P. Grant, a surgeon, who examined Mr. Cobbs and agreed that he had an intractable duodenal ulcer and that surgery was indicated. Dr. Grant explained the nature of the operation to Mr. Cobbs but did not discuss any of its inherent risks. Mr. Cobbs consented to the operation, which seemed successful. However, nine days later, the patient began to experience intense abdominal pain. Dr. Sands advised him to return to the hospital. Two hours after his return, Mr. Cobbs went into shock, and emergency surgery was performed. Internal bleeding was discovered, the result of a severed artery at the hilium of the spleen. Because of the seriousness of the hemorrhaging, Dr. Grant decided to remove the spleen (which may be taken out of an adult without adverse effects). Injuries to the spleen necessitating a subsequent operation are a risk inherent to the original type of surgery performed on Mr. Cobbs. The probability of the patient needing further surgery was approximately five percent at the time of the original operation.

A month after his second discharge from the hospital, Mr. Cobbs again experienced sharp pains in his stomach. These were traced to a developing gastric ulcer. The development of a new ulcer is another risk inherent in surgery performed to relieve a duodenal ulcer. Within four months, the patient had to be rehospitalized, and a third operation was performed, a gastrectomy removing fifty percent of Mr. Cobbs's stomach (to reduce its acid-producing capacity). Subsequent to his discharge this time, the patient had to be readmitted because of internal bleeding caused by the premature absorption of a suture, another inherent risk of surgery. The bleeding began to abate after a week, and Mr. Cobbs was discharged for the final time.

Mr. Cobbs then brought a malpractice suit against Dr. Grant on two grounds: (1) negligent performance of the operation and (2) failure to disclose the risks of the original surgery. The Supreme Court of California used expert testimony to determine that the operation was not performed negligently; all the subsequent problems Mr. Cobbs experienced were inherent risks of the surgery, not the result of negligence. The second ground, however, received extensive commentary in the court's opinion. The court reasoned that this case provides a "classic illustration" of possible negligence in disclosure. While Dr. Grant had thoroughly explained the nature of the procedure and had performed the operation exactly as described, he had not discussed the possibilities of the spleen injury, of the new ulcer and ensuing gastrectomy, or of the internal bleeding resulting from the premature absorption of a suture—all "links in a chain of low probability events inherent in the initial operation." The court reasoned that this failure to inform may have constituted a violation of the physician's duty to disclose pertinent information to patients. This violation would make the physician liable for subsequent injuries, because he withheld the facts necessary for Mr. Cobbs to consent intelligently to the proposed treatment.

Dr. Grant argued that it was uncommon medical practice to disclose hazards of such low probability and that he should be held only to the standards of disclosure operative among surgeons. The court, however, quoted a precedent case (*Canterbury* v. *Spence*), which reached a different conclusion: "To bind the disclosure obligation to medical usage is to arrogate the decision on revelation to the physician alone. Respect for the patient's right of self-determination on particular therapy demands a standard set by law for physicians rather than one which physicians may or may not impose upon themselves." The court held that in this matter physician discretion cannot be reconciled with a patient's basic right to make the ultimate informed decision about his or her own treatment. "A mini-course in medical science is not required," the court held, but "when a given procedure inherently involves a known risk of death or serious bodily harm, a medical doctor has a duty to disclose to his patient the potential of death or serious harm. . . . The patient's right of self-decision is the measure of the physician's duty to reveal." A physician is therefore required to disclose "all information relevant to a meaningful decisional process," with respect to both the proposed therapy and its inherent risks.

Given these problems, the court determined that a trial court should reach a judgment in this case after further analyzing the extent of "the doctor's duty to obtain the patient's informed consent."

This case is summarized from *Cobbs* v. *Grant*, 502 P.2d 1, decided October 27, 1972.

The language closely follows that of the court, and all direct quotations are from this source. The opinion was written by Justice Mosk.

Case 9

Mrs. Catherine Lake, who was then sixty years old, suffered from chronic brain syndrome with arteriosclerosis. As a result, she had periods of confusion and mild loss of memory, interspersed with times of mental alertness and rationality. She was hospitalized after having been found wandering on a city street; when questioned, she could not give her home address. During her third hospitalization, she petitioned for release on grounds of unlawful deprivation of liberty.

A psychiatrist who testified at her hearing claimed that she was unable to remember when her sister, her son, and her husband had died. She also showed what were diagnosed as paranoid tendencies, believing that government agencies had taken her pension away from her. (Her government pension had, indeed, been cut off several years earlier.) However, the psychiatrist was concerned mainly about Mrs. Lake's wandering, which presented a risk of harm to herself. She showed no tendency to harm others or to harm herself intentionally. Her commitment was based solely on the need for supervision because of her confused and defenseless state.

Mrs. Lake also testified at her hearing. She appeared to be fully rational and stated that she understood her condition and the risks involved in her living outside the hospital. But she preferred to accept these risks rather than endure continued hospitalization.

The district court, supported by the U.S. Court of Appeals, denied her petition. The court found that Mrs. Lake's family lacked the means to provide needed supervision for her. They claimed that she was "a danger to herself in that she has a tendency to wander about the streets, and is not competent to care for herself." The legal basis for her involuntary commitment was a statute providing for hospitalization of a person who "is mentally ill, and because of that illness, is likely to injure himself or others if allowed to remain at liberty." The court declared that *injure* ought to be construed broadly enough to include Mrs. Lake's situation.

However, about six months later, the court of appeals agreed to consider a rehearing of the case, identifying several crucial issues: How should "likely to injure himself" be interpreted? Is one who is "likely to injure himself" also automatically incompetent to choose between risk and hospitalization? Must the court consider community resources other than commitment to a mental hospital? Is equal protection denied by commitment of a person like Mrs. Lake, who would be released if her family had the means to care for her?

The case was finally returned to the district court for an inquiry into alternative courses of treatment. The court was asked to consider whether Mrs. Lake could be released if she agreed to carry an identification card, to accept public health nursing care, to live in a foster home, or to abide by other similar conditions. Judge Bazelon, presiding officer of the court of appeals, instructed the district court that the burden of finding alternatives ought to be on the court, not on Mrs. Lake, since she lacked access to the necessary information. Bazelon referred to the position of the Department of Health, Education, and Welfare (now Health and Human Services), which mandates provision of a wide spectrum of services so that the interests of both the mentally ill person and the public will be served. He also endorsed the view of the National Council on the Aging, which recommends that "care and services be provided so as to be most satisfying to the person concerned." In line with this view, Bazelon ordered that "every effort should be made to find a course of treatment which appellant might be willing to accept." However, the lower court, after conducting a further investigation of Mrs. Lake's case, concluded that her propensity to wander aimlessly made "constant supervision . . . not only proper but required for the safety of this patient." Mrs. Lake died four years later, still confined in a mental hospital.

This case was prepared by Carol Tauer from materials in Jay Katz, Joseph Goldstein, and Alan M. Dershowitz, *Psychoanalysis, Psychiatry, and Law* (New York: Free Press, 1967). It was expanded by James Tubbs from materials in *Lake v. Cameron*, 267 F. Supp. 155 (D.D.C 1967), and Robert A. Burt, *Taking Care of Strangers: The Rule of Law in Doctor-Patient Relations* (New York: Free Press, 1979), chap. 2.

Case 10

P.Z., now twenty-seven-years old, is an involuntary mental patient at Lakeland State Hospital, where he was committed in June 1971, after amputating his right hand. He had been previously committed to Lakeland for eight months in 1966 (after perforating his right eardrum) and for eighteen months in 1969 (after removing his right eye). In all, P.Z. has spent approximately eight years in hospitals undergoing medical treatment, e.g., treatment for meningitis following the perforation of his eardrum, and for psychiatric care of a custodial and involuntary nature.

For a variety of reasons, P.Z. now wishes to leave the hospital, but his family is strongly opposed. P.Z.'s father, a factory foreman whose job is in some jeopardy due to recession layoffs, points out that the family is already in debt more than thirty thousand dollars for the medical care necessitated by P.Z.'s penchant for self-mutilation. Neither P.Z.'s parents nor his siblings can control his self-destructive outbursts at home; indeed, they are very frightened that he will turn upon them as well. P.Z., on the other hand, maintains that he has been confined long enough, that he is not dangerous, and that, in any event, there is "no treatment for me in the hospital." He states repeatedly that "I believe in God and in brotherly love" and that "one man must sacrifice himself to God for the good of all men." He believes that "it is far better for one man to believe and accept an appropriate message from God to sacrifice an eye or a hand according to the sacred scriptures rather than for the present course of the world to cause even greater loss of human life." P.Z. believes that he is the only one whom God has selected for that sacrifice and maintains that he enucleated his right eye and amputated his right hand upon "direct orders from God," and that he and God thereby established a "covenant." P.Z. now wants release from the hospital in order to "carry God's love to His children"; he emphasizes his commitment to this work by stating: "I would cut off my right foot if God told me to."

What rights does P.Z. have to determine where and how he shall live, and what mental competence does he have to assert such rights? Alternatively, what rights may be asserted by his family, or by society, to restrain, isolate, or "contain" him? If others have the right ultimately to restrain P.Z., must they also provide him with treatment beyond mere containment? If so, is custodial treatment sufficient? May society compel P.Z. to undergo more drastic, irreversible treatments, with or without his consent?

This case was prepared by P. Browning Hoffman, M.D., for presentation in the series of "Medicine and Society" conferences at the University of Virginia School of Medicine and is used by permission. The longest quotation has been added by the authors.

Case 11

John K., a thirty-two-year-old lawyer, had worried for several years about developing Huntington's chorea, a neurological disorder that appears in a person's thirties or forties, bringing rapid uncontrollable twitching and contractions and progressive, irreversible dementia, and leading to death in approximately ten years. John K.'s mother died from this disease, which is autosomal dominant and afflicts fifty percent of an affected parent's offspring. Often parents have children before they are aware that one of them has the disease. John K. and his wife had a child because of contraceptive failure and an unwillingness to have an abortion because of his wife's religious convictions.

John K. had indicated to many people that he would prefer to die rather than to live and die as his mother lived and died. He was anxious, drank heavily, and had intermittent depression, for which he saw a psychiatrist. Nevertheless, he was a productive lawyer.

John K. first noticed facial twitching three months ago, and two neurologists independently confirmed a diagnosis of Huntington's. He explained his situation to his psychiatrist and requested help in committing suicide. When the psychiatrist refused, John reassured him that he did not plan to attempt suicide any time soon.

But when he went home, he ingested all his antidepressant medication after pinning a note to his shirt to explain his actions and to refuse any medical assistance that might be offered. His wife, whom he had not told about the diagnosis, found him unconscious and rushed him to the emergency room without removing the note.

This case has been adapted from Marc Basson, ed., *Rights and Responsibilities in Modern Medicine: The Second Volume in a Series on Ethics, Humanism, and Medicine* (New York: Alan R. Liss, 1981), pp. 183–84.

Case 12

Janet P., a practicing Jehovah's Witness, had refused to sign a consent for blood infusions before the delivery of her daughter. Physicians determined that the newborn infant needed transfusions to prevent retardation and possible death. When the parents refused permission for these transfusions, a hearing was conducted at the Columbia Hospital for Women to decide whether the newborn infant should be given transfusions over the parents' objections. Superior Court Judge Tim Murphy ordered a guardian appointed to sign the necessary releases, and the baby was given the transfusions. During the hearing, Janet P. began hemorrhaging, and attending physicians said she needed an emergency hysterectomy to stem the bleeding. Her husband, also a Jehovah's Witness, approved the hysterectomy but not infusions of blood. This time, Judge Murphy declined to order transfusions for the mother, basing his decision on an earlier D.C. Court of Appeals ruling. Janet P. bled to death a few hours later. Her baby survived.

This case is based on a news report by Martha M. Hamilton in the *Washington Post*, November 14, 1974. It was prepared by James J. McCartney.

Case 13

Mrs. Jones was brought to the hospital by her husband for emergency care, having lost two-thirds of her body's blood supply from a ruptured ulcer. She had no personal physician, and relied solely on the hospital staff. She was a total hospital responsibility. It appeared that the patient, age twenty-five, mother of a seven-month-old child, and her husband were both Jehovah's Witnesses, the teachings of which sect, according to their interpretation, prohibited the injection of blood into the body. When death without blood became imminent, the hospital sought the advice of counsel, who applied to the District Court in the name of the hospital for permission to administer blood. Judge Tamm of the District Court denied the application, and counsel immediately applied to me [Judge J. Skelly Wright], as a member of the Court of Appeals, for an appropriate writ.

I called the hospital by telephone and spoke with Dr. Westura, Chief Medical Resident, who confirmed the representations made by counsel. I thereupon proceeded with counsel to the hospital, where I spoke to Mr. Jones, the husband of the patient. He advised me that, on religious grounds, he would not approve a blood transfusion for his wife. He said, however, that if the court ordered the transfusion, the responsibility was not his. I advised Mr. Jones to obtain counsel immediately. He thereupon went to the telephone and returned in ten or fifteen minutes to advise that he had taken the matter up with his church and that he had decided that he did not want counsel.

I asked permission of Mr. Jones to see his wife. This he readily granted. Prior to going into the patient's room, I again conferred with Dr. Westura and several other doctors assigned to the case. All confirmed that the patient would die without blood and that there was a better than fifty percent chance of saving her life with it. Unanimously they strongly recommended it. I then went inside the patient's room. Her appearance confirmed the urgency which had been represented to me. I tried to communicate with her, advising her again as to what the doctors had said. The only audible reply I could hear was "Against my will." It was obvious that the woman was not in a mental condition to make a decision. I was reluctant to press her because of the seriousness of her condition and because I felt that to suggest repeatedly the imminence of death without blood might place a strain on her religious convictions. I asked her whether she would oppose the blood transfusion if the court allowed it. She indicated, as best as I could make out, that it would not then be her responsibility. . . .

I . . . signed the order allowing the hospital to administer such transfusions as the doctors should determine were necessary to save her life. . . .

This case is excerpted directly from *Application of the President and Directors of Georgetown College*, 331 F.2d 1000 (D.C. Cir.), certiorari denied, 377 U.S. 978 (1964).

Case 14

Carl Wells, a twenty-three-year-old Texas tenant farmer, widower, and father to two children (ages five and seven), was admitted by ambulance to St. Magdalene's Hospital in a small East Texas town following a motorcycle accident. The accident occurred as he was returning from work when a sudden burst of rain wet the highway. As Carl was rounding a turn, a pickup truck pulled into the highway ahead of him. His attempt to brake resulted in a skid into a concrete abutment, throwing him from his bike.

The rescue squad reported that when they arrived Carl was conscious, could talk, and knew where he was and what had happened. Almost immediately, he asked to be taken not to the hospital but to his home, saying that it was against his religious principles to be healed by any but the elders of his church. He knew he needed "healing," but not at the hands of doctors.

He seemed to have a fracture of his left leg and a large bleeding contusion/ laceration over the right temporal region. He was pale, sweaty, and in obvious pain. His pulse was "very rapid" and "thready." Despite his protestations, the ambulance squad started an IV and took him to the hospital. On the way to the hospital, he had a transient loss of consciousness estimated by the attendants as not more than five to six minutes in duration. By the time he arrived at the emergency room, he had recovered sufficiently to protest being admitted, to refuse all treatment, and to ask that his IV be removed and that his brother, an elder of his church, be called immediately to take him home so he could be properly healed. He refused the taking of blood, X rays, or measures to relieve pain. He was restrained from pulling out his IV line. He quieted down when told that his brother was on the way and did not resist further.

In the ensuing half-hour, he became drowsy, vomited once, and had a grand mal seizure, after which he became aphasic and his breathing became stertorous and deep. He was drowsy and difficult to arouse. His pulse was 60, and his blood pressure was 190/40. He had a left Babinski sign and left hemiparesis. A neurosurgeon making rounds in the nearby ICU was called. He made a clinical diagnosis of acute epidural hemorrhage and ordered immediate surgery. Signs of increasing intracranial pressure were obvious, and brainstem compression and temporal lobe herniation had to be prevented or the patient would die or survive in a permanent vegetative state.

At this point, Carl's brother had not yet been located. The neurosurgeon explained to Carl that he had a ruptured meningeal artery, that immediate surgery to place burr holes, locate the tear, and ligate the vessel was necessary. If done, Carl had an excellent chance of complete recovery, but a delay of even minutes was life-threatening. Carl's aphasia and drowsiness prevented his answering the question of consent to the procedure.

The hospital attorney advised against intervention, citing a judge's order in the same county forbidding intervention in the case of another member of the same church. In this fundamentalist, conservative community, nurses and other physicians were sharply divided on what to do. The neurosurgeon, however, ordered the patient taken to the operating room. Two nurses protested that they could not "participate."

The neurosurgeon argued that Carl had had a serious head injury from the outset, that he could not be competent when he refused such definitive treatment, and that he did not realize the extent of his injury or the very good possibility of amelioration by the surgical procedure. Moreover, Carl was now aphasic and could not express himself. No one could know what his choice would be. The chaplain argued that he knew the tenets of Carl's religious group and that Carl probably would rather die a martyr than violate his beliefs. The neurosurgeon argued that it was his ethical responsibility to be Carl's advocate. Besides, Carl's two children would lose his support and become a public responsibility. The chaplain argued that he had an ethical responsibility to protect Carl's wishes, and his spiritual purity, and that the neurosurgeon was incompetent to make a spiritual decision.

This case was prepared by Edmund Pellegrino and is used with slight modifications and with his permission.

Case 15

Mrs. R., a forty-five-year-old housewife, has multiple sclerosis and suffers frequent asthma attacks that require treatment in the emergency room of the local community hospital. The physician has written a "no code" order for Mrs. R. This means that no efforts will be made to resuscitate her if she were to suffer a cardiac arrest during an acute asthma attack in the hospital. As far as the nurses know, the physician's decision was made without discussion with the patient or the patient's family. Mrs. R.'s husband, a middle-management executive in a local firm, divorced her several years earlier, and Mrs. R. had been responsible for two teenage daughters (ages fourteen and sixteen), who live at home.

According to some of the nurses, Mrs. R.'s medical condition and situation at home are "intolerable." They even feel that they "certainly wouldn't want to live under those conditions." There is, however, no evidence that Mrs. R. feels this way. She usually seems depressed when she comes into the emergency room, but she has not expressed her views to the nurses. The nurses wonder what they should do if Mrs. R. suffers a cardiac arrest when they are on duty.

This case has been adapted from Anne J. Davis and Mila A. Aroskar, *Ethical Dilemmas and Nursing Practice* (New York: Appleton-Century-Crofts, 1978), pp. 207–8.

Case 16

By 1976, sixty-seven-year-old Joseph Saikewicz had lived in state institutions for more than forty years. His IQ was ten, and his mental age was approximately two years and eight months. He could communicate only by gestures and grunts, and he responded only to gestures or physical contacts. He appeared to be unaware of dangers and became disoriented when removed from familiar surroundings.

His health was generally good until April 1976, when he was diagnosed as having acute myeloblastic monocytic leukemia, which is invariably fatal. In approximately thirty to fifty percent of cases of this type of leukemia, chemotherapy can bring about temporary remission, which usually lasts between two and thirteen months. The results are poorer for patients older than sixty. In addition, chemotherapy often has serious side effects, including anemia and infections.

At the petition of the Belchertown State School, where Saikewicz was located, the probate court appointed a guardian *ad litem* with authority to make the necessary decisions concerning the patient's care and treatment. The guardian *at litem* noted that Saikewicz's illness was incurable, that chemotherapy had significant adverse effects and discomfort, and that Saikewicz could not understand the treatment or the resulting pain. For all these reasons, he concluded "that not treating Mr. Saikewicz would be in his best interests." The Supreme Judicial Court of Massachusetts upheld this decision on July 9, 1976 (although its opinion was not issued until November 28, 1977). Mr. Saikewicz died on September 4, 1976.

This case is drawn from *Superintendent of Belchertown* v. *Saikewicz*, Mass. 370 N.E. 2d 417 (1977).

Case 17

In November 1977, seventy-eight-year-old Earle Spring suffered a mild scratch on the instep of his foot. A fiercely independent outdoorsman, he left the cut unattended until his foot finally became gangrenous. Hospitalization was followed by pneumonia and then a diagnosis of kidney failure. After undergoing three five-hour dialysis sessions a week, Spring soon improved enough to return home. Meanwhile, his mental deterioration, which had been diagnosed before his injury as "chronic organic brain syndrome," became markedly pronounced.

After more than a year of treatment, the nephrologist informed Spring's son, Robert, that his father was not benefiting from dialysis. He suggested it may have been a mistake to have initiated it on a man his age and that it might be best if the treatments were ended. The son and the wife agreed with the physician and requested that the treatments be stopped. However, because of the Massachusetts Supreme Judicial Court's 1977 *Saikewicz* ruling (Case 16 in this appendix), decisions of such significance in that state have to be made by courts rather than by families and physicians.

On January 25, 1979, Robert Spring, who had been appointed temporary guardian, petitioned the Franklin County Probate Court for an order to terminate the hemodialysis treatments. They began a full adversary hearing in which the guardian *ad litem*, an attorney appointed by the court to represent the best interests of the patient, had the responsibility for presenting "all reasonable arguments in favor of administering treatment to prolong the life of the individual involved."

Mark I. Berson, Spring's guardian *ad litem,* insisted (contrary to *Saikewicz*) that the court not render a "substituted judgment" (a statement of what Spring himself would have wanted) without some evidence from Spring's lucid moments on that subject. On May 15, 1979, Judge Keedy entered a judgment permitting the temporary guardian, Robert Spring, "to refrain from authorizing further life-prolonging medical treatment" for his father. Attorney Berson was not satisfied that there was sufficient evidence that Spring would have wanted to terminate the treatments, and he appealed. Judge Keedy vacated his original order and on July 2 entered a new one to the effect that Spring's wife and son, together with the attending physician, were to make the decision. Again Berson appealed.

The court of appeals upheld the probate court's action. It rejected Berson's position on the need for an express statement of intent to withhold treatment. In its words, "Such a contention would largely stifle the very rights of privacy and personal dignity which the *Saikewicz* case sought to secure for incompetent persons." Berson appealed.

On January 10, the supreme judicial court heard the case. It concluded that the trial judge's finding that Earle Spring "would, if competent, choose not to receive the life-prolonging treatment" was correct. But, unlike the trial judge and the court of appeals, the supreme judicial court found that the facts "bring the case within the rule of *Saikewicz.*" It therefore held "it was an error to delegate the decision to the attending physician and the ward's wife and son." Once again, Spring's guardian was directed by the probate court to "refrain from authorizing any further life-prolonging treatment" for his father.

Meanwhile, it was becoming clear that the staff of the Holyoke Geriatric Center were, in their own words, "appalled over the decision to stop the dialysis treatment." Two nurses on the three P.M. to eleven P.M. shift asked Spring if he wanted to die. Reportedly, he replied, "No." Although a psychiatrist had previously evaluated Spring as "incompetent," the nurses taking his statement as proof of Spring's desires brought their story to a local newspaper, which used it as headline news. Berson responded immediately. On the basis of an affidavit filed by a right-to-life group, he petitioned Judge Keedy to reinstate the dialysis treatments until new evidence of Spring's competence could be gathered. The right-to-life activists hired a lawyer to petition the probate court to admit them as parties to the case. In the sixth judicial determination on Spring's case, Judge Keedy denied the petition to reinstate dialysis treatment. Berson appealed once more.

This appeal was granted by the supreme judicial court, which then appointed five psychiatrists and geriatric specialists to determine Spring's mental status.

During that time, Spring had been admitted to the hospital suffering from an infection and pneumonia. He responded to medical treatment and returned to the nursing home on March 25, but in an extremely weakened condition. The following Sunday, the day before the competency hearing was scheduled, Earle Spring died. The next day, the five court-appointed physicians filed their report: Spring "was suffering from such profound mental impairment that he had no idea where he was or what was going on. The dementia was not related to the kidney failure, was untreatable, and irreversible." Had he not died the day before, the responsibility for deciding to stop the dialysis treatments would have rested where it had fourteen months previously—with the court.

This case was prepared by John J. Paris, S.J. It derives from his "Death, Dying, and the Courts: The Travesty and Tragedy of the Earle Spring Case," *Linacre Quarterly* 49 (February 1982): 26–41.

Case 18

Paul E. Brophy, Sr., a firefighter and emergency medical technician in Easton, Massachusetts, suffered a ruptured brain artery on March 22, 1983. Surgery was performed in April, but it was unsuccessful, and Brophy never regained consciousness. He was transferred to the New England Sinai Hospital in a persistent vegetative state. When he developed pneumonia in August, both his physicians and Patricia Brophy, his wife and legal guardian, concurred in an order not to resuscitate him if he suffered a cardiac arrest. In December 1983, Mrs. Brophy gave the physicians permission for a surgical procedure to insert a feeding tube into his stomach. He received seven and a half hours of nursing care each day, consisting of bathing, shaving, turning, and so on. Brophy's medical bills, approximately ten thousand dollars per month, were paid entirely by Blue Cross/Blue Shield.

Brophy had often told family members that he did not want to be kept alive if he ever became comatose. In a discussion of the Karen Ann Quinlan case, he had indicated to his wife that "I don't ever want to be on a life-support system. No way do I want to live like that; that's just not living." Several years earlier, the town of Easton had given Brophy and his partner a commendation for bravery after they had pulled a man from a burning truck. When he learned that the victim had suffered a great deal before dying several months after being saved, Brophy threw his commendation into the wastebasket, exclaiming to his wife, "I should have been five minutes later. It would have been all over for him." He told his brother, Leo, "If I'm ever like that, just shoot me, pull the plug." And prior to his own neurosurgery, he told one of his daughters, "If I can't sit up to kiss one of my beautiful daughters, I may as well be six feet under."

Mrs. Brophy, a devout Catholic and a nurse who worked part-time with the mentally retarded, decided to question the continuation of artificial feeding when her husband's condition remained unchanged through the next year. There was no hope that he would regain consciousness, and, though he had never expressed a specific judgment about artificial feeding, she recalled his previously expressed wishes about "pulling the plug." She consulted with clergy, ethicists, and a lawyer before requesting withdrawal of artificial nutrition with the understanding that her husband would die in one to two weeks. Her decision received the unanimous support of their five children and other family members, including Brophy's seven brothers and sisters and his elderly mother, who was in her nineties. However, the physicians and the hospital administration refused to act on this request.

In February 1985, Mrs. Brophy asked a probate court for a declaratory judgment ordering the hospital to act affirmatively on her request. The New England Sinai Hospital responded that the physician-in-chief of the hospital could not "in good conscience, consistent with the ethical codes of the medical profession, participate in the discontinuation of all nutrition and hydration." And it requested that Brophy be transferred to another facility if the court ordered discontinuation of artificial nutrition and hydration.

The court-appointed guardian *ad litem* (a person appointed by the court to protect the interests of a ward in a legal proceeding) found that "removal of the G [gastrostomy] tube is not comparable to cessation of dialysis or removal of a respirator because removal of the aforesaid artificial mechanisms permits the illness or injury to run its natural course. Nutrition, however, is not a need required by Mr. Brophy as a result of his illness, but rather, it is a need common to all human beings." Furthermore, the guardian *ad litem* continued, "Brophy is a chronically ill patient, but is not terminally ill. He is entitled to the same fundamentals of comfort, i.e., food, shelter and bedding, as is any other chronically ill patient, and it is the duty of the medical facility to provide him with the aforesaid care." The probate judge ruled that the feeding tube must be continued, even though he found that Brophy would have preferred to be dead than to have his life prolonged in a persistent vegetative state and that if competent he would reject artificial nutrition. Mrs. Brophy appealed this verdict.

In September 1986, in a split decision (4 to 3), the Supreme Judicial Court of Massachusetts held the Brophy's feeding tube could be removed. Three U.S. Supreme Court justices declined to review the decision. The Massachusetts court did not require the hospital to compromise its principles by terminating feeding, but it did require the hospital's cooperation in transfering Brophy to Emerson Hospital in Concord, which was willing to honor Mrs. Brophy's request.

In October 1986, Brophy was transferred to Emerson Hospital under the care of a neurologist who had earlier testified that Brophy was in a persistent vegetative state. Many of the hospital staff volunteered to help care for Brophy by providing supportive care, including anticonvulsants and antacids, while he died. Brophy, age forty-nine, died of pneumonia on October 23, 1986, eight days after the feeding tube was removed. He was surrounded by his wife, who had remained with him around the clock, their children, and a grandchild. According to the attending physician, Brophy's death was an "amazing, peaceful, quiet time."

This case summary has been drawn from *Brophy* v. *New England Sinai Hospital, Inc.,* 497 N.E. 2d 626 (Mass. 1986), and Robert Steinbrook and Bernard Lo, "Artificial Feeding—Solid Ground, Not a Slippery Slope," *New England Journal of Medicine* 286 (February 4, 1988): 286–90.

Case 19

Baby girl Betsy Novick had immediately apparent physical malformations when she was born. A diagnosis of Seckel or "bird-headed" dwarfism was made. She had, in addition to low birth weight and length, large eyes, a large beaklike nose, narrow face, receding lower jaw, strabismus, and a club foot. Seckel dwarfism, an autosomal-recessive genetic disease, had affected Mr. Novick's brother as well. Life expectancy is good, but a much simplified gross cerebral structure is related to mental retardation. It was apparent that institutionalization would be necessary. The Novicks were of modest means, and the vivid memory of the devastating impact of Mr. Novick's brother immediately convinced him that the child could not be cared for at home.

The Novicks lived in the state that has the lowest per capita income spent on institutions for the retarded. Although court action promised some marginal improvements in the institutions, they promised to be bleak, understaffed, custodial institutions for the foreseeable future. The fact that Betsy had rather peculiarly repulsive features led the parents to fear that she would receive particularly poor care, yet they saw no alternative.

In the next two months, Betsy developed a persistent pyloric stenosis, a narrowing of the pylorus between the stomach and intestines, causing projectile vomiting that did not respond to phenobarbital, atropine, or special diet. If not surgically treated, death by starvation would result. The parents, at first stunned by the additional severe medical problem, considered the alternatives. They envisioned the virtually certain severe burden and suffering to be placed on the child in any institutions conceivably available in the next decade or two. They decided that it was a burden the child should not bear, even though in principle they knew society should be providing better support for them. They decided against the surgery. The child died after two weeks of deterioration.

This case was prepared by Robert M. Veatch and is used by permission.

Case 20

On May 18, 1982, the U.S. Department of Health and Human Services issued a letter to 6800 hospitals receiving federal funding, reminding the recipients that under Section 504 of the Rehabilitation Act of 1973, "it is unlawful . . . to withhold from a handicapped infant nutritional sustenance or medical or surgical treatment required to correct a life-threatening condition if: (1) the withholding is based upon the fact that the infant is handicapped; and (2) the handicap does not render treatment or nutritional sustenance medically contraindicated." HHS Secretary Richard Schweiker noted that "In providing this notice . . . we are reaffirming the strong commitment of the American people and their laws to the protection of human life."

The occasion for this reminder was the death, one month earlier, of a Bloomington, Indiana, infant identified to the public only as "Infant Doe." Baby boy Doe was born with Down syndrome (trisomy 21) and with a tracheoesophageal fistula (an opening between the breathing and swallowing tubes that prevents passage of food to the stomach). The baby's parents were informed that surgery to correct his fistula would have "an even chance of success." Left untreated, the fistula would soon lead to the baby's death from starvation or pneumonia (induced by stomach secretions reaching the lungs). The parents, who also have two healthy children, chose to withhold food and treatment and "let nature take its course."

Court action to remove the infant from his parents' custody (and permit the surgery) was sought by the county prosecutor. Such action was denied by the court, and the Indiana Supreme Court declined to review the lower court's ruling. Infant Doe died, at six days of age, as Indiana authorities were seeking intervention from the U.S. Supreme Court. The parents' lawyer commented that the mother was with the child to the end: "It wasn't a case of abandonment. It was a case of love."

This case was adapted by James Tubbs from Fred Barbash and Christine Russell, "The Demise of 'Infant Doe': Permitted Death Gives Life to an Old Debate," *Washington Post,* April 17, 1982, and from the *HHS News,* May 18, 1982.

Case 21

The patient, a 40-year-old nullipara [a woman who has never given birth to a viable infant] with an 18-month history of infertility, underwent genetic amniocentesis at 17 weeks' gestation for the indication of advanced maternal age. Her medical history was unremarkable except for hypothyroidism, for which she had received dessicated thyroid extract, 3 g daily, since 1960. An ultrasound scan before the procedure revealed a twin pregnancy with biparietal diameters of both fetuses compatible with 17.5 weeks' gestation, two clearly defined amniotic sacs, and one placenta on the posterior uterine wall. Amniotic fluid from each sac obtained separately from chromosomal studies revealed two male fetuses. Twin A had a normal male karyotype (46, XY), but chromosomal analysis of Twin B indicated trisomy 21 (47, XY + 21).

Presented with the diagnosis of carrying one normal and one affected fetus, the parents were confronted with the difficult task of making one of two decisions: to induce abortion and lose both fetuses, or to continue the pregnancy. The mother desperately wanted to have the normal child but could not face the burden of caring for an abnormal child for the rest of her life. Having been made aware of the case report from Sweden in which selective termination of an abnormal twin had been successfully performed even though the unaffected twin was delivered prematurely, she asked if a similar procedure could be offered to her. If it had been refused, she would have chosen to abort both fetuses. At that point, she was referred to us.

Extensive medical and legal counseling and an explanation of the many risks were provided. These risks included abortion of both fetuses, premature delivery of the surviving fetus, performing the procedure on the wrong twin since markers for sac A or B were lacking, and the development of disseminated intravascular coagulation in the mother as a result of fetal death in utero. After careful consideration, the patient decided to undertake the procedure anyway. In view of the fact that the procedure had never been performed in this country, we decided, out of an abundance of caution, to obtain confirmation from a court of law of the parent's right to consent on behalf of the normal fetus.

This case is reprinted with permission from *New England Journal of Medicine* 304 (June 8, 1981): 1525, where it appeared in Thomas D. Kerenyi and Usha Chitkara, "Selective Birth in Twin Pregnancy with Discordancy for Down's Syndrome."

Case 22

A 33-year-old unmarried white woman, gravida 2, para 1 [second pregnancy with the previous pregnancy resulting in viable offspring], was admitted to the hospital in labor at 0730. The patient had received no prenatal care, and although the expected date of confinement was uncertain she was thought to be near term. Membranes had ruptured spontaneously 2 hours before admission. Early in the pregnancy the patient had been hospitalized twice for gallbladder disease, at which time cholecystectomy and subsequent reexploration for removal of a common duct stone were performed. While the patient recovered uneventfully from both of these procedures, it was not recognized that she was pregnant. Significant past history included the delivery of twins 3 years before admission and a lifelong problem of morbid obesity (estimated weight 157.5 kg).

The patient was noted to be angry and uncooperative. Vital signs included blood pressure, 140/100 mmHg; pulse, 100 beats/min; and temperature, 36.5C. With the exception of obesity, the general physical findings were essentially normal. Estimated fetal weight was 3000 g, regular contractions were occurring every 5 to 7 minutes, and fetal heart tones were 140 beats/min. The cervix was 2 cm dilated and not well effaced, and amniotic fluid was clear, but the exact presentation and position of the fetus were difficult to ascertain because of the high and unidentifiable presenting part.

. . . Ninety minutes after admission the amniotic fluid was noted to be meconium stained. Later the fetal heart rate (FHR) tracing demonstrated late decelerations, which were confirmed by internal FHR monitoring showing a loss of baseline variability as well. Because of these findings suggesting fetal hypoxia, the high station of the fetal presenting part, and the desultory progress of labor, the patient was advised of the dangers to the infant, and delivery by cesarean section was recommended. Because of her fear of surgery, the patient refused; furthermore, she requested permission to leave the hospital against medical advice. The patient's mother and sister, with whom she lived, and the father of the baby were fully informed of the circumstances. All involved attempted to persuade the patient to accept the advice of the physicians, but to no avail. The obstetric psychiatric consultant interviewed the patient and was convinced that she was neither delusional nor mentally incompetent. The patient was capable of understanding the circumstances and making a rational decision.

At this point the hospital administration was advised of the situation, and the hospital attorney interviewed the patient. Convinced of the intransigence of the patient's position and advised by the physicians that there was evidence of persistent, even worsening fetal distress, the legal staff requested intervention by the juvenile court. Attorneys were appointed by the court to represent the patient and the unborn infant, and a hearing was convened in the patient's room with the judge presiding. Testimony from the professional staff and from the patient, including cross-examination by the attorneys for the mother and the fetus was heard, after which the court found that the unborn baby of the patient was a dependent and neglected child within the meaning of the Colorado Children's Code. It was then ordered that a cesarean section be performed to safeguard the life of the unborn child.

Following the court's decision, the patient, although still reluctant, became more cooperative and agreed to the induction of general anesthesia. At 1830 hours, 11 hours after admission, a 3500-g female infant was delivered by low transverse cesarean section. . . .[1]

The infant responded promptly to resuscitation, which included direct endotracheal suctioning to remove meconium. Except for transient respiratory dis-

[1]Apgar scores were 2 and 8 at 1 and 5 minutes, respectively; umbilical artery blood gases (cord specimen) were pH, 7.20; PCO2, 59 mmHg; PO2, 4mmHg; and base excess, −7.

tress, attributed to intrapartum asphyxia, the infant had an uneventful neonatal course and at 8 months of age was growing normally. The patient's postoperative recovery was uncomplicated except for delayed healing of the superficial portion of the abdominal incision.

Following the delivery, the physicians, nurses, social workers, and consultants from the Department of Psychiatry met on a regular basis to discuss concerns about this patient's relationship with her newborn infant. Initially the patient demonstrated affectionate and caring behavior toward the infant. Several months later, however, the court assigned all 3 of her children to foster care when case workers found significant evidence of neglect of the infant and siblings. The court's decision to remove the children from the custody of the mother was independent of events that occurred in the second pregnancy.

This case is reprinted by permission from Watson Bowes, Jr., and Grad Selgestad, "Fetal versus Maternal Rights: Medical and Legal Perspectives," *Obstetrics and Gynecology* 58 (August 1981); 209–11.

Case 23

Mrs. Mary Beth Whitehead, a twenty-nine-year-old housewife from Brick Township, New Jersey, signed a contract on February 6, 1985, to bear a child for William and Elizabeth Stern. As part of the sixteen-page contract, arranged by the Infertility Center of New York, Mrs. Whitehead agreed "that in the best interests of the child, she will not form or attempt to form a parent-child relationship with any child . . . she may conceive . . . and shall freely surrender custody to William Stern, Natural Father, immediately upon birth of the child; and terminate all parental right to said child pursuant to this agreement." Mrs. Whitehead was to receive ten thousand dollars for "compensation for services and expenses" from the Infertility Center as part of the total of approximately twenty-five thousand dollars Mr. Stern agreed to pay the center. Of the remainder, five thousand dollars went to Mrs. Whitehead's medical, legal, and insurance costs during pregnancy, and seventy-five hundred to ten thousand dollars went to the center as its fee.

When the child, conceived through artificial insemination with Mr. Stern's sperm, was born on March 27, 1986, Mrs. Whitehead and her husband, who already had two children, were reluctant to part with the child. They turned her over to the Sterns on March 30, but Mrs. Whitehead would not accept the ten thousand dollars, and within a few days she went to the Stern residence and begged to be allowed to take the child for a week. The Sterns agreed. But by early May, it was clear that Mrs. Whitehead would not willingly return the child, and the Sterns filed a successful petition for temporary custody with the family court. Mrs. Whitehead managed to hand the baby out a bedroom window to her husband when six policemen arrived to take the baby. The husband left with the baby, and Mrs. Whitehead was able to join them later without detection. The Whiteheads were able to elude law enforcement officials in Florida for three months. When the infant, known in the court records as "Baby M," was finally located, she was turned over to the Sterns, and Family Judge Harvey R. Sorkow's temporary custody order was extended, along with limited visitation rights to Mrs. Whitehead.

A court-ordered paternity test established that Mrs. Whitehead's husband, Richard Whitehead, who had had a vasectomy, could not have fathered the child. After a thirty-two-day trial, Judge Sorkow declared the surrogacy contract valid and enforceable, terminated Mrs. Whitehead's parental rights, and awarded sole custody of Baby M to Mr. Stern. Judge Sorkow required specific performance of the surrogate contract on the grounds that it was in Baby M's best interests. He also immediately granted Mrs. Stern an order of adoption.

Upon appeal, the New Jersey Supreme Court (February 3, 1988) held that a surrogacy contract that provides money to the surrogate mother and requires her irrevocable agreement to surrender her child at birth is invalid and unenforceable. The surrogacy contract in the case of Baby M violates New Jersey statutes that prohibit the use of money in connection with adoptions, that limit termination of parental rights to situations in which there has been a valid showing of parental unfitness or abandonment of the child, and that allow a mother to revoke her consent to surrender her child in private-placement adoption. In addition, the surrogacy contract conflicts with New Jersey's public policy that custody be determined on the basis of the child's best interests (the surrogacy contract makes a determination of custody prior to the child's birth), that children be brought up by their natural parents (the surrogacy contract guarantees the separation of the child from its natural mother), that the rights of the natural father and the natural mother are equal (the surrogacy contract elevates the natural father's right by destroying the natural mother's right), that a natural mother receive counseling before agreeing to surrender her child (the surrogacy contract in this case did not have such a provision), and that adoptions not be influenced by the payment of money (the surrogacy contract was based on such a payment).

Regarding the point that Mrs. Whitehead "agreed to the surrogacy arrangement, supposedly fully understanding the consequences," the court responded: "Putting aside the issue of how compelling her need for money may have been, and how significant her understanding of the consequences, we suggest that her consent is irrelevant. There are, in a civilized society, some things that money cannot buy. In America, we decided long ago that merely because conduct purchased by money was 'voluntary' did not mean that it was good or beyond regulation and prohibition." In addition, the court expressed concern about the unknown long-term effects of surrogacy contracts on various parties: "Potential victims include the surrogate mother and her family, the natural father and his wife, and most importantly, the child." However, the court did not find any legal prohibition of surrogacy "when the surrogate mother volunteers, without any payment, to act as a surrogate and is given the right to change her mind and to assert her parental rights."

The New Jersey Supreme Court affirmed the lower court's grant of custody to the natural father, reversed the lower court's termination of the natural mother's parental rights, and required the lower court to determine the terms of the natural mother's visitation with Baby M.

Matter of Baby M, 537 A. 2d. 1227 (N.J. 1988).

Case 24

A forty-year-old widow with chronic glomerulonephritis has been on maintenance hemodialysis for ten years. Over the past two years she has been progressively deteriorating from multiple complications which have included severe renal osteodystrophy, inability to obtain adequate blood access, and malnutrition from intermittent depression. Peritoneal dialysis cannot be accomplished because of multiple abdominal surgical procedures with adhesions. Her physician has recommended transplantation because he feels she will not survive four to six months on dialysis.

The patient has four children (ages eleven to fourteen years) and wants a transplant to allow her to live and provide for the future well-being of her children.

The patient's forty-four-year-old brother is a farmer with eight children. He refused to donate or be tissue typed. The patient has a forty-two-year-old sister who was willing to donate but was not tissue typed because she has been an insulin-requiring diabetic for ten years.

The patient also has a thirty-five-year-old mentally retarded brother who has been institutionalized since age eight. This brother is an A match with four antigens being identified. He is so severely retarded that he cannot comprehend or understand any of the risks of nephrectomy. He is able to take care of his own personal needs and ambulate with guidance. He neither recognizes his own family members nor interacts with medical staff. The patient would regularly drive three hundred miles to see her brother four times per year until twelve years ago, when her own personal and family needs reduced the frequency to one to two times per year. She has not seen her brother for three years, because of her own medical illnesses. At the present time she feels she has a duty to her brother, but there is no particular closeness.

Her fourteen-year-old daughter would like to donate a kidney, even though she is a two-antigen mismatch. The daughter has demonstrated a perceptive, thorough, and reasonably unemotional grasp of her mother's situation and needs and of the seriousnesses of her own potential donation. ABO blood types for the retarded brother and the daughter are compatible.

The patient's older brother and sister feel the donor should be the younger, mentally retarded brother. The diabetic sister is the legal guardian of the retarded brother. Both parents are dead. The patient has been on the cadaveric transplant waiting list for two years.

The following statements are reasonable projections based on known data:

	2-yr. kidney survival	2-yr. patient survival
Retarded brother to patient	70%	85%
Minor child to patient	60%	75%
Cadaveric to patient	40%	65%

This case was written from a case history at St. Francis Hospital, Honolulu, by Dr. Arnold W. Seimsen, Institute of Renal Diseases, St. Francis Hospital.

Case 25

In June 1978, Robert McFall, thirty-nine years old and a Pittsburgh asbestos worker, entered Mercy Hospital with an uncontrollable nosebleed. Physicians diagnosed his condition as aplastic anemia, a rare and usually fatal disease in which the bone marrow fails to produce enough red and white blood cells and platelets. McFall's physician recommended a bone marrow transplant on the grounds that it would increase his patient's chance of surviving for one year from twenty-five percent to forty to sixty percent. The search for a compatible transplant donor began with McFall's six brothers and sisters. After they were located in various parts of the country, none turned out to be compatible.

The search continued, and McFall's first cousin, David Shimp, age forty-three, agreed to undergo some preliminary tests. He was a perfect match for tissue compatibility, but then suddenly he refused to be tested for genetic compatibility. He had decided that he would not donate bone marrow to his cousin, even if he was a perfect match. Apparently, some family discussions and disagreements had influenced Shimp's decision. He told his cousin that his wife was angry because he had undergone the first tests without telling her. Shimp's mother also appeared to be bitter about a decades-old disagreement in the family, and she, too, asked him to stop the testing.

Some friends and other relatives believed that disagreements of the past should not affect the present, and they tried to persuade Shimp to change his mind. When McFall called his cousin and told him, "You're killing me," Shimp responded that his wife had to come first. Even Shimp's four children tried to persuade him that he would be responsible for his cousin's early death, and they volunteered to be tested themselves, but Shimp would not be moved.

McFall then filed suit to compel his cousin to undergo the bone marrow transplant. McFall's attorney argued in court that the procedure is essentially harmless to the donor and that the marrow would be replenished, just as blood is replenished after donation. He also cited English common law, dating back to the thirteenth century, which upheld society's right to force an individual "to help secure the well-being of other members of society." Shimp's attorney argued that his client's right to refuse could not be invaded and that "no one could be forced to submit to an operation." Shimp told reporters that he refused to be a donor because he was afraid of becoming paralyzed during the procedure and feared that his marrow might fail to regenerate.

Judge John Flaherty denied McFall's request to force Shimp to undergo the transplant. The judge based his decision on U.S. common-law precedents, which do not recognize a legal duty to take action to save another person's life. "This would defeat the sanctity of the individual. It would require forcible submission to the medical procedure. Forcible extraction of bodily tissues causes revulsion to the judicial mind. The rights of the individual must be upheld, even though it appears to be a harsh decision." The judge also declared irrelevant the argument by McFall's attorney that in English law, court-ordered transplants are permitted. Although he thus held that Shimp had no legal obligation to donate his marrow, Judge Flaherty nevertheless called Shimp's refusal "morally indefensible."

After the ruling, McFall told the press, "I feel sorry for my cousin because he and I are friends and he was under a lot of pressure." Shimp made no comment, but his mother said, "He's not a coward the way they are trying to make him out to be. When you get on the table, there is no guaranteeing how much bone marrow they will take. It could be my son's death sentence. The doctors don't care about the donors; they care about patients."

On August 10, 1978, Robert McFall died of a cranial hemorrhage. His last request was that his family forgive his cousin, whose actions he found understandable even if not justifiable. A hospital spokesperson said that cranial hemorrhage is a common complication for people with aplastic anemia and that it might have occurred even with the bone marrow transplant. The day after his cousin died, Shimp said, "I could throw up right now. I feel terrible about Robert dying, but he asked me for something I couldn't give. That's all I can say now. I feel sick."

Sources for this case include Barbara J. Culliton, "Court Upholds Refusal to Be Medical Good Samaritan," *Science 201* (August 18, 1978): 596–97; "Bone Marrow Transplant Plea Rejected," *American Medical News* 21 (August 11, 1978): 13; "Anemia Victim Dies, Asks Forgiveness for Cousin," *International Herald Tribune*, August 12–13, 1978; "Judge Upholds Transplant Denial," *New York Times*, July 27, 1978, p. A10; Dennis A. William and Lawrence Walsh, "The Law: Bad Samaritan," *Newsweek* 92 (August 7, 1978): 35; Alan Meisel and Loren H. Roth, "Must a Man Be His Cousin's

Keeper?'' *Hastings Center Report* 8 (October 1978): 5–6. The case is *McFall* v. *Shimp*, no. 78-1771 in Equity (C.P. Allegheny County, Penn., July 26, 1978).

Case 26

The Willowbrook State School is an institution for mentally retarded children on Staten Island, New York. The number of its residents increased from two hundred in 1949 to more than six thousand in 1963. Hepatitis was first noticed among the children in 1949, and in 1954 Dr. Saul Krugman and his associates, including Dr. Joan Giles and Dr. Jack Hammond, began to study the disease in the institution. Of the fifty-two hundred residents at Willowbrook during one part of their study, thirty-eight hundred were severely retarded, with IQs of less than 20. In addition, at least three thousand of the children were not toilet-trained. Because infectious hepatitis is transmitted via the fecal-oral route, and because susceptible children were constantly admitted to the institution, contagious hepatitis was persistent and endemic.

As Dr. Krugman (1971) describes the situation, "viral hepatitis is so prevalent that newly admitted susceptible children become infected within 6 to 12 months after entry in the institution. These children are a source of infection for the personnel who care for them and for their families if they visit with them. We were convinced that the solution of the hepatitis problem in this institution was dependent on the acquisition of new knowledge leading to the development of an effective immunising agent. The achievements with small pox, diptheria, poliomyelitis, and more recently measles represent dramatic illustrations of this approach.''

Krugman continues, "It is well known that viral hepatitis in children is milder and more benign than the same disease in adults. Experience has revealed that hepatitis in institutionalized, mentally retarded children is also mild, in contrast to measles which is a more severe disease when it occurs in institutional epidemics involving the mentally retarded. Our proposal to expose a small number of newly admitted children [ultimately seven hundred fifty to eight hundred children were involved altogether] to the Willowbrook strains of hepatitis virus was justified in our opinion for the following reasons: (1) they were bound to be exposed to the same strains under the natural conditions existing in the institution; (2) they would be admitted to a special, well-equipped, and well-staffed unit where they would be isolated from exposure to other infectious diseases which were prevalent in the institution—namely, shigellosis, parasitic infections, and respiratory infections—thus, their exposure in the hepatitis unit would be associated with less risk than the type of institutional exposure where multiple infections could occur; (3) they were likely to have a subclinical infection followed by immunity to the particular hepatitis virus; and (4) only children with parents who gave informed consent would be included.''

Critics have leveled several charges against the Willowbrook hepatitis studies. First, some contend that it is "indefensible to give potentially dangerous infected material to children, particularly those who were mentally retarded, with or without parental consent, when no benefit to the child could conceivably result" (Goldby). Hence, these critics reject the claim by Krugman and Giles that "the artificial induction of hepatitis implies a 'therapeutic' effect because of the immunity which is conferred." The ground for rejecting this claim is that most of the children would have become infected anyway and that this therapeutic effect is not different from what the natural environment would have bestowed. Thus, one major question is whether this experiment offered some therapeutic benefit to the subjects themselves or only to others. The aim of the study was to determine the period of infectivity of infectious hepatitis. Even if the experiment produced good results, as it did (see Krugman 1986), critics contend that an experiment is justified not by its results but "is ethical or not at its inception" (Beecher). In this case, "immunisation was not the purpose of these Willowbrook experiments but merely a by-product that incidentally proved beneficial to the victims" (Pappworth).

Second, critics contend that there were alternative ways to control hepatitis in the institution. According to the head of the State Department of Mental Hygiene in New York, for much of the period of the experiment a gamma-globulin inoculation program had already reduced the incidence of viral hepatitis in Willowbrook by eighty to eighty-five percent (Beecher). And the pediatrician's duty is to improve the situation, not to take advantage of it for experimental purposes (Goldby).

Third, questions have been raised about whether the parents' consent for their children to participate in the research was informed and voluntary. Originally, information was conveyed to individual parents by letter or personal interview, but later information was disclosed through a detailed discussion of the project with groups of six to eight parents who were invited to enroll their children in the research. Krugman and Giles contend that the "group method" enabled them "to obtain more thorough informed consent." In either setting, "it was not clear whether any or all parents were told that hepatitis sometimes progresses to fatal liver destruction or that there is a possibility that cirrhosis developing later in life may have had its origin in earlier hepatitis" (Beecher). Serious questions emerged about the voluntariness of parental consent when parents of prospective residents of Willowbrook were told in late 1964 that overcrowding prevented further admissions but were subsequently informed, often within a week or so, that there were some vacancies in the hepatitis unit and that if the parents wanted to volunteer their children for the research project the children could be admitted to Willowbrook.

Defenders of Willowbrook reject most of these criticisms and ask, "is it not proper and ethical to carry out experiments in children, which would apparently incur no greater risk than the children were likely to run by nature, in which the children generally receive better medical care when artificially infected than if they had been naturally infected, and in which the parents as well as the physician feel that a significant contribution to the future well-being of similar children is likely to result from the studies?'' (Edsall).

Saul Krugman and Joan P. Giles, "Viral Hepatitis: New Light on an Old Disease," *Journal of the American Medical Association* 212 (May 10, 1970): 1019–29; Henry Beecher, *Research and the Individual* (Boston: Little, Brown, 1970); letters to the editor of *Lancet* by Stephen Goldby (April 10, 1971), Saul Krugman (May 8, 1971), Edward N. Willey (May 22, 1971), Benjamin Pasamanick (May 22, 1971), Joan Giles (May 29, 1971), M. H. Pappworth (June 5, 1971), Geoffrey Edsall (July 10, 1971); F. J. Ingelfinger, "Ethics of Experiments on Children," *New England Journal of Medicine* 288 (April 12, 1973): 791–92; Saul Krugman, "The Willowbrook Hepatitis Studies Revisited: Ethical Aspects," *Reviews of Infectious Diseases* 8 (January–February 1986): 157–62).

Case 27

On August 11, 1977, Richard Whitley et al. reported in the *New England Journal of Medicine* that a new drug, adenine arbinoside (ara-A), had been tested and found to be highly useful in the treatment and cure of biopsy-proved herpes simplex encephalitis, a disease that often leads to severe brain and nerve damage or death. Prior to ara-A, standard treatment consisted mainly of palliative care and was not considered effective. Some critics of the research insisted that it is not necessary to have a randomized clinical trial of therapy for a disease that has such high rates of mortality and severe damage and that is currently treated by ineffective therapy. In such cases, they argue, it is sufficient to use historical controls. Furthermore, they insist, in previous tests ara-A had been found to be effective in treating some herpes infections and to have no demonstrable hepatic, renal, or hematologic toxicity. They claim that scientific knowledge did not require a controlled trial, which would deprive some patients of a promising drug. Furthermore, they note, brain biopsy may be risky for such seriously ill patients and perhaps put the control group at greater risk than standard treatment.

Defenders of the research respond that previously scientists did not know the mortality and long-term morbidity rates of herpes simplex encephalitis because it is difficult to diagnose with certainty apart from a brain biopsy and that scientists did not know whether ara-A would have serious toxic effects when administered in large doses along with large volumes of intravenous fluid to patients suffering from this disease.

The collaborative study, supported by the National Institute of Allergy and Infectious Disease, was a controlled, double-blind trial. Of the twenty-eight patients involved, ten received the placebo (standard treatment), while the others received the experimental drug.

Ara-A

Number of recipients	18
Deaths	5
Severe damage	6
Reasonably normal recovery	7

Placebo

Number of recipients	10
Deaths	7
Severe damage	1
Reasonably normal recovery	2

The trial was stopped when these statistics emerged because of the greater chance of surviving the disease with ara-A. All patients were then treated with ara-A. Some critics, however, contend that the research was stopped too soon. They note that the number of recipients of both treatments is very small and that the figures about reasonably normal recovery may be misleading: thirty-eight percent for recipients of ara-A and twenty percent for recipients of the placebo. If the next recipient of the placebo had recovered to a reasonably normal level, the results would then have been "not significant." I. J. Good, a statistician, argues that "if having severe sequelae is regarded as just as bad as being dead, the ara-A treatment is barely significantly better than the placebo." Thus, some critics claim, the research did not definitely establish the superiority of ara-A in the treatment of herpes simplex encephalitis.

This case was prepared on the basis of information in the following sources: Richard J. Whitley et al., "Adenine Arbinoside Therapy of Biopsy-Proved Herpes Simplex Encephalitis," *New England Journal of Medicine* 297 (August 11, 1977): 289–94; correspondence, *New England Journal of Medicine* 297 (December 8, 1977): 1288–90; James J. McCartney, "Encephalitis and Ara-A: An Ethical Case Study," *Hastings Center Report* 8 (December 1978): 5–7; R. J. Whitley and C. A. Alford, "Encephalitis and Adenine Arabinoside: An Indictment without Fact," *Hastings Center Report* 9 (August 1979): 4, 44–47; and I. J. Good, "Adenine Arabinoside Therapy," *Journal of Statistical Computation and Simulation* 6 (1978): 314–15.

Case 28

The realization that AIDS (acquired immunodeficiency syndrome) will probably affect and kill millions of people worldwide has prompted massive research on potential treatments or cures. In the United States, a screening program was conducted by the National Cancer Institute (NCI) to find a drug that would kill, or at least inactivate or inhibit, the human immunodeficiency virus (HIV), the retrovirus that causes AIDS. In a cooperative program between NCI and private industry, Burroughs Wellcome discovered that AZT (azidothymidine), which had been synthesized by Dr. Jerome Horwitz in 1964 and shelved when it proved to be ineffective in the treatment of cancer, inhibits animal viruses in tissue culture. Then scientists at NCI and elsewhere demonstrated that AZT inhibits duplication of the AIDS virus in the test tube. What followed raises major questions about starting and stopping placebo-controlled, double-blind trials; about distributing scarce, life-prolonging treatments; about costs of treatments, including whether a company is charging excessive prices and whether society should cover those costs; and about governmental regulation of therapeutic drugs.

The promising laboratory tests were followed by a (phase 1) trial to determine the safety of AZT for AIDS patients; during that trial, several patients showed clinical improvement. Because AIDS is believed to be universally fatal and there is no promising alternative treatment, many people argued that "compassion" dictated making it immediately available to all AIDS patients and even to patients who have ARC (AIDS-related complex) or who are antibody positive for exposure to the AIDS virus but have no symptoms. Not only did the company have an inadequate supply of the drug for all such patients, but it set up, as federal regulations require, a placebo-controlled trial of AZT to determine its effectiveness and its toxicity for certain groups of HIV-infected patients—AIDS patients within one hundred twenty days of their first diagnosis of *Pneumocystis carinii* pneumonia, a rare form of pneumonia that affects many immunocompromised patients and patients with advanced AIDS-related complex.

Critics such as scientist Mathilde Krim argued that a placebo-controlled trial under such circumstances was "morally unacceptable": "AZT currently appears to be the most promising treatment. Ten thousand victims are being denied the drug that they and their doctors believe holds the most hope. It should be possible to resolve the need for scientific data with justice and compassion." However, defenders of the placebo-controlled trial insisted that it was necessary to determine whether AZT is effective and whether its side effects would be tolerable or outweighed by its benefits. Dr. Samuel Broder of NCI denies that "compassion and science are in conflict," for "we have to be concerned with people who have AIDS both now and in the future." He notes that "serious errors—irredeemable errors . . . can be introduced if we don't undertake appropriately controlled studies. It would be a catastrophe if we dismissed a 'good drug' or if we allowed a 'bad drug' to become the standard of therapy."

The multicenter trial began in February 1986, and a computer randomly assigned some patients to AZT and others to a placebo, an inactive pill. This was a double-blind study; neither clinicians nor subjects knew who received AZT and who received the inactive pill. An independent data and safety monitoring board had the task of examining the data periodically before the planned end of the trial. According to Dr. David Barry, director of research at Burroughs Wellcome, "Should either the placebo or drug-treated group do either so poorly or so well that it would be unethical to continue that study as designed, this outside review board will inform us and the study will be stopped." For a few months, no major differences emerged, but then suddenly patients in one arm of the trial began dying at a much higher rate. At this point, the data and safety monitoring board broke the code and recommended that the trial be terminated earlier than scheduled because of the statistically significant differences in the death rates of the patients receiving AZT and the patients receiving the placebo: Only one of the 144 patients receiving AZT died; 19 of the 137 patients receiving the placebo died. The p value is 0.0001; thus, the probability of these results occurring solely by chance is one in ten thousand. Patients in the AZT group had a probability of 0.98 of surviving twenty-four weeks; patients in the placebo group had a probability of 0.78 of surviving twenty-four weeks. Balancing the interests of present patients and the interests of future patients, the monitoring board determined that it would be unfair to present patients to continue the trial even if it could produce more information about the effectiveness and benefit-risk ratio of AZT versus a placebo over time. Subjects in the trial who had received the placebo were, as promised, the first to receive the drug, and researchers praised all the participants in the trial for their contribution to the development of scientific knowledge that could benefit numerous patients.

AZT also significantly reduced the patients' probability of acquiring opportunistic infections and the severity of those infections when they occurred. In addition to improving immune status as measured by T helper (T4) cell counts and skin tests, AZT improved the patients' general health as measured by Karnofsky performance scores (an index of ability to perform activities of daily life), by the number of symptoms related to HIV infection, and by body weight, in comparison to the placebo group. AZT is not a "magic bullet"; it does not rid the body of the virus. Its toxic side effects can often be quite severe, particularly on the bone marrow which produces red and white blood cells. AZT often lowers red-blood-cell production, resulting in severe anemia that frequently requires blood transfusions. Little can be done for reduced production of white cells, a condition that increases the risk of bacterial infections, except to reduce the dosage or terminate the drug regimen altogether. Thus, over time, because of AZT's toxicity, many recipients stop the treatment, while others receive reduced doses. Some patients also experience other adverse events such as nausea, myalgia, insomnia, and moderate to severe headaches.

Once AZT emerged as effective for some AIDS and ARC patients, U.S. regulations require that AZT, rather than a placebo, serve as a control in future clinical trials for groups of patients for whom AZT has been shown to be effective. However, double-blind, placebo-controlled trials have been set up for categories of subjects for whom it has not been determined that AZT is effective and that its benefits outweigh its risks—for example, patients with Kaposi's sarcoma, a cancer that affects many AIDS patients; patients with AIDS-related neurological problems; and people with HIV infection but no symptoms. In addition, trials without placebos are now being conducted to determine the best dosage of AZT for groups of patients for whom it has been determined to be effective.

When the placebo-controlled AZT trial was stopped on September 19, 1986, the Food and Drug Administration (FDA) agreed to a special distribution of AZT to selected AIDS patients, while considering the drug for approval for commercial distribution. The supply of the drug was limited because of its rapid development and its complex production process—originally, AZT was made from fish sperm, mainly herring, but it is now produced by synthetic methods. Thus, Burroughs Wellcome, with assistance from experts from the Infectious Disease Society of America, set strict criteria to ensure the best utilization of AZT and a continuous supply of AZT for patients who had the greatest need and the greatest probability of benefit. The eligibility rules required that patients document one or more bouts of *Pneumocystis carinii* pneumonia, not be on drug therapy for AIDS or on chemotherapy or other drugs that are toxic to the kidneys or bone marrow, and have adequate liver and kidney function and sufficiently high red and white blood cell counts. Among the categories excluded were children, pregnant women, and nursing mothers, because of the lack of information about the drug's effects on children, newborns, and fetuses. In addition, patients with AIDS-related complex were excluded—even though they had been in the original trial—because their disease is at an early stage and it was unclear whether the benefits outweighed the risks of AZT's toxicity for this group of patients.

The FDA moved to license AZT for commercial distribution on March 20, 1987. Some critics charge that this decision was too rapid and failed to protect consumer health; others charge that the FDA moved too slowly and, in any event, inappropriately restricted patients' freedom in desperate circumstances. Still others stress the remarkable speed of approval in comparison with other drugs: In less than thirty months, AZT went from laboratory experiments to clinical trials to federal approval.

One result of NCI's mass drug trials was the award of sole license (for a limited time) to Burroughs Wellcome for the production of AZT, now marketed as Retrovir (zidovudine). During the period between the termination of the trial in September 1986 and the issue of a license for commercial distribution in March 1987, approximately five thousand patients received the drug for free—roughly five hundred in continuing clinical trials and forty-five hundred in the categories identified above. Once the drug was approved for commercial distribution, the latter patients had to start paying in what was described as a "rea-

sonable period,'' whereas those in clinical trials did not have to pay. Furthermore, Burroughs Wellcome continued to limit distribution to selected categories
of patients for months after FDA approval because of scarcity of the drug and
concerns about its severe side effects. The categories of eligible patients were
expanded to include advanced ARC. For all interested patients, physicians had
to provide information to Burroughs Wellcome, which had to approve distribution.

Because there is no competition in the sale of the drug, in accordance with
the sole licensing agreement, the pharmaceutical company is free to charge
whatever price the market will bear. In 1987, Burroughs Wellcome charged
pharmacies about eight thousand dollars for a year's supply of AZT, but then
patients had to pay pharmacies about ten thousand dollars, sometimes even
more. In December 1987, the company announced a twenty percent price reduction to pharmacies. Many argue that the price is still unreasonably high and
creates a major hardship for patients who lack any real alternative treatment.
Stressing that it committed eighty million dollars to producing the drug, Burroughs Wellcome refuses to disclose its profit margin. But some analysts believe that the drug was originally priced to produce profit margins up to forty
percent so that the company could make a quick return on its investment because of the possibility that better treatments would emerge within a few years.
NCI's Dr. Samuel Broder, who helped develop the drug, said that ''the inability of many people to afford to pay for this drug makes me very sad. I'm not
sure they [Burroughs Wellcome] needed to recoup all their costs in a year.
They should have had the same faith in the drug that those of us who developed
it have.'' At eight thousand dollars per patient per year, the company's revenues would rise by four hundred million dollars if fifty thousand patients were
treated. By December 1987, approximately twenty thousand patients worldwide
were being treated with AZT, and the number of AIDS cases continues to
increase.

Even at the reduced price, an AIDS patient would spend approximately twenty-
two dollars a day for the usual dosage. Moreover, many AIDS patients are
young, indigent, and uninsured. Thus, much of the financial burden for treatment falls on public programs such as Medicaid, and it has been estimated that
as many as forty percent of AIDS patients will be on Medicaid. But such
programs do not always pay for prescriptions, and, if they do, they often place
a dollar limit on drug benefits. However, Burroughs Wellcome notes that the
use of AZT could reduce the average first-year treatment costs for an AIDS
patient from $43,500 to approximately $32,500 and could reduce the costs of
treatment for patients with ARC by sixty percent. Hence, public programs,
insurance companies, and individuals, Burroughs Wellcome estimates, could
save approximately $386 million in the first year of treatment of twenty thou-
sand patients. Nevertheless, the debate about the provision of funds for the

care of AIDS patients, including the coverage of AZT, is forcing reconsideration of the society's obligation to provide health care.

This case study has been prepared, with the assistance of Jeff Kahn, from various materials, including Marilyn Chase, "AIDS Research Stirs Bitter Fight over Use of Experimental Drugs," *Wall Street Journal*, June 18, 1986, p. 29; Denise Grady, "Look, Doctor, I'm Dying. Give Me the Drug," *Discover* (August 1986): 78–86; Philip J. Hilts, "Methods of Testing AIDS Drug Raises Ethical Questions," *Washington Post*, September 14, 1986, pp. A1, A17; "A Failure Led to Drug against AIDS," *New York Times*, September 19, 1986; Erik Eckholm, "AIDS Test Drug Prolongs Lives in Some Cases," *New York Times*, September 20, 1986, pp. 1, 7; Erik Eckholm, "AIDS Drug Is Raising Host of Thorny Issues," *New York Times*, September 28, 1986, sec. 1, p. 38; Philip J. Hilts, "AZT Distribution Rules Announced," *Washington Post*, October 1, 1986, p. A14; Dale Gieringer, "Twice Wrong on AIDS," *New York Times*, January 12, 1987, p. A21; Erik Eckholm, "License Move Nears for AIDS Drug," *New York Times*, January 16, 1987; Philip J. Hilts, "FDA Panel Urges Sales of AZT," *Washington Post*, January 17, 1987, pp. A1, A11; Sally Squires, "The High Cost of Treating AIDS," *Washington Post/Health*, March 19, 1987, p. 7; Irvin Molotsky, "U.S. Approves Drug to Prolong Lives of AIDS Patients," *New York Times*, March 21, 1987, pp. 1, 32; Barnaby J. Feder, "Drug Expected to Spur Growth and Profit of Its Maker," *New York Times*, March 21, 1987, p. 32; M. A. Fischl, D. D. Richman, M. H. Grieco, et al., "The Efficacy of Azidothymidine (AZT) in the Treatment of Patients with AIDS and AIDS-Related Complex: A Double-Blind, Placebo-Controlled Trial," *New England Journal of Medicine* 317 (1987): 185–91; D. D. Richman, M. A. Rischl, M. H. Grieco, et al., "The Toxicity of Azidothymidine (AZT) in the Treatment of Patients with AIDS and AIDS-Related Complex: A Double-Blind, Placebo-Controlled Trial," *New England Journal of Medicine* 317 (1987): 192–97; Sandra G. Boodman, "Costly Drug Brings Hope to AIDS Patients," *Washington Post*, July 20, 1987, p. B1; Michael Specter, "AIDS Drug's Price to Be Cut 20%," *Washington Post*, December 15, 1987, p. A3; Gina Kolata, "Doctors Stretch Rules on AIDS Drug," *New York Times*, December 21, 1987, pp. A1, A20.

Case 29

Patients and their physicians try several different methods to control gross obesity, including repeated dieting, psychiatric treatment, anorectic drugs, and surgery. Despite widespread support for surgical procedures, no randomized clinical trial had been conducted prior to 1973 to compare their effectiveness to medical treatments or no treatments. A group of Danish investigators wondered whether it was justifiable to continue to use intestinal bypass in the treatment of gross obesity without a careful assessment of its risks and benefits through a randomized clinical trial. Having completed some initial trials, the investigators decided to do a randomized clinical trial to compare the effects of the surgical procedure (jejunoileostomy) and medical treatments in order to assess their respective effects on mortality, morbidity, weight loss, and quality of life.

The potential subjects had heard about the operation through the media and wanted it because their obesity had not responded to such conventional medical treatments as diet, fasting, exercise, and anorectics. After a physical examination, they received a detailed explanation of the surgical procedure, particularly its risks, side effects, and uncertainties. If they met the conditions for the surgery, they were "randomly allocated to either a medical management or to an end-to-site jejunoileostomy group. . . . We [the researchers] did not ask for informed consent for randomisation. Patients allocated to medical treatment were told that surgery had to be postponed for an undetermined period primarily because liver-biopsy findings showed fatty infiltration. . . . After randomisation all patients were seen frequently for 36 months; thereafter the individual departments were free to choose type of treatment." The study established that after twenty-four months median weight loss was 42.9 kg in the bypass group but only 5.9 kg in the control group. Even though complications of surgery were common and occasionally severe, no deaths occurred, and the surgical patients had a higher degree of patient satisfaction and a higher quality of life than the control subjects.

Because the potential subjects wanted the surgery so badly, the researchers believed that they would not be able to persuade them to enter a trial that involved a control group receiving only conventional medical treatment; thus, they decided to bypass informed consent and to deceive the subjects. The editor of *The Lancet*, which published the results of the research, noted that "at first sight this seems a breach of the rules of informed consent (though, curiously it is a question of consent *not* to have an operation). The patients were misinformed, and a good rule in clinical trials is that relations between patient and doctor should be open and honest. At second sight, too, *The Lancet* takes the view that the end did not justify the means and that this trial was ethically unsound. Would an ethics committee (if such there had been in Denmark at the time) have passed the protocol? *The Lancet*'s guess is No; the Danish group's is Yes. At this point, according to the World Medical Association's Declaration of Helsinki, an editor is supposed to retire to his corner and decline the paper, but we believe that this disagreement is better aired publicly than buried in a filing cabinet."

See the Danish Obesity Project, "Randomised Trial of Jejunoileal Bypass versus Medical Treatment in Morbid Obesity," *Lancet* (December 15, 1979): 1255–57; editorial, "Bypassing Obesity," *Lancet* (December 15, 1979): 1275–76.

Case 30

State Bill 529 calls for the establishment of community-based homes for the care and education of the mentally retarded. The bill provides one home for every fifteen persons presently institutionalized in four state institutions for the mentally retarded at a cost of $55.8 million. The estimated costs for the new care for the present population of 7600 will be $70 million a year.

The bill was introduced by Representative John Sheehan who spoke in favor of it. He painted a dismal picture of antiquated institutions bereft of basic human necessities or amenities. Thousands of human beings, many unclothed, spend their lives huddled in dark, drab rooms, where they are supervised by an overworked staff, many of whom have no professional training. Sheehan, who has the support of the parents' organization, the State Department of Mental Health, the local ACLU, and the religious leadership, concluded his case by pleading, ''Justice requires that we extend this token contribution to these citizens, burdened by physical and psychological suffering, and by the degradation of our society's past inhumanity to its fellow humans.''

Representative James Hudson and Dr. Robert Simmons, while emphasizing their concern for care of the retarded, spoke in opposition to the bill. Representative Hudson, noting that he was the elected representative of all the citizens in his district, argued that he had an obligation to examine the alternative uses for the $14 million in additional funds called for by the bill. But first, he pointed out that the new total sum of $70 million equalled 1.5 percent of the state's budget, a budget raised by all its citizens, while the institutionalized population equalled only one-tenth of one percent of the state's population. The proposed increase of $14 million could buy hot lunches for all the state's school children; it could also provide job training for productive members of society. Hudson argued that the fairest thing to do would be to spread the money evenly among those who would be productive. ''Our task as legislators,'' he concluded, ''must be to serve the greatest good of the greatest number.''

Dr. Simmons, as a physician, argued that the money could be used more efficiently in providing health care for three groups: normal or more nearly normal children (thousands of whom could be reached for every mentally retarded child), those potentially engaged in productive labor, and pregnant women. He showed that much mental retardation can be eliminated, through prenatal diagnosis which he estimated to cost $200 per case for Down syndrome compared to $60,000 for each institutionalized child. Even allowing that some of the institutionalized retarded might be gainfully employed if they were in high-quality, community-based homes, the saving from spending the funds on detection rather than on more expensive forms of institutionalized care are enormous.

The legislative committee must now make its decision on the bill.

This case, written by Robert M. Veatch, appeared as Case 529 in ''Who Has First Claim on Health Care Resources?'' *Hastings Center Report* 5 (August 1975): 13, and is used by permission.

Case 31

Thomas Merriam was Director of Budget Planning at the National Institutes of Health and chief advisor to the Assistant Secretary for formulating the congres-

sional message on the 1976 fiscal year NIH budget. He was under a great deal
of pressure from Dr. Alan Sanders, Director of the National Institute of Arthritis, Metabolism, and Digestive Disease, to increase the budget for research on
arthritis.

Dr. Sanders argued that in 1974, 3,377,000 persons in the United States
suffered from arthritis severe enough that their activity was limited. There were
almost 4 million hospital days attributable to arthritis and 57 million days of
bed disability. There was anger in Dr. Sanders' voice during the meeting Merriam had with the Institute director. It was as if he could not get anyone to take
arthritis seriously. He claimed that because there were virtually no deaths attributable to arthritis, the government policy analysts were grossly underem-
phasizing the disease that produced the second largest number of persons with
limitation of activity in the United States. The suffering was enormous, yet the
planners were using formulas that calculated number of days of life likely to
be added for research dollar invested. This meant that arthritis would receive
virtually no funding if Merriam and his associates relied exclusively on the
formula.

Sanders claimed that the National Cancer Institute and the Heart and Lung
Institute were getting more money than they could use because of the excessive
emphasis on death prevention rather than suffering prevention. Sanders conceded that cancer and heart disease also produce some disability. The cancer
institute was less the target of his attack since the cancer budget was not part
of the NIH planning, it being separated out by the Nixon administration as part
of the war on cancer. He emphasized the inequality between the heart institute
and the funds for arthritis. The number of persons with limitation of activity is
about the same in the two cases (3.9 million for heart disease compared with
3.4 million for arthritis). Yet the heart institute budget was $290,511,000, while
the arthritis portion of Sanders' institute's budget was only $14,076,000. Ex-
pressed in days of disability, there were 93 million days for heart disease and
57 million for arthritis. How, Sanders asked, can that difference justify the
much larger difference in the budgets?

Merriam was frustrated after his conversation with Sanders. He wanted an
objective, statistically certain way of allocating the research funds between a
condition like heart disease that produces some disability, but is the primary
cause of death, and a condition like arthritis that is also a serious debilitator,
but causes no death. He considered his options:

1. Use cost/benefit ratios to maximize the number of days of life added per
   dollar invested.
2. Use cost/benefit analysis to calculate the dollars lost to the economy from
   work lost from the two conditions, and use that ratio to propose funds for
   the two programs.

3. Use cost/benefit analysis to calculate both costs of the diseases and costs of the potential research, and use dollars most efficiently.
4. Survey people asking them how they would like their money to be spent, and allocate the funds by calculating the average apportionment.
5. Allocate funds in proportion to the number of people suffering from the two conditions regardless of deaths, costs of treatment, costs of research, or any other variables.
6. Ask experts working on research in the two areas what the likelihood of a breakthrough might be, and use those estimates as a basis for allocating funds.
7. Turn the matter over to the politicians to decide what the priorities ought to be.

Merriam needed a principle for dealing with Dr. Sanders' complaint. What should he do?

This case is based on actual data but does not reflect actions or positions taken by employees of the National Institutes of Health during the period described in this case. It is Case 570 in "Arthritis and Heart Disease: Where Should Research Funds Go?" prepared by Robert M. Veatch, and is used by permission.

Case 32

The totally implantable artificial heart, including a totally implantable power source, has long been a therapeutic hope for patients with end-stage heart disease. According to P. Simmons, "at a symbolic level, the [artificial] heart is a sign of the expectations of the American public and of medical and scientific researchers." The effort to develop the artificial heart, especially the total artificial heart (TAH), has raised questions about human experimentation, including patient risk-benefit ratios and informed consent, about initiating and discontinuing experimental life-prolonging procedures, about quality of life, about research priorities, and about the provision of funds for experimental and expensive life-prolonging technologies.

Progress has been slow and costly since the first artificial heart was successfully implanted into a dog in 1957. Dr. Denton Cooley implanted the first TAH in a human being in 1969 (and then again in 1981) as a bridge to cardiac transplantation, but the first TAH implantation intended to be permanent was performed by Dr. William DeVries and his colleagues at the University of Utah in December 1982; the patient, Barney Clark, survived 112 days.

As a new experimental procedure, the TAH was evaluated by the University of Utah institutional review board (IRB), which focused mainly on risk-benefit ratio and informed consent, as well as by the Food and Drug Administration (FDA). In the Barney Clark case, the IRB worried about whether recognizing

the patient's right to withdraw—as stated in virtually all research protocols—
would imply the legitimacy of suicide; a patient's decision to remove himself
or herself from the drive system would result in immediate death. However,
without freedom to withdraw without prejudice and loss of care, the patient
might believe that he or she had to follow every recommendation or be subject
to discontinuation of the experimental TAH.

In 1988, Dr. DeVries, who had subsequently relocated at Humana Hospital
in Louisville, Kentucky, reported the results of four implanted permanent TAHs,
with one patient living only 10 days and another (William Schroeder) living
620 days. All of these patients were selected on the basis of several criteria:
They were referred by their personal physicians, were symptomatic during bed
rest with more severe symptoms such as shortness of breath or chest pain during any physical activity, and had been rejected for cardiac transplantation by
at least three centers. In addition, they had a history of compliance with medical advice and understood their illness and the TAH. Finally, they had a stable
psychological profile and "strong, reliable family-support systems."

As DeVries noted, the quality of life—even for the patient who lived the
longest—was not what had been hoped for by the patient or his family, as
clotting, infection, and other problems were common. And yet, DeVries continued, the patient and his family in each of the three long-term survivors
"communicated to us that life of an acceptable quality was realized for significant periods of time, if not the entirety of their postoperative days." His overall assessment is that the four implants with the Jarvik 7 show that "TAH is
feasible, practical, and durable and offers life to those who would not otherwise
be able to continue living," but that "if the (Jarvik) device is to become a
viable medical therapy, extensive financial commitment and sophisticated human research are required."

Serious questions have been raised about the artificial heart program. First,
some who support the program in general raise questions about particular approaches or devices; for example, some oppose the pneumatically powered TAH,
such as the Jarvik 7, recommending instead electrically or thermally powered
TAHs that would permit more independence and mobility. Others would assign
priority to partial over total artificial hearts, stressing the promise of the left
ventricular assist device (LVAD), a partial artificial heart. A controversy erupted
in 1988 when the National Heart, Lung and Blood Institute, which had awarded
four centers contracts for a term of six years to work on the TAH, decided to
withdraw those contracts after one year in order to reassign the funds to ventricular assist devices, which could be ready for clinical testing within three
years. An advisory council to the National Heart, Lung and Blood Institute
agreed that the ventricular assist devices should have priority but also supported
additional funding for the TAH on the grounds that it is "technically feasible,
clinically important and timely," that canceling the contracts would break up

valuable research groups that would be needed later, and that competitors in other countries would pursue the project. Political pressure reportedly forced a restoration of the TAH program.

A second criticism has been directed at developing or using *permanent* TAHs when cardiac transplantation has become so successful (see Case 33). However, many patients suffering from end-stage heart disease will not be candidates for cardiac transplantation, at least as long as there is a shortage of donor hearts, and in 1987 there were approximately fifteen hundred heart transplants, far short of the number with clinical need. Since the shortage of donor hearts appears to be persistent, the TAH may offer a real therapeutic alternative if it can be improved.

In addition, *temporary* TAHs (and assist devices) have been used as bridges to cardiac transplantation. However, George Annas and others have raised serious questions about this use of TAHs, in part because it gives a patient priority for scarce donor hearts on the basis of medical need even though his or her chances for success may be minimal. Critics charge that the temporary TAH does not save lives; it only changes the identities of the lives saved by giving very sick patients priority for heart transplantation and may even result in fewer lives being saved because the patients are so ill when they receive heart transplants.

A final criticism focuses on the whole program to develop the artificial heart, particularly the TAH. Years ago, there was concern that the development of a nuclear-powered TAH would pose a threat to others who came into contact with the recipient. Albert Jonsen, an ethicist who has been involved in several public assessments of the artificial heart, notes an analogous concern about all artificial hearts in today's society: The artificial heart, particularly the TAH, "creates a distinct and direct threat to the health of others," because "it threatens to deprive many persons of access to needed medical care." Under conditions of scarcity, where the society cannot or will not fund all needed or beneficial medical care, Jonsen fears that the experimental artificial heart program will consume excessive resources. These resources could meet other medical needs, which may be less visible and less urgent: health education, screening, prevention, community clinics, and hospital stays.

In addition, the TAH may not be and probably is not the most cost-effective way to reduce morbidity and mortality from heart disease; prevention is more effective for more people as well as less expensive. Since 1957, the federal government has spent more than two hundred million dollars on research on the artificial heart. And it is estimated that between seventeen thousand and thirty-five thousand patients below age seventy could benefit each year from a total or partial artificial heart (though some estimates are as high as sixty-six thousand). It is difficult to predict the probable cost per patient if the TAH achieves a level of clinical adequacy. A 1985 report of the National Heart,

Lung and Blood Institute projected as plausible an average survival at 4.5 years with an average lifetime cost of one hundred fifty thousand dollars, including both implantation and maintenance. The total cost of the program was estimated to be two and a half to five billion dollars per year. The report stresses that "these costs and the level of cost effectiveness are not outside the range reimbursed for such therapies as heart transplantation, renal dialysis, and bone marrow transplants. However, addition of another high cost technology increases the need to evaluate its cost effectiveness and to address questions of how it will be paid for and what might be displaced." As DeVries himself notes, "When we first started the artificial heart program, the question was simply, 'Would it support life?' Now that we know it can, we can address other important questions, including whether it is worth doing and can we afford it."

This case was developed from several sources, including William C. DeVries et al., "Clinical Use of the Total Artificial Heart," *New England Journal of Medicine* 310 (February 2, 1984): 273–78; F. Ross Woolley, "Ethical Issues in the Implantation of the Total Artificial Heart," *New England Journal of Medicine* 310 (February 2, 1984): 292–96; National Heart, Lung, and Blood Institute Working Group on Mechanical Circulatory Support, *Artificial Heart and Assist Devices: Directions, Needs, Costs, Societal and Ethical Issues* (Bethesda, Md.: NIH Publication No. 85-2723, 1985); George Annas, "No Cheers for Temporary Artificial Hearts," *Hastings Center Report* 15 (October 1985); Albert R. Jonsen, "The Artificial Heart's Threat to Others," *Hastings Center Report* 16 (February 1986); George Annas, "Death and the Magic Machine: Informed Consent to the Artificial Heart," *Western New England Law Review* 9 (1987): 89–112; Dale Jamieson, "The Artificial Heart: Reevaluating the Investment," in *Organ Substitution Technology: Ethical, Legal, and Public Policy Issues*, ed. Deborah Mathieu (Boulder, Colo.: Westview Press, 1988): and several articles in *Journal of the American Medical Association* 259 (February 12, 1988): 785, 849–95, including William C. DeVries, "The Permanent Artificial Heart: Four Case Reports"; Philip M. Boffey, "Panel Appeals for Funds in Artificial Heart Work," *New York Times*, May 20, 1988, p. A12.

Case 33

In 1967, Dr. Christian Barnard performed the first heart transplant on a human being. After a brief flurry of heart transplants over the next several months, an informal moratorium occurred because the early results were so dismal. However, a few centers, most notably the one at Stanford University, continued heart transplantation programs, and by the early 1980s Dr. Norman Shumway and his colleagues at Stanford had achieved good success rates—sixty-five percent of their carefully selected heart transplant patients could be expected to survive at least one year, and they had a better than fifty percent chance of surviving five years. Because of these successes, proponents of cardiac transplantation argued that it should be made widely available, but critics were not convinced that the problem of tissue rejection had been sufficiently solved or that the benefits of cardiac transplantation outweighed its costs.

On February 1, 1980, the twelve lay trustees of the Massachusetts General Hospital announced that they had voted not to permit heart transplants at that institution "at the present time." Their explanatory statement noted that "to turn away even one potential cardiac transplantation patient is a very trying course to follow," but that "in an age where technology so pervades the medical community, there is a clear responsibility to evaluate new procedures in terms of the greatest good for the greatest number." In June 1980, Patricia Harris, then secretary of the Department of Health and Human Services (HHS), withdrew an earlier tentative authorization for Medicare to cover heart transplants. She held that authorization of funds can no longer depend solely on the safety, effectiveness, and acceptance of a technology by the medical community. In addition, a technology must be evaluated in terms of its "social consequences." Cost is one factor, and the specter of another program like the one for kidney dialysis and transplantation has created bureaucratic and congressional caution. For example, heart transplants at Stanford then averaged more than one hundred thousand dollars per patient. If two thousand transplants were performed, the cost would thus be more than two hundred million dollars. If thirty thousand transplants were performed, the cost would thus be more than three billion dollars. Estimates vary, but some reports suggest that each year in the United States there may be as many as thirty-five thousand victims of heart disease whose condition is hopeless without cardiac transplantation and who could possibly benefit from cardiac transplantation (if we assume that it would be possible to locate enough hearts for transplantation).

HHS was also concerned about Stanford's screening criteria, which included "a stable, rewarding family and/or vocational environment to return to post-transplant; a spouse, family member or companion able and willing to make the long-term commitment to provide emotional support before and after the transplant; financial resources to support travel to and from the transplant center accompanied by the family member for final evaluation." "Contraindications" for selection as a cardiac recipient at Stanford included "a history of alcoholism, job instability, antisocial behavior, or psychiatric illness." While some of these criteria may be medically relevant, others may incorporate unarticulated, undefended, and even indefensible criteria of "social worth." In any event, patient selection criteria raise serious issues of "distributive justice."

As a result of the uncertainty surrounding cardiac transplantation, HHS ordered a major National Heart Transplant Study, prepared by the Battelle Institute, to assess the "social consequences" before deciding whether to provide funds to pay for the operation. This study, which was submitted in 1984, determined that heart transplantation's success rates in length and quality of life, including rehabilitation for work, warranted viewing the procedure as nonexperimental. In 1986, the federal Task Force on Organ Transplantation also emphasized the successes of heart transplantation, noting that cyclosporine in the last couple of years had improved the one-year survival rate of heart transplant recipients to seventy-five to eighty-five percent. Because of such successes, the Massachusetts General Hospital reconsidered its decision and joined a consortium of Boston hospitals to provide cardiac transplantation, and the Health Care Financing Administration of HHS in 1987 agreed to provide funds for a few heart transplants for Medicare-eligible patients at selected centers on the grounds that heart transplants are a medically reasonable and necessary service.

Some individuals can afford the one hundred thousand dollars required for a heart transplant and the expensive follow-up care, and some insurance policies cover heart transplants. However, many patients lack these resources and cannot meet the Medicare criteria. As a result, the decision about whether society should pay for heart transplants has fallen to the states. The most publicized decision not to provide state funds for heart transplants (and other transplants except for corneas and kidneys) occurred in Oregon. The Oregon legislature voted in 1987 to discontinue its Medicaid organ transplant coverage for an estimated thirty-four recipients over two years at an estimated cost of 2.2 million dollars in order to provide basic health care for approximately fifteen hundred low-income children and pregnant women. The governor, Neil Goldschmidt, stated when he signed the bill into law: ''We all hate it, but we can't walk away from this issue any more. It goes way beyond transplants. How can we spend every nickel in support of a few people when thousands never see a doctor or eat a decent meal?'' The Oregon Senate president, John Kitschaber, a physician, asked, ''Is the human tragedy and the personal anguish of death from the lack of an organ transplant any greater than that of an infant dying in an intensive care unit from a preventable problem brought about by a lack of prenatal care?''

Three features of the context of the Oregon decision are important. First, Oregon voters have approved limits on state revenues and expenditures, and Oregon has a constitutional mandate for a balanced budget. Second, in an experiment that has increasing parallels elsewhere, an effort was made beginning in 1982 to develop public awareness and consensus on bioethical issues through the involvement of local communities. The effort focused on two fundamental questions: (1) ''How does society value expensive curative medical care relative to preventive services being progressively curtailed in government budgets? (2) Can the present implicit rationing of health care be made explicit and congruent with community values?'' A series of approximately three hundred town meetings with more than five thousand citizens was followed by a statewide parliament in fall 1984, which produced a document, ''Society Must Decide: Oregon Health Decisions Final Report.'' A major conclusion of that report was that ''collective financing of health care should be accomplished by

community responsibility for the ethics of allocation and rationing policies.''
A third relevant factor is that Oregon's experience with organ transplants other
than kidneys and corneas had involved great expenses and limited success for
a very few patients; the state had spent one million dollars for nineteen transplants in 1985–1987, and only nine of the nineteen recipients still survived in
1987. The cost of follow-up care for each patient was twenty-four thousand
dollars a year.

In addition to these debates about the "green screen"—the criterion of ability to pay—patient selection criteria are still controversial. The supply of donated organs is limited, and in 1987 there were approximately fifteen hundred
heart transplants. The United Network for Organ Sharing (UNOS) is developing criteria for distributing hearts and other organs, considering such factors as
urgency of medical need, probability of successful transplantation, and time on
the waiting list. There is vigorous debate about how to make these factors
operational (e.g., how many points to assign to each factor) and about the
relevance of other factors, such as age, contribution of person's lifestyle to
end-stage organ failure, and social network of support.

This case has been prepared from the following sources: Alexander Leaf, "The MGH
Trustees Say No to Heart Transplants," *New England Journal of Medicine* 302 (May
8, 1980): 1087–88; Richard A. Knox, "Heart Transplants: To Pay or Not to Pay,"
Science 209 (August 1, 1980): 570–75; Lois K. Christopherson, "Heart Transplants,"
Hastings Center Report 12 (February 1982): 18–21; John Iglehart, "The Politics of
Transplantation," *New England Journal of Medicine* 310 (1984): 864–68; Roger W.
Evans et al., *The National Heart Transplantation Study: Final Report* (Seattle: Battelle
Human Affairs Research Centers, 1984); Task Force on Organ Transplantation, *Organ
Transplantation: Issues and Recommendations* (Washington, D.C.: U.S. Department of
Health and Human Services, April 1986); Ward Casscells, "Heart Transplantation: Re-
cent Policy Developments," *New England Journal of Medicine* 315 (1986): 1365–68;
H. Gilbert Welch and Eric B. Larson, "Dealing with Limited Resources: The Oregon
Decision to Curtail Funding for Organ Transplantation," *New England Journal of Med-
icine* 319 (1988): 171–73; Richard Rettig, "The Politics of Organ Transplantation,"
Journal of Health Politics, Policy and Law, forthcoming.

Case 34

In June 1985, Luiza Magardician, a twenty-year-old Rumanian citizen, came
to New York City hoping to obtain a kidney transplant. The priest at the Rumanian Orthodox Church in Manhattan indicated that she had come in desperation because "all available methods of treatment were tried unsuccessfully in
her country." An official of the National Kidney Foundation in New York–
New Jersey indicated that Ms. Magardician had only a slim chance of obtaining
a kidney because "there is a bad shortage of donors in the United States, and
U.S. citizens would usually come first." Ms. Magardician's case was also

complicated because she lacked the funds to cover the hospital costs if a donor kidney were available.

Some media reports have suggested that some transplant centers have made donated organs available to foreign nationals ahead of U.S. citizens and residents, perhaps, according to the charges, because of financial incentives. Apart from the question of the ability to pay—or to pay more—clinicians and policymakers have to face the question of the relevance of accidents of national residence in providing scarce medical resources to needy patients, particularly when those resources are organs donated in the United States (occasionally, of course, by foreign nationals in the United States) and the donated organs are inadequate to meet the needs of all U.S. citizens and residents on the waiting list. In 1985, approximately eight thousand to ten thousand patients were on the active waiting list for a kidney transplant, and there were just eighty-seven hundred transplants in the United States (more than seventeen hundred of those from living donors). (It has been argued that the waiting list has been kept artificially low because of the shortage of kidneys for transplantation and that many more—perhaps a total of twenty thousand altogether—of the eighty thousand or so on dialysis in 1985 would have chosen a kidney transplant if it had been an option.) In that same year, approximately three hundred foreign nationals received kidney transplants in the United States, and approximately two hundred to two hundred fifty kidneys were shipped abroad. Critics have charged that such practices cost U.S. taxpayers millions of dollars because the end-stage renal disease program of Medicare ensures access to dialysis for patients with end-stage renal disease.

One question is whether the decision to transplant foreign nationals should be made by individual transplant centers or whether procedures and standards should be set at other levels, perhaps even at the national level. A second question is what procedures and standards should be used. Several policy options are available: let individual transplant centers and physicians transplant whom they will; exclude all foreign nationals; admit some foreign nationals to the waiting list, setting a maximum number such as ten percent and treating all candidates on the waiting list equally according to medical criteria and time on the list; admit some foreign nationals to the waiting list after informing them that they will not be eligible for any organ until it is clear that no U.S. citizen or resident on the list could use that organ. In 1988, the United Network for Organ Sharing (UNOS) proposed a compromise policy: It would allow transplant centers some discretion, while reserving the right to audit records of all foreign nationals receiving organ transplants and automatically auditing the records of any center transplanting more than ten percent of its organs to foreign nationals. It also recommends a local board including lay participants to evaluate the program. However, the debate continues about which policy would best satisfy the competing moral principles in the face of organ scarcity and accidents of geography.

This case has been developed, with amplifications, from "In Organ Transplants, Americans First?" *Hastings Center Report* 16 (October 1986): 23–24.

Case 35

In the mid-1970s, two professors at Harvard, Milton Weinstein and William B. Stason, became interested in facts and policies pertaining to high blood pressure in American society. Few people in the United States know about or pay much attention to the fact that they themselves may have high blood pressure. The Harvard researchers noted that seventeen percent of the adult American population, or twenty-four million persons, have problems with high blood pressure, that even minimally adequate treatment for these persons would cost more than five billion dollars annually (if all were treated), that close to fifty percent of the affected population are not even aware of the fact that they have problems, and that only about one-sixth of that group are receiving proper medical treatment and control.

The investigators became concerned with determining the most cost-effective way to tackle the problem of controlling hypertension in the American population. Data from screening programs that identify people who do not know that they have high blood pressure revealed that it is not cost-efficient to try to inform persons of their problem unless they are already under a physician's care. In general, people who were informed of their condition through massive screening and education programs were not likely to report to a physician for treatment. Among those who did subsequently see a physician, adherence to the recommended therapy turned out to be extremely poor.

As they further developed their research, Weinstein and Stason discovered (somewhat surprisingly) that, rather than launching a communitywide campaign, it is more cost-effective to treat three classes of persons in the attempt to reduce the general public health problem of high blood pressure: (1) younger men, (2) older women, and (3) those patients with very high blood pressure. When the researchers combined these findings with their previous findings that large-scale public screening and informational programs are not medically effective (and not cost-effective), they were led to conclude: "A community with limited resources would probably do better to concentrate its efforts on improving adherence of known hypertensives, even at a sacrifice in terms of the numbers screened. This conclusion holds even if such proadherence interventions are rather expensive and only moderately effective, and even if screening is very inexpensive. . . . Finally, screening in the regular practices [of physicians] is more cost-effective than public screening."

These investigators were bothered by their own recommendation because it implicitly meant that, if acted on by public policy experts in the government, the poorest sector of the country, which is also in greatest need of medical attention, would not be provided with any benefits of high blood pressure education and management. Public screening would be sacrificed in order to do a larger good for the whole community, where only persons known to have high blood pressure who were already in contact with a physician about their problem would be recontacted and new education attempts made. These investigators were concerned because there seemed to them to be a possible injustice in excluding the poor and minorities by a public health endeavor aimed expressly at the economically better-off sector of society. Yet their statistics were very compelling: No matter how carefully planned the efforts, nothing worked except programs directed at those already in touch with physicians. They also discovered that a certain amount of money devoted to the education of physicians was quite cost-effective. Moreover, they knew that it was most unlikely, and perhaps undeserved in light of other health needs, that there would be new allocations of public health money to control high blood pressure. Yet it would take massive new allocations even to begin to affect the poorer sectors of society.

These investigators therefore recommended what they explicitly referred to as a ''utilitarian'' set of criteria for allocation.

This case was prepared by consulting Milton Weinstein and William B. Stason, *Hypertension* (Cambridge: Harvard University Press, 1976), and their articles in *New England Journal of Medicine* 296 (1977): 716–21, and *Hastings Center Report* 7 (October 1977): 24–29.

Case 36

You are the physician in a small community and spend fifty percent of your time working for a local company. The company employs most of the workers in the community, and you are the private physician for many of the workers also. Work at the company involves exposure to a particular hazardous compound, and the government is now considering lowering the standard for exposure to that compound. Exposure to the compound is associated with COPD (chronic obstructive pulmonary disease). It is considered that compliance with the new standard will be quite costly but will reduce deaths from COPD in the industry by two per year nationwide. There have been no deaths attributable to exposure at your company, but there have probably been cases of new or exacerbated COPD; the new standard might be expected to reduce these and save one death from COPD at your company over your lifetime. The cost of compliance will most likely force your company out of business and increase unemployment in your community significantly.

1. You support the standard because your primary responsibility is to reduce occupational disease at any cost.
2. You oppose the standard: Your primary responsibility is the health and welfare of your patients, and that includes their economic well-being.
3. You support the standard: Your responsibility for the physical health of your patients would outweigh any economic consequences, however devastating.
4. You oppose the standard, reasoning that economic consequences nationwide exceed the benefits in workers' health.

This case was prepared by Paul Brandt-Rauf and Paul Andreini and is reprinted with permission.

Case 37

In June 1985, G. R. Lafon, a fifty-six-year-old uninsured Dallas laborer, received third-degree burns on his side and back from a grease fire at a fish fry. Doctors at the first three emergency rooms he visited, after determining that he could not pay a deposit ranging from five hundred dollars to fifteen hundred dollars, decided he was not an emergency case. At the second of these hospitals, North Texas Medical Center, doctors inserted an intravenous tube and a catheter in Lafon, to stabilize his liquids (a critical factor for burn patients). But without a deposit, they would not admit him.

Lafon slung the IV bottle over the coat hook of his sister's 1976 Oldsmobile and headed off. Finally, after seven hours and seventy miles of trekking around, he wound up at Parkland Memorial, a public teaching hospital. "It was starting to hurt real bad," Lafon said. At Parkland, he ran up a bill of $22,189 for nineteen days of hospitalization and a skin graft.

"Our doctors here . . . think that maybe the course of treatment [at Parkland] was a little bit excessive," said Steven Woerner, administrator of North Texas Medical Center.

"He was definitely an emergency case, with third-degree burns that would not heal on their own," said Dr. John Hunt, director of the Parkland burn unit. "I would question whether those doctors had the experience to determine this was a third-degree burn. I also find it grossly inappropriate for them to insert an IV and a catheter and then send him on his way."

Lafon recovered and received a $353.75 bill from North Texas Medical Center for the catheter and IV.

In April 1986, the "Texas transfer law," which became the model for national legislation regulating patient transfers from one hospital to another, went into effect.

This case was prepared by Bethany Spielman on the basis of Paul Taylor, "Ailing, Uninsured and Turned Away," *Washington Post,* June 30, 1985, p. A1, A15.

Case 38

Having recently completed his Ph.D. in chemistry, George has not been able to find a job. His family has suffered from his failure, since they are short of money, his wife has had to take a full-time job, and their small children have been subjected to considerable strain, uncertainty, and instability. An established chemist can get George a position in a laboratory that pursues research in chemical and biological warfare. Despite his perilous financial and familial circumstances, George feels that he cannot accept this position because of his conscientious opposition to chemical and biological warfare. The older chemist notes that although he is not enthusiastic about this project, the research will continue whatever George decides. Furthermore, if George does not take the position, it will be offered to another young man who would probably pursue the research with alacrity and promptitude. Indeed, the older chemist confides, his concern about this other candidate's nationalistic fervor and uncritical zeal for research in chemical and biological warfare in part led him to recommend George. George's wife is puzzled and hurt by George's reaction, since she sees nothing wrong with such research. She is mainly concerned about the instability of their family and their children's problems.

Adapted from Bernard Williams, "A Critique of Utilitarianism," in J. J. C. Smart and Bernard Williams, *Utilitarianism For and Against* (Cambridge: Cambridge University Press, 1973), pp. 97–98.

Index